Clinical Laboratory Case Studies

100 Progressive Diagnostic Reasoning Cases for MLS, MLT, and Medical Students

A Progressive-Disclosure Case-Based Approach to Laboratory Testing, Clinical Correlation, and ASCP Certification Preparation

Mandel Willie Henson

First Edition

ISBN: 978-1-923604-87-2

DISCLAIMER

Educational and Informational Purposes Only

This book is intended for educational and informational purposes only and is designed to support the learning of medical laboratory science students, medical laboratory technicians, medical laboratory scientists, medical students, and healthcare professionals. It is NOT intended to replace formal education, clinical training, or professional medical advice.

Not Medical Advice

The information contained in this book does not constitute medical advice and should not be used to diagnose or treat any medical condition. Readers should consult qualified healthcare providers for diagnosis and treatment of medical conditions. The case presentations, while based on realistic clinical scenarios, are educational constructs and should not be applied directly to patient care without proper clinical context and professional judgment.

No Patient-Physician or Laboratory-Patient Relationship

Nothing in this book creates or should be construed as creating a patient-physician relationship, laboratory-patient relationship, or any professional healthcare relationship between the author, publisher, and readers.

Fictional Case Presentations

All cases presented in this book are educational scenarios created for teaching purposes. While cases are based on realistic clinical presentations and authentic laboratory findings, they are composite educational examples. Any resemblance to actual patients, living or deceased, is coincidental. Patient names, demographic details, and identifying information have been fictionalized to protect privacy.

No Endorsement of Products, Institutions, or Individuals

References to specific laboratory instruments, reagent manufacturers, medical devices, pharmaceutical products, healthcare institutions, or individuals mentioned in case scenarios are for educational illustration only and do not constitute endorsement or recommendation by the author or publisher. Trade names and trademarks are the property of their respective owners.

Laboratory Standards and Guidelines

Laboratory reference ranges, testing methodologies, and clinical guidelines presented in this book reflect current standards at the time of publication but may change. Readers should consult current published guidelines from organizations such as CLSI (Clinical and Laboratory Standards Institute), CAP (College of American Pathologists), CLIA (Clinical Laboratory Improvement Amendments), FDA (Food and Drug Administration), and relevant professional societies for the most up-to-date recommendations.

Certification Examination Preparation

While this book is designed to support preparation for ASCP (American Society for Clinical Pathology) and other laboratory certification examinations, it does not guarantee success on certification exams. Readers should consult official examination content outlines and additional study resources as part of comprehensive exam preparation.

Professional Judgment Required

Laboratory medicine is a complex field requiring integration of analytical skills, clinical knowledge, and professional judgment. The diagnostic approaches and clinical reasoning demonstrated in this book represent educational frameworks and may not be the only appropriate approaches in actual clinical practice. Healthcare professionals must exercise independent professional judgment based on specific patient circumstances, institutional protocols, and current evidence.

Accuracy of Information

While every effort has been made to ensure the accuracy and completeness of information presented in this book, the author and publisher make no warranties, express or implied, regarding errors, omissions, or the accuracy of content. Medical knowledge evolves continuously, and laboratory testing methodologies, reference ranges, and clinical interpretations may change over time.

Limitation of Liability

The author, publisher, and any affiliated organizations or individuals shall not be liable for any direct, indirect, incidental, consequential, or punitive damages arising from the use of this book or reliance on information contained herein. Readers assume all risks associated with the use of information in this book.

Regulatory and Licensing Requirements

Practice of medical laboratory science is regulated by federal, state, and local laws. Readers are responsible for complying with all applicable regulatory requirements, licensing laws, scope of practice restrictions, and institutional policies in their jurisdiction.

Quality Control and Laboratory Safety

While this book discusses quality control procedures and laboratory practices, readers must follow their institution's specific standard operating procedures (SOPs), safety protocols, and quality management systems. Laboratory safety information provided is general in nature and does not replace comprehensive safety training and OSHA compliance.

Continuing Education

This book may be used as part of continuing education activities for laboratory professionals. However, readers should verify with their certifying organization and employer regarding specific continuing education credit requirements and approval processes.

Updates and Revisions

Information in this book is current as of the publication date (2025). Readers are encouraged to consult current literature, clinical guidelines, and professional resources for the most recent developments in laboratory medicine.

Table of Contents

Chapter 1: Introduction to Clinical Reasoning in Laboratory Medicine

Welcome, and in this book, I will work through real patient cases that will teach you how to think like a laboratory professional. Not just memorize facts—actually *think* through diagnostic puzzles.

Here's what makes this book different from your typical laboratory medicine textbook. Instead of reading page after page of theory, you'll face actual clinical scenarios. A patient walks in with symptoms. Lab tests get ordered. Results come back. Now what? That's where you come in.

Laboratory professionals don't just run tests and report numbers. You interpret patterns, spot abnormalities, suggest additional testing, and help clinicians reach the right diagnosis. This book trains you to do exactly that through 100 carefully selected cases that mirror what you'll encounter in real practice.

Why Case-Based Learning Works Better

Think about how you learned to ride a bike. Did someone hand you a manual explaining the physics of balance and the biomechanics of pedaling? No. You got on the bike, wobbled, maybe fell, tried again, and eventually figured it out through experience.

Medical diagnosis works the same way. Reading about anemia types helps, sure. But working through a case where a 28-year-old woman has fatigue, low hemoglobin, low MCV, and you need to figure out if it's iron deficiency or thalassemia—that's where real learning happens.

Research shows case-based learning produces better retention and problem-solving skills than traditional lectures (Thistlethwaite et al., 2012). One study found that medical students using case-based methods scored 15% higher on diagnostic reasoning tests compared to those using standard textbooks (Srinivasan et al., 2007). The cases stick with you because they tell stories, not just facts.

You'll remember the diabetic patient who came in confused with a glucose of 850 mg/dL and pH of 7.15. The numbers mean something when attached to a real person, real symptoms, real consequences.

How This Book Actually Works

Each chapter focuses on one laboratory discipline—hematology, chemistry, microbiology, and so on. Within each chapter, you'll find multiple cases arranged from simpler to more challenging.

Here's the structure of every case:

The case opens with a brief clinical presentation. A patient's age, gender, chief complaint, and relevant history. Just like real life—you don't get all the information upfront. You get what the doctor noticed and what prompted them to order lab work.

Then come the **initial laboratory findings**. The first round of test results that hit the chart. Your job? Start thinking. What do these numbers tell you? What patterns do you see? What additional tests might you need?

Before you jump to conclusions (and we all do this, don't worry), you'll encounter **diagnostic reasoning questions**. These make you pause and think through the case systematically:

- What's the most likely diagnosis based on current findings?

- What other conditions should you consider?

- What additional tests would you order next?

- What's the pathophysiology behind these results?

Then comes the fun part. **Sequential test results** appear, mimicking how real clinical workups unfold. You don't get all the answers at once. A complete blood count leads to a peripheral smear. Chemistry panel abnormalities trigger endocrine testing. You follow the diagnostic trail step by step.

Finally, the case reveals the **final diagnosis** with a detailed explanation. This is where theory meets practice. You learn not just *what* the diagnosis was, but *how* the laboratory findings pointed toward it and *why* other possibilities got ruled out.

Teaching points wrap up each case. These highlight the most important lessons—the patterns you should recognize, the pitfalls to avoid, the clinical pearls that will serve you for years.

Related cases at the end connect to similar scenarios elsewhere in the book. If you enjoyed (or struggled with) a particular case, you'll find others that build on those concepts.

The Progressive Disclosure Format

Most textbooks give you everything at once. Diagnosis, symptoms, lab findings, treatment—all on the same page. That's not how medicine works.

This book uses *progressive disclosure*, meaning information appears gradually. Just like in clinical practice, you start with limited data and gather more as you go.

A patient presents with fatigue and pallor. You see a hemoglobin of 8.5 g/dL. Stop. What are you thinking? Anemia, obviously, but what kind? You need more information.

The MCV comes back low at 72 fL. Okay, now you're narrowing it down. Microcytic anemia. Your differential list shortens. Iron deficiency, thalassemia, anemia of chronic disease, lead poisoning. What's next?

You check iron studies. Ferritin is low, iron saturation is low, TIBC is high. Classic iron deficiency picture. But wait—the patient's been taking iron supplements for months with no improvement. Now it gets interesting.

This is how diagnostic reasoning actually flows. One finding leads to another question, which leads to another test, which leads to a diagnosis. The progressive format trains your brain to think this way naturally.

Clinical Reasoning Frameworks for Laboratory Diagnosis

Let's talk about the mental processes you'll develop working through these cases. Good laboratory professionals use systematic approaches, not hunches or guesses.

Pattern Recognition comes first. After you've seen enough cases, certain combinations jump out immediately. Low platelets plus schistocytes plus elevated LDH? Your brain should whisper "TTP or HUS." Markedly elevated alkaline phosphatase with normal ALT and AST? Think bone disease or biliary obstruction, not hepatocellular damage.

These patterns develop through exposure. The more cases you work through, the faster you'll recognize them. It's like learning to read—at first you sound out each letter, but eventually you see whole words instantly.

Hypothesis-Driven Testing is your next tool. When lab results don't fit a clear pattern, you generate hypotheses and test them systematically. A patient has elevated calcium at 12.5 mg/dL. Your hypotheses might include hyperparathyroidism, malignancy, vitamin D toxicity, or milk-alkali syndrome. You order PTH, vitamin D, PTHrP, and review medications. Each result either supports or refutes a hypothesis.

The cases in this book teach you to generate smart hypotheses based on initial findings, then select appropriate follow-up tests. Not just ordering everything (expensive and often confusing), but choosing tests that will actually help you distinguish between competing diagnoses.

Bayesian Reasoning sounds fancy but it's simple. Pre-test probability + test characteristics = post-test probability. In plain English: how likely is this diagnosis before testing, how good is the test at detecting it, and how does the result change your level of certainty?

A 65-year-old man with a 40 pack-year smoking history has a lung nodule on chest X-ray. His pre-test probability of lung cancer is high. A positive biopsy essentially confirms it. But if the same nodule appears in a 25-year-old nonsmoker, the pre-test probability is much lower, and even a suspicious biopsy might warrant additional testing before assuming cancer.

The cases here will train you to consider pre-test probability. Not every elevated PSA means prostate cancer. Not every positive D-dimer means pulmonary embolism. Context matters enormously.

Ruling In vs. Ruling Out strategies depend on your clinical question. Sometimes you need tests with high sensitivity to rule out dangerous conditions. A negative highly-sensitive troponin in a low-risk chest pain patient effectively rules out myocardial infarction (Pickering et al., 2018). Sometimes you need high specificity to confirm a diagnosis before starting risky treatment.

You'll practice both approaches throughout these cases. When do you need more tests? When can you stop testing? These judgment calls separate good laboratory professionals from great ones.

Getting the Most from Individual Study

Here's how to use this book if you're working alone (maybe preparing for boards, maybe just expanding your knowledge).

Don't peek ahead. I know it's tempting. You see the initial findings and want to flip to the answer. Resist. Cover the diagnosis section with your hand or a piece of paper. Force yourself to think through the case first.

Write down your thoughts. Literally grab a notebook or open a document and type out your thinking:

- Initial impression based on symptoms
- Interpretation of first lab results

- Differential diagnosis list

- What tests you'd order next

- Reasoning behind each test choice

This active engagement beats passive reading by miles. Studies show students who actively work problems retain information three times longer than those who just read examples (Freeman et al., 2014).

After you've thought it through, reveal the next section. See if your reasoning matched the case progression. Don't feel bad if you missed it—that's how you learn. Figure out where your thinking went wrong and why.

Keep a **"mistake journal"** if you're really serious. When you misdiagnose a case or miss a key finding, write down:

- What you thought initially

- What you missed or misinterpreted

- The correct diagnosis

- The key learning point

After working through 20-30 cases, review your mistake journal. You'll see patterns in your own thinking—maybe you consistently forget to consider medication effects, or you overlook subtle differences between similar conditions. Identifying your weak spots lets you strengthen them deliberately.

Timing matters too. Don't try to cram five cases in one sitting. Your brain needs time to process and consolidate learning. One or two cases per day works better than marathon sessions. Space your learning out over weeks, not days.

And here's something interesting—come back to cases you've already solved. Wait a week, then try the same case again without looking at your notes. You'll be surprised how much you've forgotten or how your reasoning has sharpened. Spaced repetition is one of the most powerful learning techniques in existence (Cepeda et al., 2006).

Making Group Discussion Even More Powerful

If you're using this book as part of a study group or teaching session, the cases become even more valuable. Different people see different angles, catch different details, miss different clues.

Start with independent thinking. Don't jump straight into group discussion. Give everyone 10-15 minutes to read the case and form their own impressions first. If you discuss immediately, the loudest or most confident person dominates and quieter members don't develop their own reasoning skills.

After individual thinking time, go around the room. Each person shares their initial impression and reasoning. No interrupting, no judging. Just listen to how different brains approach the same problem.

You'll hear things like: "I thought iron deficiency immediately because of the low MCV." Someone else says: "I actually considered thalassemia first because the patient's ferritin wasn't *that* low." A third person chimes in: "I was worried about lead toxicity because the patient works in construction."

All reasonable thoughts. All worth exploring. The discussion reveals multiple valid pathways to diagnosis and helps everyone see their blind spots.

Assign roles to make discussions more structured. One person plays the laboratory director who must justify test ordering decisions to administration. Another plays the clinician who needs quick answers. A third plays devil's advocate, poking holes in proposed diagnoses. Rotating roles keeps discussions dynamic and helps you see cases from multiple professional perspectives.

Use whiteboards or shared screens. Draw out thought processes visually. Create tables comparing differential diagnoses. Sketch pathophysiology mechanisms. Visual mapping helps cement concepts in ways that verbal discussion alone can't achieve.

Don't rush. One case can easily generate 30-45 minutes of rich discussion. That's good. Deep exploration beats superficial coverage every time. Better to thoroughly discuss three cases than skim through ten.

And here's something groups often skip—**debrief the process**, not just the content. After solving a case, talk about how the group worked through it. What questions led to breakthroughs? Where did the group get stuck? What thinking patterns helped or hindered? This meta-cognition—thinking about thinking—accelerates learning dramatically.

Tackling Unknown or Difficult Cases

Some cases in this book will stump you completely. You'll stare at the findings, read them three times, and still have no idea what's happening. Good. That's when the deepest learning occurs.

Start with the basics. When you're lost, return to fundamentals. Is this pattern consistent with increased production, decreased destruction, or redistribution? Is the primary problem in the bone marrow, peripheral blood, or reticuloendothelial system? Is this acute or chronic? Simple questions often point you in the right direction.

Make lists. When diagnostic possibilities seem overwhelming, literally write out every condition you can think of that might produce these findings. Don't self-censor. Include common things and rare things. Then work through each one systematically, asking: "Does this fit all the findings? What would I expect to see if this were the diagnosis? Do I see those things?"

This exhaustive approach feels slow, but it prevents you from missing diagnoses due to premature closure (jumping to the first plausible explanation without considering alternatives).

Look for the outlier. Most test results will fit together, but often one or two findings seem weird. That weird finding is frequently the key to the whole case. Don't ignore it or explain it away. Investigate it. Why is the platelet count normal when you expected it to be low? Why is the alkaline phosphatase elevated when liver enzymes are normal? The answer to "why is this finding unexpected?" often unlocks the diagnosis.

Consider the clinical context always. Laboratory medicine doesn't exist in isolation. A slightly elevated troponin means something very different in a marathon runner versus a dialysis patient versus someone with chest pain. The patient's age, gender, medications, comorbidities, and presenting symptoms guide interpretation. Cases that seem impossible based on lab values alone often make perfect sense with clinical context.

Accept uncertainty. In real practice, you won't always know the diagnosis immediately. Sometimes you'll say "I need more information" or "several diagnoses remain possible" or "let's repeat this in a week." That's not failure—that's good medicine. The cases here will sometimes leave you uncertain until the final results appear. Get comfortable with that uncertainty because it's how clinical medicine actually works.

Use resources smartly. When you're genuinely stuck, it's okay to look things up. Check reference ranges, review disease pathophysiology, read about test characteristics. The goal isn't to memorize everything— it's to learn how to find answers and apply them. Knowing that spherocytosis causes indirect hyperbilirubinemia is less important than knowing how to recognize spherocytes on a smear and understanding why they lead to hemolysis.

What You'll Gain from This Approach

After working through these 100 cases, your diagnostic thinking will be different. Not just more knowledge—though you'll definitely have that—but different mental habits.

You'll develop **pattern recognition** that helps you spot diagnoses quickly. That immediate "this looks like..." feeling that comes from experience.

You'll build **structured reasoning skills** that let you work through unfamiliar cases systematically when pattern recognition fails.

You'll gain **practical knowledge** about which tests to order when, how to interpret results in context, and what findings warrant urgent attention versus routine follow-up.

You'll understand **test limitations** and learn not to over-interpret small abnormalities or trust single data points without confirmation.

You'll see **how laboratory disciplines integrate**. Hematology findings affect chemistry values. Microbiology results guide immunology testing. Real patients don't fit neatly into separate categories, and these cases reflect that reality.

Most importantly, you'll develop **confidence**. The kind that comes from successfully navigating complex cases, making mistakes, learning from them, and gradually getting better. You'll walk into clinical practice or board exams feeling prepared, not just educated.

Moving Forward

The next chapters contain the cases themselves. Hematology cases come first—anemia, bleeding disorders, thrombosis, leukemias, and more. Then chemistry and metabolic disorders. Then transfusion medicine, microbiology, molecular diagnostics, and specialized areas.

Each chapter builds on previous ones. Concepts introduced early reappear in more complex forms later. The cases aren't arranged by difficulty within each chapter—they're mixed, reflecting real clinical practice where simple and complex cases arrive randomly.

Take your time. Work carefully through each case. Think before you read ahead. Write down your reasoning. Discuss with colleagues when possible. Review cases you found difficult. Use this book as a tool, not just a text.

And remember—every expert was once a beginner who felt overwhelmed by all this. The difference between experts and beginners isn't some innate talent. It's deliberate practice, thoughtful reflection, and persistence through confusion until understanding emerges.

You're ready. Turn the page and meet your first patient.

What You'll Take Away

By working through this book thoughtfully, you'll gain diagnostic skills that transfer directly to clinical practice. You'll learn to recognize patterns quickly while maintaining systematic thinking for complex cases. You'll understand not just what tests show, but what they mean for patient care. You'll develop the confidence that comes from solving real diagnostic puzzles, making mistakes in a safe environment, and learning from them. Most importantly, you'll bridge the gap between theoretical knowledge and practical application—the gap that separates students from practicing professionals. These cases will challenge you, occasionally frustrate you, and ultimately prepare you for the real work of laboratory medicine: helping clinicians reach accurate diagnoses that improve patient outcomes.

Chapter 2: Hematology Cases

Blood tells stories. Every cell count, every morphology finding, every coagulation result reveals something about what's happening inside a patient's body. Your job is learning to read those stories accurately.

Hematology intimidates many laboratory professionals at first. Anemia alone has dozens of causes. Throw in thrombocytopenia, abnormal white cells, coagulation disorders, and rare conditions, and the complexity seems overwhelming.

Here's the secret though—hematology follows patterns. Master the patterns, and you'll solve most cases. Miss the patterns, and you'll drown in the details.

These 15 cases will teach you those patterns through actual clinical scenarios. You'll work through common presentations like unexplained anemia and unusual ones like thrombotic thrombocytopenic purpura. Some cases will feel straightforward. Others will twist in unexpected directions.

Before we start, let's establish a framework that applies to nearly every hematology case.

The Hematology Diagnostic Framework

When you face any hematology case, ask yourself four fundamental questions:

What's abnormal? Is it red cells (anemia or polycythemia), white cells (leukopenia or leukocytosis), platelets (thrombocytopenia or thrombocytosis), or coagulation (bleeding or thrombosis)? Sometimes multiple cell lines are affected. Identify the abnormalities clearly before jumping to diagnoses.

Is it production or destruction? Are cells not being made properly (bone marrow problem), or are they being made normally but destroyed too quickly (peripheral destruction)? This distinction guides your entire workup. The reticulocyte count is your best friend here—high retic count suggests destruction, low retic count suggests production failure.

Is it acquired or inherited? New onset in adulthood usually means acquired. Lifelong history or family patterns suggest inherited. Don't assume though—some inherited conditions don't manifest until adulthood, and not everyone knows their family medical history.

What's the mechanism? Once you've narrowed things down, understand the pathophysiology. Why are the cells abnormal? What process caused this? Understanding mechanism helps you anticipate complications, plan treatment, and recognize related conditions.

Keep these questions in mind as you work through each case. They'll guide you through the diagnostic reasoning process.

Now let's meet the first patient.

Case 1: The Tired Graduate Student

Clinical Presentation

A 23-year-old female graduate student presents to student health services complaining of increasing fatigue over the past three months. She initially attributed it to her demanding coursework and late-night study sessions, but the exhaustion has worsened to the point where she struggles to climb the stairs to her apartment. She also mentions feeling lightheaded when she stands up quickly.

Her past medical history is unremarkable. She doesn't take any medications. She's been vegetarian for five years and vegan for the past year. Menstrual periods are heavy, lasting 7-8 days with significant cramping.

Physical examination reveals pale conjunctivae and nail beds. Her heart rate is 95 beats per minute, and blood pressure is 108/70 mmHg. The rest of the examination is normal.

Initial Laboratory Findings

The physician orders a complete blood count (CBC):

- Hemoglobin: 9.2 g/dL (normal: 12.0-16.0 g/dL)

- Hematocrit: 28% (normal: 36-46%)

- MCV: 72 fL (normal: 80-100 fL)

- MCH: 23 pg (normal: 27-31 pg)

- MCHC: 31 g/dL (normal: 32-36 g/dL)

- RDW: 18% (normal: 11.5-14.5%)

- White blood cell count: 7,200/μL (normal)

- Platelet count: 385,000/μL (normal: 150,000-400,000/μL)

Stop and Think

What's your initial impression? Look at the pattern here. The hemoglobin is clearly low—that's anemia. But what kind?

The MCV at 72 fL tells you this is **microcytic anemia** (small red cells). The elevated RDW indicates significant size variation among red blood cells, which is common in developing anemias.

What causes microcytic anemia? Your differential diagnosis should include:

1. **Iron deficiency** (most common)

2. **Thalassemia** (inherited)

3. **Anemia of chronic disease** (sometimes microcytic)

4. **Lead poisoning** (rare)

5. **Sideroblastic anemia** (rare)

Based on this patient's presentation, what's most likely? She's a young woman with heavy menstrual periods and a vegan diet (limited dietary iron). Iron deficiency seems obvious, right?

Maybe. But don't jump to conclusions yet. Let's gather more data.

Diagnostic Reasoning Questions

Before ordering more tests, think through these questions:

What additional laboratory tests would help distinguish between these possibilities?

Iron studies are essential here. You'd want:

- Serum iron
- Total iron-binding capacity (TIBC)
- Ferritin
- Transferrin saturation

What would you expect to see in iron deficiency?

Classic iron deficiency shows:

- Low serum iron
- High TIBC (the body makes more transferrin trying to capture any available iron)
- Low ferritin (iron storage is depleted)
- Low transferrin saturation (<20%)

What about thalassemia?

Thalassemia would show:

- Normal or elevated ferritin
- Normal iron studies
- More severe microcytosis (MCV often <75 fL) relative to the degree of anemia
- Family history of anemia
- Certain ethnic backgrounds (Mediterranean, Southeast Asian, Middle Eastern, African)

Should you order a peripheral blood smear?

Yes. The smear would show characteristic findings. In iron deficiency, you'd expect hypochromic (pale) microcytic red cells with significant variation in size and shape. In thalassemia, you'd see more uniform microcytic cells, often with target cells and basophilic stippling.

Sequential Test Results

The physician orders iron studies and a peripheral blood smear.

Iron Studies:

- Serum iron: 25 µg/dL (normal: 60-170 µg/dL) - LOW

- TIBC: 450 µg/dL (normal: 250-450 µg/dL) - HIGH

- Ferritin: 8 ng/mL (normal: 12-150 ng/mL) - LOW

- Transferrin saturation: 5.5% (normal: 20-50%) - LOW

Peripheral Blood Smear: Microcytic, hypochromic red blood cells with marked anisocytosis (variation in size) and poikilocytosis (variation in shape). Occasional pencil cells and target cells. No basophilic stippling or schistocytes. Platelets appear adequate and morphologically normal. White blood cells are unremarkable.

What Do These Results Tell You?

The iron studies confirm **iron deficiency anemia**. Every parameter points toward this diagnosis:

- Low serum iron (not enough circulating iron)

- High TIBC (body responds by making more transferrin)

- Very low ferritin (iron stores are depleted)

- Very low transferrin saturation (transferrin is mostly empty)

The ferritin of 8 ng/mL is particularly telling. Ferritin reflects iron stores, and a level this low virtually guarantees iron deficiency. Some sources suggest ferritin below 15 ng/mL in women confirms iron deficiency even without other tests (Lopez et al., 2016).

The peripheral smear supports this diagnosis with hypochromic, microcytic cells and the characteristic shape changes seen in iron deficiency.

But Why Is She Iron Deficient?

Finding iron deficiency isn't the end of the investigation—it's the beginning. You need to understand *why* she's iron deficient. In this patient, two factors likely contribute:

1. Chronic blood loss from heavy menstrual bleeding. Women lose approximately 30-40 mL of blood per menstrual period normally. Heavy periods (menorrhagia) can double or triple that amount. Each milliliter of blood contains about 0.5 mg of iron. With heavy periods lasting 7-8 days, she could be losing 100+ mL of blood monthly, depleting her iron faster than diet can replace it (Muñoz et al., 2017).

2. Inadequate dietary iron intake. She became vegan a year ago. Plant-based iron (non-heme iron) is absorbed much less efficiently than iron from meat (heme iron). While vegetarians and vegans *can* meet iron requirements through careful dietary planning, many don't. Without attention to iron-rich plant foods and absorption enhancers like vitamin C, deficiency develops gradually (Hunt, 2003).

The combination of increased iron loss (menstruation) plus decreased iron intake (vegan diet) created the perfect conditions for iron deficiency.

Final Diagnosis

Iron deficiency anemia secondary to menorrhagia and inadequate dietary iron intake.

Treatment and Follow-up

The physician prescribes ferrous sulfate 325 mg daily (65 mg elemental iron) to be taken with orange juice (vitamin C enhances absorption) on an empty stomach. She's advised about side effects (constipation, dark stools, nausea) and counseled on iron-rich plant foods: beans, lentils, tofu, fortified cereals, dark leafy greens, dried fruits.

She's also referred to gynecology to evaluate her heavy menstrual bleeding. Menorrhagia has underlying causes—hormonal imbalances, uterine fibroids, bleeding disorders—that should be addressed.

The reticulocyte count should increase within one week of starting iron supplementation as the bone marrow responds. Hemoglobin typically rises by 1-2 g/dL over 3-4 weeks. Complete correction takes 2-3 months.

If her hemoglobin doesn't improve despite iron supplementation, additional investigation would be needed. Non-response to iron suggests either ongoing blood loss, malabsorption (celiac disease, inflammatory bowel disease, H. pylori infection), non-compliance, or an incorrect diagnosis (Camaschella, 2019).

Teaching Points

Microcytic anemia isn't always iron deficiency. Although iron deficiency is the most common cause globally, always consider thalassemia, especially in patients of Mediterranean, African, Middle Eastern, or Southeast Asian descent. The "Mentzer index" (MCV/RBC count) can help distinguish—a value <13 suggests thalassemia, while >13 suggests iron deficiency, though this rule has exceptions (Urrechaga et al., 2015).

Ferritin is the single best test for iron deficiency in otherwise healthy people. Values below 15 ng/mL confirm deficiency. However, ferritin is an acute phase reactant—it rises during inflammation, infection, liver disease, or malignancy. In patients with inflammatory conditions, higher ferritin thresholds (50-100 ng/mL) may be needed to diagnose iron deficiency (Lopez et al., 2016).

Always investigate the cause. Finding anemia is just step one. Understanding *why* is step two. In premenopausal women, menstrual blood loss is common. In men and postmenopausal women, assume gastrointestinal blood loss until proven otherwise—they may need colonoscopy and upper endoscopy to rule out bleeding ulcers or colon cancer.

Dietary history matters. Ask about meat consumption, vegetarian/vegan diets, and unusual eating habits (pica—craving ice, clay, or cornstarch—is a classic but underrecognized symptom of iron deficiency). Diet modification plus supplementation works better than either alone.

Monitor response to treatment. Failure to respond to iron supplementation requires investigation. Check for malabsorption, ongoing blood loss, or incorrect diagnosis. Some patients need intravenous iron if oral supplementation fails or causes intolerable side effects.

Related Cases

This case connects to:

- **Case 9: Iron Deficiency vs. Thalassemia** (explores how to distinguish these similar presentations)

- **Case 13: Factor V Leiden Thrombophilia** (mentions menorrhagia as a bleeding manifestation)

- **Case 2: Persistent Thrombocytopenia in Young Woman** (another case involving menstrual issues)

Case 2: The Unexplained Bruising

Clinical Presentation

A 32-year-old woman presents to her primary care physician concerned about easy bruising that she's noticed over the past month. She reports developing large bruises on her arms and legs from minor bumps that wouldn't normally cause bruising. She also mentions increased bleeding from her gums when brushing her teeth and heavier menstrual periods than usual.

She feels otherwise well—no fevers, no weight loss, no fatigue. Her past medical history includes seasonal allergies treated with loratadine. No recent illnesses, infections, or new medications. No family history of bleeding disorders.

Physical examination reveals multiple ecchymoses (bruises) in various stages of healing on her extremities, ranging from fresh purple marks to fading yellow-green areas. Petechiae (tiny red spots) are visible on her lower legs. No lymphadenopathy, no hepatosplenomegaly. The rest of the examination is normal.

Initial Laboratory Findings

A CBC is ordered:

- Hemoglobin: 13.1 g/dL (normal: 12.0-16.0 g/dL)

- Hematocrit: 39% (normal: 36-46%)

- MCV: 88 fL (normal: 80-100 fL)

- White blood cell count: 7,800/µL (normal: 4,000-11,000/µL)

- Platelet count: 22,000/µL (normal: 150,000-400,000/µL) - VERY LOW

Stop and Think

One abnormality jumps out immediately: **severe thrombocytopenia** (platelet count of 22,000/µL). Normal platelet counts range from 150,000-400,000/µL. This patient's count is dramatically reduced.

Thrombocytopenia explains all her symptoms. Platelets are essential for hemostasis—they plug small breaks in blood vessels and prevent bleeding. When platelet counts drop below 50,000/µL, bleeding risk increases. Below 20,000/µL, spontaneous bleeding becomes a real concern (Neunert et al., 2011).

The petechiae and easy bruising are classic manifestations of thrombocytopenia. Petechiae develop from tiny capillary bleeds. Ecchymoses form from minor trauma that normally wouldn't cause bruising. Gingival bleeding and menorrhagia also stem from inadequate platelet numbers.

But why is her platelet count so low? Thrombocytopenia has three basic mechanisms:

1. Decreased production (bone marrow not making enough platelets) **2. Increased destruction** (platelets are destroyed faster than normal) **3. Sequestration** (platelets are trapped in an enlarged spleen)

How do we determine which mechanism is operating here?

Diagnostic Reasoning Questions

What additional history would you want?

Ask about:

- Recent viral infections (viruses can trigger immune thrombocytopenia)
- Alcohol use (causes bone marrow suppression and sequestration)
- Medication exposure including over-the-counter drugs and supplements
- Tick bites or travel (some infections cause thrombocytopenia)
- Symptoms of lupus or other autoimmune diseases
- Family history of blood disorders

What additional laboratory tests would you order?

Start with a **peripheral blood smear**. This is the most important next step. The smear tells you:

- Are the platelets truly decreased, or is this pseudothrombocytopenia (platelets clumping in the test tube)?
- Are the remaining platelets normal in size and morphology?
- Is there evidence of platelet destruction (large platelets suggest increased production trying to compensate)?
- Are there any abnormalities in red or white blood cells?

Other useful tests:

- HIV and Hepatitis C (chronic viral infections cause thrombocytopenia)
- Thyroid function (hypothyroidism and hyperthyroidism can affect platelets)
- Bone marrow biopsy (if production failure is suspected)

What would make you think of immune thrombocytopenic purpura (ITP)?

ITP is a diagnosis of exclusion, meaning you rule out other causes first. It typically presents as:

- Isolated thrombocytopenia (other cell lines normal)

- No clear secondary cause

- Large platelets on smear (bone marrow making new platelets rapidly)

- Young to middle-aged adults (though it can occur at any age)

- Often preceded by viral infection

Sequential Test Results

Peripheral Blood Smear: Markedly decreased platelet count confirmed. The platelets that are present appear large (megathrombocytes), suggesting increased platelet production. Red blood cells are normal in appearance. White blood cells show normal morphology and differential. No schistocytes, no atypical cells, no evidence of leukemia or lymphoma.

Additional Laboratory Tests:

- HIV: Negative

- Hepatitis C antibody: Negative

- TSH: 2.1 mIU/L (normal: 0.4-4.0 mIU/L)

- ANA: Positive at 1:80 with speckled pattern

- Direct antiglobulin test (Coombs): Negative

The positive ANA is mildly elevated but not highly specific. Many healthy people have low-titer positive ANA without autoimmune disease. However, it does raise the possibility of underlying autoimmune predisposition.

No bone marrow biopsy was performed. Why not? The peripheral smear showed large platelets (indicating the bone marrow is responding appropriately by making platelets), and other cell lines were normal. Bone marrow examination is usually reserved for cases where the diagnosis is unclear, when other cytopenias are present, or in older patients where primary bone marrow disorders are more likely (Neunert et al., 2011).

What's Happening Here?

The clinical picture points to **primary immune thrombocytopenic purpura (ITP)**, formerly called idiopathic thrombocytopenic purpura.

In ITP, the immune system produces antibodies against platelet surface antigens. These antibody-coated platelets are then recognized and destroyed by macrophages in the spleen and liver. The bone marrow tries to compensate by increasing platelet production, which is why you see large, young platelets on the smear. However, destruction outpaces production, resulting in severe thrombocytopenia (Rodeghiero et al., 2009).

The exact trigger for ITP is often unknown. In some cases, a viral infection precedes the development of ITP by a few weeks—molecular mimicry may cause the immune system to cross-react with platelet antigens. Other cases occur without any identifiable trigger.

ITP is a diagnosis of exclusion. You've ruled out:

- HIV and Hepatitis C (can cause immune thrombocytopenia)
- Drug-induced thrombocytopenia (no suspicious medications)
- Leukemia or lymphoma (normal blood smear and no concerning clinical features)
- Bone marrow failure (large platelets suggest adequate production)
- Thrombotic thrombocytopenic purpura (no schistocytes, no hemolytic anemia)

The low-titer positive ANA doesn't necessarily indicate lupus. About 10-20% of ITP patients have positive ANA without meeting criteria for systemic lupus erythematosus. However, it does warrant monitoring for development of other autoimmune symptoms over time (Zufferey et al., 2017).

Final Diagnosis

Primary immune thrombocytopenic purpura (ITP)

Treatment and Management

Treatment of ITP depends on platelet count, bleeding symptoms, and patient factors. This patient has:

- Platelet count <30,000/μL
- Active bleeding (easy bruising, gingival bleeding, menorrhagia)

She requires treatment. Options include:

First-line treatments:

- **Corticosteroids** (prednisone 1 mg/kg daily for 2-4 weeks, then taper)
- **IV immunoglobulin (IVIG)** for rapid platelet increase if needed
- **Anti-D immunoglobulin** (in Rh-positive patients)

Her physician starts prednisone 60 mg daily with plans to recheck her platelet count in one week. He advises avoiding NSAIDs and aspirin (increase bleeding risk), avoiding contact sports, and seeking immediate care for severe headache, abdominal pain, or excessive bleeding.

Expected Response: Most patients respond to corticosteroids within 1-2 weeks with platelet counts rising above 50,000/μL. Some achieve durable remission after steroid treatment. Others relapse when steroids are tapered, requiring additional therapy.

Second-line options (if steroids fail or she relapses):

- Thrombopoietin receptor agonists (romiplostim, eltrombopag)
- Rituximab (anti-CD20 antibody)
- Splenectomy (removing the site of platelet destruction)

Follow-up

One week later, her platelet count is 78,000/μL—a significant improvement. Her bruising has stopped progressing, and gingival bleeding has resolved. The prednisone is gradually tapered over the next month.

At three months, off steroids, her platelet count remains stable at 145,000/μL. She achieved durable remission, which occurs in about 60-70% of adults treated for ITP. She'll need periodic monitoring as late relapses can occur even years after initial diagnosis (Neunert et al., 2011).

Teaching Points

Isolated thrombocytopenia with normal red and white cells suggests a platelet-specific problem. When all three cell lines are low (pancytopenia), think bone marrow failure, leukemia, or hypersplenism. When only platelets are low, consider ITP, drug-induced thrombocytopenia, or other platelet-specific disorders.

Always review the peripheral smear. Pseudothrombocytopenia (platelet clumping) occurs in about 0.1% of CBC samples, usually due to EDTA-dependent antibodies that cause platelets to clump in the collection tube. The automated counter doesn't count clumped platelets, reporting falsely low counts. A smear reveals the clumps and saves the patient from unnecessary anxiety and treatment (Bizzaro, 1995).

Large platelets (megathrombocytes) indicate increased platelet production. This suggests the bone marrow is responding appropriately, which points away from production failure and toward increased destruction or consumption.

ITP severity correlates with bleeding risk, not just platelet count. A patient with 20,000 platelets and no bleeding may need less aggressive treatment than someone with 40,000 platelets and significant bleeding. Treatment decisions balance bleeding risk against treatment side effects.

Secondary ITP must be excluded. HIV, Hepatitis C, lupus, lymphoma, and medications can all cause immune-mediated thrombocytopenia. Distinguishing primary ITP from secondary causes is important because treating the underlying condition can resolve the thrombocytopenia.

Platelet transfusions are generally avoided in ITP except for life-threatening bleeding. Transfused platelets get destroyed just as quickly as the patient's own platelets, so they don't provide lasting benefit. They're reserved for emergencies like intracranial hemorrhage.

Related Cases

This case connects to:

- **Case 7: Thrombotic Thrombocytopenic Purpura** (another cause of severe thrombocytopenia but with a very different pathophysiology)

- **Case 12: Disseminated Intravascular Coagulation** (consumption of platelets)

- **Case 1: The Tired Graduate Student** (mentions menorrhagia in a different context)

Case 3: The Athletic Young Man with Fatigue

Clinical Presentation

A 19-year-old male college soccer player presents to the athletic training clinic complaining of unusual fatigue during practice over the past two weeks. He reports that he "runs out of gas" much faster than his teammates and has been experiencing mild dizziness during intense drills. His coach noticed his performance declining and suggested he get checked out.

He denies chest pain, shortness of breath at rest, or palpitations. No recent illnesses or injuries. He takes no medications and has no known medical conditions. Family history is significant—his father is from Sicily and has "some kind of blood condition" that requires occasional monitoring but no treatment.

Physical examination reveals a well-developed athlete in no acute distress. Heart rate is 58 beats per minute (expected for an athlete). Blood pressure is 118/72 mmHg. Examination is otherwise unremarkable except for very slight pallor.

Initial Laboratory Findings

The athletic trainer orders a CBC as part of routine evaluation:

- Hemoglobin: 10.8 g/dL (normal: 13.5-17.5 g/dL for males) - LOW

- Hematocrit: 33% (normal: 41-53% for males) - LOW

- MCV: 68 fL (normal: 80-100 fL) - VERY LOW

- RBC count: 5.9 million/μL (normal: 4.5-5.9 million/μL) - HIGH NORMAL

- RDW: 14.2% (normal: 11.5-14.5%)

- White blood cell count: 6,500/μL (normal)

- Platelet count: 290,000/μL (normal)

Stop and Think

Here's an interesting pattern. The hemoglobin is low (anemia), but look closely at the other values. The MCV is **markedly low** at 68 fL—more severe microcytosis than you'd typically see with iron deficiency. Yet the RBC count is at the high end of normal (5.9 million).

Think about that combination: lots of red blood cells, but they're very small, resulting in low total hemoglobin. It's like having many small buckets instead of fewer larger buckets—the total volume is reduced even though you have plenty of buckets.

Also notice the RDW is only slightly elevated at 14.2%. In iron deficiency, you typically see higher RDW values (often >16%) because the red cells vary widely in size. Here the cells are uniformly small.

Your differential for microcytic anemia includes:

1. Iron deficiency

2. Thalassemia

3. Anemia of chronic disease

4. Lead poisoning

But that family history detail—father from Sicily with a blood condition requiring monitoring—that's a huge clue. Sicily is in the Mediterranean region where thalassemia is common. Thalassemia is inherited, which would explain why his father has it too.

Diagnostic Reasoning Questions

What's the Mentzer index, and how does it help?

The Mentzer index is calculated as MCV divided by RBC count (in millions). It helps distinguish iron deficiency from thalassemia:

- Mentzer index **>13** suggests iron deficiency

- Mentzer index **<13** suggests thalassemia

For this patient: $68 \div 5.9 = 11.5$

A Mentzer index of 11.5 strongly suggests thalassemia rather than iron deficiency (Urrechaga et al., 2015).

What additional tests would you order?

Iron studies are still important to rule out coexisting iron deficiency. But the key tests here are:

- **Hemoglobin electrophoresis** (separates different types of hemoglobin)

- **Peripheral blood smear** (looking for characteristic findings)

- Iron studies (to rule out iron deficiency)

What do you expect to find in thalassemia?

Thalassemia involves decreased production of either alpha or beta globin chains that make up hemoglobin. The imbalance leads to ineffective red blood cell production and hemolysis.

On hemoglobin electrophoresis:

- **Beta thalassemia minor** (trait) shows elevated HbA2 (>3.5%) and sometimes elevated HbF

- **Alpha thalassemia trait** often shows normal electrophoresis (requires genetic testing for confirmation)

On peripheral smear, you'd expect:

- Microcytic, hypochromic cells (but more uniform than iron deficiency)

- Target cells (cells with a bull's-eye appearance)

- Basophilic stippling (blue dots representing ribosomal RNA)

- Normal or increased reticulocyte count (bone marrow is working hard)

Sequential Test Results

Iron Studies:

- Serum iron: 95 µg/dL (normal: 60-170 µg/dL) - NORMAL

- TIBC: 310 µg/dL (normal: 250-450 µg/dL) - NORMAL

- Ferritin: 85 ng/mL (normal: 12-300 ng/mL) - NORMAL

- Transferrin saturation: 31% (normal: 20-50%) - NORMAL

Peripheral Blood Smear: Microcytic, hypochromic red blood cells with uniform small size. Numerous target cells present. Occasional basophilic stippling noted. Mild polychromasia (suggesting increased reticulocyte production). No evidence of iron deficiency morphology.

Hemoglobin Electrophoresis:

- HbA: 94.8% (normal: 96-98%)

- HbA2: 5.2% (normal: 2.5-3.5%) - **ELEVATED**

- HbF: <1% (normal: <1%)

The elevated HbA2 confirms the diagnosis.

What's Happening Here?

This patient has **beta thalassemia minor** (also called beta thalassemia trait). He inherited one normal beta globin gene and one abnormal beta globin gene—one from each parent.

In beta thalassemia minor, the body produces less beta globin than normal. To compensate, more HbA2 (which uses delta chains instead of beta chains) is produced. The elevated HbA2 on electrophoresis is the diagnostic hallmark of beta thalassemia trait (Weatherall, 2010).

The decreased beta globin production results in:

- Microcytic red cells (less hemoglobin per cell)

- Increased RBC count (body tries to compensate by making more cells)

- Mild anemia (the compensation isn't quite enough)

- Minimal symptoms in most cases

His fatigue during athletic performance makes sense. Elite athletes operate at the margins of physiologic capacity. Even mild anemia that wouldn't bother a sedentary person can significantly impact athletic performance due to reduced oxygen-carrying capacity (Peeling et al., 2008).

Final Diagnosis

Beta thalassemia minor (beta thalassemia trait)

Management and Counseling

Unlike iron deficiency, beta thalassemia trait doesn't require treatment. The anemia is typically mild and stable. However, several important points need discussion:

Athletic Performance: His coaches and trainers should understand this is a chronic, stable condition. He may not perform at the absolute peak level of athletes without thalassemia trait, but many successful athletes have thalassemia trait. Adjusting training intensity and ensuring adequate hydration and rest may help.

Iron Supplementation Is NOT Indicated: This is crucial. His iron stores are normal. Taking iron supplements won't improve his anemia and could potentially lead to iron overload over time. Many people with thalassemia trait are mistakenly given iron for years before the correct diagnosis is made (Camaschella, 2019).

Genetic Counseling: Thalassemia trait is inherited. If his future partner also carries a thalassemia gene, their children could inherit thalassemia major (two abnormal genes), which causes severe anemia requiring lifelong transfusions. Genetic counseling before having children is recommended. His siblings should also be tested since they have a 50% chance of carrying the trait.

Medical Awareness: He should inform all healthcare providers about his thalassemia trait. In certain situations (pregnancy, surgery, critical illness), it becomes relevant to medical care. He should wear a medical alert bracelet or carry a card stating his diagnosis.

Family Testing: His father likely has beta thalassemia trait as well (explaining the "blood condition requiring monitoring"). If his father hasn't been formally diagnosed, testing would be appropriate. His mother should also be tested—if she's a carrier, his siblings need screening.

Follow-up

At his three-month follow-up, his hemoglobin remains stable at 10.9 g/dL. His athletic performance has improved somewhat after adjusting his training regimen and ensuring he stays well-hydrated. He's accepted that he may not have quite the endurance of his teammates but has found ways to compensate with superior technical skills.

He scheduled genetic counseling and educated his girlfriend about thalassemia inheritance patterns. His younger sister was tested and also found to have beta thalassemia trait.

Teaching Points

Think thalassemia when you see severe microcytosis (MCV <75) with minimal or mild anemia. The degree of microcytosis is often disproportionate to the severity of anemia in thalassemia. Iron deficiency typically produces more severe anemia before reaching such low MCV values.

Family history and ethnicity provide critical diagnostic clues. Thalassemia is most common in people of Mediterranean (Italian, Greek), Middle Eastern, Southeast Asian, Indian, and African descent. Always ask about family history of anemia and ethnic background when evaluating microcytic anemia.

The Mentzer index is a useful screening tool but not definitive. While a Mentzer index <13 suggests thalassemia, iron studies and hemoglobin electrophoresis are needed for confirmation. Some patients have both thalassemia trait and iron deficiency, complicating the picture (Urrechaga et al., 2015).

Don't give iron to thalassemia patients unless iron deficiency is documented. Inappropriate iron supplementation is common and potentially harmful. Always check iron studies before prescribing iron, especially in patients with microcytic anemia and certain ethnic backgrounds.

Thalassemia trait is clinically benign but genetically important. Individuals with trait are generally healthy and don't require treatment. However, two carrier parents have a 25% chance with each pregnancy of having a child with thalassemia major, a severe disease requiring lifelong transfusions and chelation therapy. Genetic counseling is essential.

Target cells and basophilic stippling are characteristic of thalassemia. While not 100% specific, these findings on peripheral smear strongly suggest thalassemia rather than iron deficiency. Target cells result from excess cell membrane relative to hemoglobin content.

Alpha thalassemia trait often shows normal hemoglobin electrophoresis. Unlike beta thalassemia trait (which shows elevated HbA2), alpha thalassemia trait typically requires DNA testing for definitive diagnosis. Suspect it when you see microcytic anemia with normal iron studies and normal hemoglobin electrophoresis, especially in Southeast Asian or African patients (Harteveld & Higgs, 2010).

Related Cases

This case connects to:

- **Case 1: The Tired Graduate Student** (iron deficiency—the other major cause of microcytic anemia)

- **Case 9: Iron Deficiency vs. Thalassemia** (directly compares these two conditions)

- **Case 15: Hereditary Spherocytosis** (another inherited hemolytic anemia)

Case 4: The Teenager with Night Sweats

Clinical Presentation

A 17-year-old female high school student presents to her pediatrician with complaints of persistent fatigue, unintentional weight loss of 12 pounds over two months, and drenching night sweats that require changing her pajamas. She initially thought she had the flu that "wouldn't go away."

She also reports itching all over her body (pruritus) that's worse after hot showers. Occasionally she experiences low-grade fevers. Her appetite has decreased, and she feels generally unwell.

Her past medical history is unremarkable. She takes no medications. She denies drug use, smoking, or alcohol consumption. No recent travel or sick contacts. Family history is noncontributory.

Physical examination reveals a thin, pale teenage girl who appears chronically ill. Vital signs show temperature of 37.8°C (100°F), heart rate of 92 beats per minute. The most striking finding is **bilateral cervical and supraclavicular lymphadenopathy**—multiple enlarged, firm, non-tender lymph nodes palpable on both sides of her neck and above her collarbones. Examination also reveals splenomegaly (enlarged spleen extending 4 cm below the left costal margin).

Initial Laboratory Findings

Her pediatrician orders a CBC with differential:

- Hemoglobin: 9.8 g/dL (normal: 12.0-16.0 g/dL) - LOW

- Hematocrit: 29% (normal: 36-46%) - LOW

- MCV: 88 fL (normal: 80-100 fL) - NORMAL

- White blood cell count: 13,500/μL (normal: 4,000-11,000/μL) - **ELEVATED**

- Platelet count: 485,000/μL (normal: 150,000-400,000/μL) - **ELEVATED**

WBC Differential:

- Neutrophils: 68% (normal: 40-70%)

- Lymphocytes: 18% (normal: 20-40%) - slightly low

- Monocytes: 10% (normal: 2-8%) - elevated

- Eosinophils: 3% (normal: 1-4%)

- Basophils: 1% (normal: 0-1%)

- **Atypical lymphocytes: noted on differential**

Stop and Think

This case presents a very different pattern from the previous anemia cases. Let's break down what we're seeing:

The combination of constitutional symptoms (fever, night sweats, weight loss—called "B symptoms" in hematology), lymphadenopathy, splenomegaly, and abnormal blood counts raises immediate red flags. This isn't simple iron deficiency or a benign condition.

The white blood cell count is elevated with an interesting differential. The presence of **atypical lymphocytes** is particularly concerning. Atypical lymphocytes are activated lymphocytes that look abnormal under the microscope—larger than normal with abundant cytoplasm and irregular nuclei.

The mild anemia could be explained by chronic disease or bone marrow infiltration. The elevated platelet count (thrombocytosis) is reactive—the body produces more platelets in response to inflammation or malignancy.

What conditions produce this constellation of findings?

Key Differential Diagnosis:

1. **Lymphoma** (Hodgkin or non-Hodgkin)

2. **Infectious mononucleosis** (EBV infection)

3. **Other malignancies** (leukemia, metastatic disease)

4. **Chronic infections** (tuberculosis, HIV)

5. **Autoimmune conditions** (rare presentations)

The B symptoms (fever, night sweats, weight loss) are classic for lymphoma. However, infectious mononucleosis can cause similar symptoms with lymphadenopathy and atypical lymphocytes. You can't distinguish these based on symptoms alone.

Diagnostic Reasoning Questions

What's the most important next test?

While blood work helps, the definitive diagnosis requires **tissue biopsy**. An excisional lymph node biopsy (removing an entire enlarged lymph node) provides tissue for pathologic examination, immunophenotyping, and molecular studies.

What additional blood tests would you order?

Before the biopsy:

- **Monospot test** or **EBV antibodies** (to rule out infectious mononucleosis)
- **Lactate dehydrogenase (LDH)** (elevated in lymphoma and hemolysis)
- **Erythrocyte sedimentation rate (ESR)** (typically markedly elevated in Hodgkin lymphoma)
- **Comprehensive metabolic panel** (assess organ function)
- **HIV test** (lymphoma risk is increased)

What would you see on peripheral smear?

The smear would show those atypical lymphocytes in detail. In infectious mononucleosis, you'd see reactive lymphocytes (Downey cells)—large lymphocytes with abundant deep blue cytoplasm that molds around adjacent red blood cells.

In lymphoma, you might see circulating lymphoma cells, though this is less common in Hodgkin lymphoma than in some non-Hodgkin lymphomas.

Sequential Test Results

Additional Laboratory Tests:

- Monospot test: **Negative**
- EBV VCA IgM: Negative (acute infection marker)
- EBV VCA IgG: Positive (past infection marker)
- EBV EBNA: Positive (past infection marker)
- LDH: 425 U/L (normal: 122-222 U/L) - **ELEVATED**
- ESR: 68 mm/hr (normal: 0-20 mm/hr) - **MARKEDLY ELEVATED**
- HIV: Negative

The EBV antibody pattern shows past EBV infection (like most adults), but not acute infection. The negative monospot rules out infectious mononucleosis.

Peripheral Blood Smear: Mild normocytic anemia. White blood cells show increased neutrophils and monocytes. Occasional atypical lymphocytes present but not in large numbers. Platelets are increased. No blasts or obvious malignant cells seen (though this doesn't rule out lymphoma—the malignant cells typically stay in the lymph nodes in Hodgkin lymphoma).

Imaging Studies:

Chest X-ray shows widening of the mediastinum (middle of chest), suggesting enlarged lymph nodes in the chest.

CT scan of neck, chest, abdomen, and pelvis reveals:

- Extensive cervical, supraclavicular, and mediastinal lymphadenopathy
- Enlarged lymph nodes throughout the abdomen
- Splenomegaly
- No liver involvement

Excisional Lymph Node Biopsy:

This is the definitive test. A cervical lymph node is removed and sent to pathology.

Microscopic examination reveals:

- Disrupted lymph node architecture
- Mixed cellular infiltrate with lymphocytes, eosinophils, neutrophils, and histiocytes
- Large, abnormal cells with bilobed nuclei resembling "owl eyes"
- **Reed-Sternberg cells identified** (the diagnostic hallmark)

Immunohistochemistry shows:

- Reed-Sternberg cells are positive for CD15 and CD30
- Reed-Sternberg cells are negative for CD45 (leukocyte common antigen)

This confirms **classical Hodgkin lymphoma**.

What's Happening Here?

Hodgkin lymphoma is a cancer of the lymphatic system characterized by the presence of Reed-Sternberg cells—large malignant cells thought to arise from B lymphocytes. These cells are surrounded by an inflammatory infiltrate of normal immune cells (Shanbhag & Ambinder, 2018).

The disease typically presents in young adults (peak incidence in the 20s) or older adults (over 55). About 40% of patients present with B symptoms—fever, night sweats, and weight loss. The pruritus (itching) she experienced is less common but characteristic when present.

Hodgkin lymphoma usually begins in a single lymph node region (most commonly cervical or mediastinal lymph nodes) and spreads predictably to adjacent lymph node groups. This is why staging is important—it determines treatment approach.

The elevated ESR, elevated LDH, and reactive blood changes (anemia, thrombocytosis, leukocytosis) all reflect the body's response to the malignancy. None of these are specific for Hodgkin lymphoma, but they support the diagnosis and help assess disease burden.

Final Diagnosis

Classical Hodgkin lymphoma, nodular sclerosis subtype (most common subtype), Stage III (involvement of lymph nodes on both sides of the diaphragm plus spleen) with B symptoms

Staging and Treatment

Staging determines treatment intensity. Hodgkin lymphoma is staged I-IV:

- Stage I: Single lymph node region

- Stage II: Two or more regions on same side of diaphragm

- Stage III: Lymph nodes on both sides of diaphragm

- Stage IV: Involvement of organs outside lymph system (bone marrow, liver, lung)

Each stage is further classified as A (no B symptoms) or B (B symptoms present).

This patient is **Stage IIIB** (lymph nodes above and below diaphragm plus spleen involvement, with B symptoms).

Treatment for classical Hodgkin lymphoma typically involves:

- **Chemotherapy**: ABVD regimen (Adriamycin, Bleomycin, Vinblastine, Dacarbazine) for 6 cycles

- **Radiation therapy**: To initially involved lymph node regions after chemotherapy

- **PET-CT scans**: To assess treatment response after 2-4 cycles

Prognosis for Hodgkin lymphoma is generally excellent, even in advanced stages. Five-year survival rates exceed 85% overall. Young patients with classical Hodgkin lymphoma and good prognostic factors (like this patient—young age, nodular sclerosis subtype, good performance status) have even better outcomes, with cure rates approaching 90-95% (Shanbhag & Ambinder, 2018).

Follow-up

She begins ABVD chemotherapy. After two cycles, a PET-CT scan shows dramatic reduction in lymph node size and metabolic activity—a positive response. She experiences typical chemotherapy side effects (nausea, fatigue, hair loss) but tolerates treatment reasonably well.

After completing six cycles of chemotherapy, she receives radiation therapy to the areas that were initially involved. Follow-up scans six months after completing treatment show complete remission—no evidence of active lymphoma.

She'll need long-term monitoring for potential late effects of treatment (cardiac toxicity from Adriamycin, pulmonary toxicity from bleomycin, secondary malignancies from radiation) and for lymphoma recurrence, though her prognosis is excellent.

Teaching Points

Constitutional symptoms (B symptoms) plus lymphadenopathy should always raise concern for lymphoma. Weight loss, fever, and night sweats aren't specific, but combined with persistent lymph node enlargement, they warrant urgent evaluation. Don't dismiss these as "just a virus" without thorough workup.

Reed-Sternberg cells are pathognomonic for classical Hodgkin lymphoma. These large, binucleated or multinucleated cells with prominent nucleoli create the characteristic "owl eye" appearance. They're necessary for diagnosis, though their presence alone isn't sufficient—you need the appropriate immunophenotype and clinical context (Shanbhag & Ambinder, 2018).

Atypical lymphocytes don't always mean mononucleosis. While atypical lymphocytes are classic for EBV infection, they appear in many viral infections, some drug reactions, and occasionally with malignancies. Always confirm infectious mononucleosis with monospot or EBV serology rather than assuming atypical lymphocytes equal mono.

Lymph node biopsy is essential for definitive diagnosis. You cannot reliably diagnose lymphoma with blood tests alone (except for some leukemias). Excisional biopsy provides tissue architecture and sufficient material for immunohistochemistry and molecular studies. Fine needle aspiration is usually inadequate for initial lymphoma diagnosis.

Hodgkin lymphoma has an excellent prognosis with modern treatment. This distinguishes it from many other cancers. Most patients are cured. However, long-term survivors face risks of late treatment effects that require ongoing monitoring—secondary cancers (breast, lung, thyroid), cardiovascular disease, and pulmonary complications (Ng et al., 2017).

The ESR is often markedly elevated in Hodgkin lymphoma. While ESR is a nonspecific inflammatory marker, values >50 mm/hr in young patients without obvious infection should prompt consideration of malignancy or serious inflammatory conditions. ESR >50 mm/hr is also a poor prognostic factor in Hodgkin lymphoma.

Enlarged lymph nodes in young adults deserve evaluation. Benign reactive lymphadenopathy is common after infections, but nodes that persist for >4-6 weeks, continue enlarging, or are associated with B symptoms or abnormal blood counts need biopsy. Supraclavicular lymphadenopathy is particularly concerning—about 90% of supraclavicular node enlargement in adults represents serious pathology (Gaddey & Riegel, 2016).

Related Cases

This case connects to:

- **Case 10: Acute Leukemia Presentation** (another hematologic malignancy in a young person)
- **Case 11: Atypical Lymphocytes in Adolescent** (infectious mononucleosis—the benign cause of atypical lymphocytes)
- **Case 14: Myelodysplastic Syndrome** (another bone marrow disorder causing cytopenias)

Case 5: The Man Who Couldn't Stop Bleeding

Clinical Presentation

A 34-year-old man presents to the emergency department with persistent bleeding from a minor cut on his finger that occurred three hours ago while cooking. He's applied pressure and multiple bandages, but the bleeding continues to ooze. This seems unusual to him since the cut isn't deep.

Further questioning reveals a lifelong history of easy bruising and prolonged bleeding after dental extractions. He recalls bleeding for several hours after a tooth extraction five years ago. He doesn't have spontaneous bleeding into joints or muscles, and he's never required blood transfusions. His father and paternal uncle have similar bleeding tendencies.

He takes no medications and denies use of aspirin, NSAIDs, or anticoagulants. No recent illnesses. He works as an accountant and lives a relatively sedentary lifestyle.

Physical examination shows a well-appearing man with a small laceration on his left index finger that continues to ooze blood despite pressure. Multiple ecchymoses in various stages of healing are noted on his arms and legs. No petechiae. No joint swelling or deformities. The rest of the examination is unremarkable.

Initial Laboratory Findings

The emergency physician orders coagulation studies:

- PT (Prothrombin Time): 12.5 seconds (normal: 11-13 seconds) - NORMAL

- INR: 1.0 (normal: 0.8-1.2) - NORMAL

- **aPTT (Activated Partial Thromboplastin Time): 48 seconds (normal: 25-35 seconds) - PROLONGED**

- Platelet count: 245,000/μL (normal) - NORMAL

- Hemoglobin: 14.2 g/dL (normal) - NORMAL

Stop and Think

Here's a patient with a clear bleeding tendency—prolonged bleeding from minor trauma, easy bruising, family history of similar problems. The laboratory results point you in a specific direction.

The normal platelet count rules out thrombocytopenia. The normal PT but prolonged aPTT narrows your differential considerably. Let's think about what these tests measure:

PT (Prothrombin Time) measures the extrinsic and common pathways of coagulation. It reflects factors VII, X, V, II (prothrombin), and fibrinogen. Warfarin prolongs PT. Liver disease prolongs PT. This patient's PT is normal.

aPTT (Activated Partial Thromboplastin Time) measures the intrinsic and common pathways. It reflects factors XII, XI, IX, VIII, X, V, II, and fibrinogen. Heparin prolongs aPTT. Deficiencies in factors VIII, IX, XI, or XII prolong aPTT.

When aPTT is prolonged but PT is normal, you're looking at a problem with the **intrinsic pathway**—specifically factors XII, XI, IX, or VIII.

The family history (father and uncle affected) suggests an inherited disorder. The pattern of inheritance matters here:

- **X-linked inheritance**: Hemophilia A (factor VIII deficiency) and Hemophilia B (factor IX deficiency)

- **Autosomal dominant**: von Willebrand disease (most common inherited bleeding disorder)

- **Autosomal recessive**: Factor XI deficiency

Since both his father and uncle are affected, this isn't X-linked (males don't pass X-linked disorders to their sons). This pattern suggests either **von Willebrand disease** (most likely) or **factor XI deficiency** (less common).

Diagnostic Reasoning Questions

What's the next step in evaluation?

You need specific factor assays to determine which clotting factor is deficient. For a prolonged aPTT with clinical bleeding, order:

- **Factor VIII activity level**

- **Factor IX activity level**

- **Factor XI activity level**

- **von Willebrand factor antigen** (vWF:Ag)

- **von Willebrand factor activity** (ristocetin cofactor activity or vWF:RCo)

- **Factor VIII:C** (coagulant activity)

What about mixing studies?

A mixing study helps distinguish factor deficiency from factor inhibitors. Patient plasma is mixed 1:1 with normal pooled plasma. If the aPTT corrects (normalizes), it indicates factor deficiency. If it doesn't correct, it suggests an inhibitor (antibody) against a clotting factor.

In this case, mixing study would likely correct the aPTT, supporting factor deficiency rather than an inhibitor.

How do you distinguish von Willebrand disease from hemophilia?

- **Hemophilia A**: Low factor VIII, normal vWF, normal platelet function, X-linked inheritance

- **Hemophilia B**: Low factor IX, normal vWF, normal platelet function, X-linked inheritance

- **von Willebrand disease**: Low vWF (usually), low factor VIII (because vWF stabilizes factor VIII), abnormal platelet function, autosomal dominant inheritance

Von Willebrand disease is tricky because factor VIII levels may be low (since vWF protects factor VIII from degradation). This can make it look like mild hemophilia A initially.

Sequential Test Results

Mixing Study: Patient aPTT: 48 seconds Normal plasma aPTT: 30 seconds 1:1 Mix aPTT: 32 seconds - **CORRECTS**

This confirms factor deficiency rather than an inhibitor.

Factor Assays:

- Factor VIII activity: 38% (normal: 50-150%) - **LOW**

- Factor IX activity: 105% (normal: 50-150%) - NORMAL

- Factor XI activity: 92% (normal: 50-150%) - NORMAL

- von Willebrand factor antigen (vWF:Ag): 35% (normal: 50-150%) - **LOW**

- von Willebrand factor activity (vWF:RCo): 32% (normal: 50-150%) - **LOW**

- Blood type: Type O

Platelet Function Analysis (PFA-100): Closure time with collagen/epinephrine: Prolonged (>300 seconds; normal: <193 seconds)

This pattern is diagnostic.

What's Happening Here?

This patient has **Type 1 von Willebrand disease**, the most common inherited bleeding disorder, affecting about 1% of the population (though most cases are mild and undiagnosed) (Leebeek & Eikenboom, 2016).

Von Willebrand factor (vWF) is a large protein that serves two critical functions:

1. It helps platelets stick to damaged blood vessel walls (platelet adhesion)

2. It carries and protects factor VIII in the circulation

In Type 1 von Willebrand disease, the body produces less vWF than normal (quantitative deficiency). This leads to:

- Reduced platelet adhesion (causing mucosal bleeding, easy bruising, prolonged bleeding from cuts)

- Reduced factor VIII levels (because factor VIII is degraded faster without vWF protection)

- Prolonged aPTT (due to low factor VIII)

The bleeding pattern in von Willebrand disease differs from hemophilia:

- **von Willebrand disease**: Mucosal bleeding (nosebleeds, gum bleeding, heavy menstrual periods in women), prolonged bleeding from cuts, easy bruising, bleeding after dental work or surgery

- **Hemophilia**: Bleeding into joints (hemarthrosis), bleeding into muscles, spontaneous bleeding episodes (in severe cases)

This patient's presentation—prolonged bleeding from minor cuts and dental work, easy bruising, but no joint bleeding—fits von Willebrand disease perfectly.

His blood type O is relevant. People with type O blood naturally have lower vWF levels (about 25% lower than other blood types), which can make Type 1 von Willebrand disease more apparent (Leebeek & Eikenboom, 2016).

Final Diagnosis

Type 1 von Willebrand disease

Classification of von Willebrand Disease

There are three main types:

Type 1 (70-80% of cases): Partial quantitative deficiency of vWF. vWF is normal in structure but reduced in amount. Usually mild bleeding. This patient's type.

Type 2 (15-20% of cases): Qualitative deficiency—normal or near-normal vWF levels, but the vWF doesn't function properly. Several subtypes exist. Variable bleeding severity.

Type 3 (<1% of cases): Complete absence of vWF. Severe bleeding similar to severe hemophilia. Very rare, autosomal recessive.

Treatment and Management

Acute Bleeding Episodes:

For his finger laceration:

- Direct pressure and local hemostatic measures (thrombin-soaked gauze, fibrin glue)
- **Desmopressin (DDAVP):** Releases vWF from storage sites in endothelial cells. Typically raises vWF and factor VIII levels 2-4 fold within 30-60 minutes. Can be given intravenously, subcutaneously, or intranasally.

The finger bleeding was controlled with DDAVP and prolonged pressure.

Perioperative Management:

Before dental work or surgeries:

- DDAVP 30 minutes before procedure
- Tranexamic acid (antifibrinolytic drug) to prevent clot breakdown
- Avoid aspirin and NSAIDs (impair platelet function)
- For major surgeries, may need vWF/factor VIII concentrate infusions

Long-term Management:

- Medical alert bracelet identifying von Willebrand disease
- Education about avoiding aspirin and NSAIDs
- Genetic counseling (autosomal dominant—50% chance of passing to each child)

- Women with von Willebrand disease may need special management during pregnancy and delivery (hemorrhage risk)

Monitoring:

Patients with mild Type 1 von Willebrand disease like this patient usually don't need regular monitoring. They live essentially normal lives with precautions during procedures and prompt treatment of bleeding episodes.

Follow-up

He was prescribed intranasal DDAVP (Stimate) to keep at home for minor bleeding episodes. He successfully used it before a dental cleaning six months later without excessive bleeding. He was counseled to inform all healthcare providers about his diagnosis and to avoid medications that impair clotting.

His two children (ages 8 and 11) were screened for von Willebrand disease. His daughter tested positive with similarly mild Type 1 disease. His son tested negative.

Teaching Points

Von Willebrand disease is the most common inherited bleeding disorder but often goes undiagnosed. Many people with mild Type 1 von Willebrand disease don't realize they have a bleeding disorder—they just think they "bruise easily" or "bleed more than other people." The diagnosis is often made when excessive bleeding occurs after dental work, surgery, or childbirth.

Prolonged aPTT with normal PT and platelets points to intrinsic pathway deficiency. The differential includes hemophilia A (factor VIII deficiency), hemophilia B (factor IX deficiency), factor XI deficiency, and von Willebrand disease. Family history and specific factor assays distinguish these.

Von Willebrand disease can lower factor VIII levels. This causes confusion because low factor VIII suggests hemophilia A. Always check vWF levels when evaluating low factor VIII to rule out von Willebrand disease. The distinction matters for treatment, genetic counseling, and prognosis (Leebeek & Eikenboom, 2016).

The bleeding pattern helps distinguish von Willebrand disease from hemophilia. Mucosal bleeding, prolonged bleeding from cuts, and menorrhagia suggest von Willebrand disease. Joint and muscle bleeding suggests hemophilia. This isn't absolute—severe von Willebrand disease (Type 3) can cause joint bleeding—but the pattern is useful.

DDAVP is first-line treatment for Type 1 von Willebrand disease. It's effective in 80-90% of Type 1 patients. However, it doesn't work for all subtypes—Type 2B patients may worsen with DDAVP, and Type 3 patients lack vWF to release. A trial dose should be given to assess response before relying on DDAVP for procedures (Castaman & Linari, 2017).

Blood type influences vWF levels. Type O individuals have 25-30% lower vWF than non-O blood types due to faster vWF clearance. This means Type O individuals with von Willebrand disease may have more pronounced symptoms, while borderline von Willebrand disease might only manifest in Type O individuals (Leebeek & Eikenboom, 2016).

Factor VIII and vWF levels can fluctuate. Stress, exercise, pregnancy, estrogen use, and inflammation can raise vWF and factor VIII levels. Testing should ideally be done when patients are at baseline. Sometimes repeat testing is needed to confirm diagnosis, especially in mild cases.

Related Cases

This case connects to:

- **Case 12: Disseminated Intravascular Coagulation** (acquired coagulation disorder with very different presentation)

- **Case 13: Factor V Leiden Thrombophilia** (hereditary clotting disorder but causing thrombosis rather than bleeding)

- **Case 2: Unexplained Bruising** (ITP—another bleeding disorder but due to thrombocytopenia)

Case 6: The Older Man with Increasing Fatigue

Clinical Presentation

A 68-year-old retired postal worker presents to his primary care physician complaining of increasing fatigue, shortness of breath with exertion, and decreased exercise tolerance over the past six months. He used to walk two miles daily but now becomes winded after just one block.

He denies chest pain, but mentions occasional lightheadedness. His appetite has been good, and he hasn't lost weight. No fever, night sweats, or bleeding. He takes medications for hypertension (lisinopril) and high cholesterol (atorvastatin). He's a former smoker (quit 15 years ago, 30 pack-year history).

Physical examination reveals a well-nourished older man in no acute distress. His face appears somewhat ruddy and flushed. Blood pressure is 152/88 mmHg. Heart rate is 88 beats per minute. Cardiovascular examination reveals no murmurs. Lung examination is clear. Abdominal examination reveals splenomegaly—the spleen tip is palpable 3 cm below the left costal margin. No hepatomegaly or lymphadenopathy.

Initial Laboratory Findings

A CBC is ordered:

- **Hemoglobin: 19.2 g/dL (normal: 13.5-17.5 g/dL for males) - ELEVATED**

- **Hematocrit: 58% (normal: 41-53% for males) - ELEVATED**

- RBC count: 7.2 million/µL (normal: 4.5-5.9 million/µL) - ELEVATED

- MCV: 88 fL (normal: 80-100 fL) - NORMAL

- White blood cell count: 14,500/µL (normal: 4,000-11,000/µL) - elevated

- Platelet count: 625,000/µL (normal: 150,000-400,000/µL) - elevated

Stop and Think

Wait—elevated hemoglobin and hematocrit? All the previous cases involved low hemoglobin (anemia). This patient has the opposite problem: **polycythemia** (increased red blood cell mass).

His hemoglobin of 19.2 g/dL and hematocrit of 58% are significantly elevated. Normal hematocrit for men is 41-53%, so 58% represents a substantial increase. This means his blood has more red cells than normal, making it thicker and more viscous.

But look at the other cell lines—his white blood cells and platelets are also elevated. This is **pancytosis** (increased numbers of all cell lines), which is unusual. Most conditions cause selective increases in one cell line.

The combination of elevated red cells, white cells, and platelets plus splenomegaly suggests a **myeloproliferative neoplasm**—a group of bone marrow disorders where the marrow produces too many cells.

His symptoms make sense with polycythemia. Thick blood flows sluggishly through small vessels, impairing oxygen delivery despite high hemoglobin. This causes fatigue and shortness of breath. The increased blood viscosity also increases cardiovascular workload and thrombosis risk.

The ruddy, flushed appearance is classic for polycythemia—increased red cells make the skin appear darker and more flushed, especially on the face.

Diagnostic Reasoning Questions

What causes polycythemia?

Polycythemia can be:

Primary (intrinsic bone marrow problem):

- Polycythemia vera (a myeloproliferative neoplasm)

Secondary (appropriate response to hypoxia):

- Chronic lung disease (COPD)

- Living at high altitude

- Sleep apnea

- Right-to-left cardiac shunts

- High-affinity hemoglobin variants

Secondary (inappropriate erythropoietin production):

- Renal tumors or cysts

- Hepatocellular carcinoma

- Uterine fibroids

- Other tumors

Relative polycythemia (decreased plasma volume, not truly increased red cell mass):

- Dehydration

- Diuretic use

- Gaisbock syndrome (stress polycythemia)

How do you distinguish primary from secondary polycythemia?

Key tests include:

- **Erythropoietin (EPO) level**: Low in polycythemia vera (the bone marrow doesn't need EPO to produce red cells), high or normal in secondary polycythemia

- **JAK2 mutation testing**: Present in >95% of polycythemia vera cases

- **Oxygen saturation**: Normal in polycythemia vera, low in secondary polycythemia due to lung disease

- **Abdominal imaging**: Looking for renal tumors or other causes of inappropriate EPO production

What makes you think this is polycythemia vera rather than secondary polycythemia?

Several clues:

1. Elevation of all three cell lines (red cells, white cells, platelets)—secondary polycythemia usually only elevates red cells

2. Splenomegaly—common in polycythemia vera, rare in secondary polycythemia

3. No obvious cause of hypoxia (he's a former smoker but has clear lungs on exam)

Sequential Test Results

Additional Laboratory Tests:

- **Erythropoietin level: 2.8 mU/mL (normal: 4.0-25.0 mU/mL) - LOW**

- Oxygen saturation: 98% on room air - NORMAL

- Comprehensive metabolic panel: Normal kidney and liver function

- **JAK2 V617F mutation: POSITIVE - Detected**

Bone Marrow Biopsy: Hypercellular marrow (95% cellularity) with increased numbers of all three cell lines—erythroid precursors, myeloid cells, and megakaryocytes. No increase in blast cells. No dysplasia. No evidence of leukemia or other malignancy. Morphology consistent with a myeloproliferative neoplasm.

The low EPO level is the key finding here. Normal kidneys produce EPO in response to tissue hypoxia. If this patient had secondary polycythemia due to lung disease or living at altitude, his EPO would be elevated (appropriately stimulating red cell production). Instead, his EPO is suppressed because his body recognizes the hemoglobin is too high.

The positive JAK2 V617F mutation clinches the diagnosis. This mutation occurs in about 96% of polycythemia vera patients and is highly specific for myeloproliferative neoplasms (Tefferi & Barbui, 2020).

What's Happening Here?

This patient has **polycythemia vera**, a myeloproliferative neoplasm caused by a mutation in the JAK2 gene. The JAK2 V617F mutation causes constitutive (continuous) activation of the JAK-STAT signaling pathway, leading to growth factor-independent proliferation of blood cells.

In polycythemia vera:

- Red blood cell production is increased (causing polycythemia)

- White blood cell production is often increased

- Platelet production is often increased

- The spleen enlarges (extramedullary hematopoiesis and congestion)

- Blood viscosity increases (raising thrombosis and bleeding risks)

The median age at diagnosis is 60-65 years. The disease progresses slowly but is associated with significant complications:

Thrombosis is the major concern. About 20-30% of patients experience thrombotic events—stroke, myocardial infarction, deep vein thrombosis, pulmonary embolism, or unusual site thromboses (portal vein, splenic vein) (Tefferi & Barbui, 2020). The combination of elevated red cells (increased viscosity), elevated platelets (thrombocytosis), and elevated white cells creates a hypercoagulable state.

Hemorrhage can occur paradoxically, especially with very high platelet counts (>1,000,000/μL). The platelets function abnormally, and acquired von Willebrand syndrome can develop.

Progression to myelofibrosis occurs in about 10-15% of patients over 10-15 years. The bone marrow becomes scarred, and blood cell production moves to the spleen.

Transformation to acute leukemia occurs in about 5% of patients, especially those treated with certain chemotherapy agents.

Final Diagnosis

Polycythemia vera with JAK2 V617F mutation

Treatment and Management

Goals of treatment are to:

1. Reduce thrombosis risk

2. Control symptoms

3. Prevent progression

Immediate Management:

Phlebotomy (bloodletting) is first-line therapy. Removing 500 mL of blood weekly reduces the hematocrit quickly. Target hematocrit is <45% in men, <42% in women. Lower hematocrit significantly reduces thrombosis risk (Marchioli et al., 2013).

This patient undergoes phlebotomy of 500 mL. His hematocrit drops from 58% to 54%. Weekly phlebotomies continue until hematocrit reaches the target range.

Aspirin 81 mg daily is started. Low-dose aspirin reduces thrombosis risk by about 60% in polycythemia vera patients without significantly increasing bleeding risk (Landolfi et al., 2004).

Long-term Management:

Risk stratification determines who needs cytoreductive therapy:

Low risk (age <60 and no thrombosis history): Phlebotomy + aspirin usually sufficient

High risk (age ≥60 or prior thrombosis): Need cytoreductive therapy to reduce cell counts

This patient is 68 years old, placing him in the high-risk category. Cytoreductive options include:

- **Hydroxyurea**: Oral chemotherapy agent that reduces blood cell production. First-line cytoreductive therapy. Target is to keep hematocrit <45%, white cells 4,000-10,000/μL, platelets 100,000-400,000/μL.

- **Interferon-alpha**: Alternative for younger patients or those intolerant of hydroxyurea. Particularly useful in women of childbearing age.

- **Ruxolitinib**: JAK2 inhibitor approved for patients intolerant of or resistant to hydroxyurea. Expensive but effective.

He's started on hydroxyurea 500 mg daily along with continued phlebotomy as needed and aspirin. His symptoms improve within weeks as his blood counts normalize.

Follow-up

At three months, on hydroxyurea and aspirin:

- Hemoglobin: 15.8 g/dL

- Hematocrit: 46%

- White blood cells: 9,200/μL

- Platelets: 385,000/μL

His exercise tolerance has improved dramatically. He's back to walking a mile daily without dyspnea. His skin appears less ruddy. No thrombotic events have occurred.

He'll need lifelong therapy and monitoring. Regular follow-up every 3-6 months tracks blood counts, assesses for disease progression, and monitors for complications.

Teaching Points

Polycythemia is not always pathologic but always needs investigation. While mild increases in hemoglobin can be normal (especially in people living at high altitude), hemoglobin >18.5 g/dL in men or

>16.5 g/dL in women warrants evaluation. Don't dismiss elevated hemoglobin as "not a problem" like you might with slightly low values.

Low EPO levels distinguish polycythemia vera from secondary causes. If EPO is low or low-normal with elevated hemoglobin, think primary polycythemia (polycythemia vera). If EPO is elevated, look for secondary causes—chronic hypoxia, sleep apnea, renal tumors, high-affinity hemoglobin. If EPO is normal, consider relative polycythemia (dehydration, diuretics).

JAK2 V617F mutation is present in >95% of polycythemia vera cases. Testing for this mutation has revolutionized diagnosis. A positive result essentially confirms polycythemia vera (assuming other criteria are met). A negative result doesn't completely rule it out—test for JAK2 exon 12 mutations in V617F-negative cases with suspected polycythemia vera (Tefferi & Barbui, 2020).

Thrombosis is the major cause of morbidity and mortality in polycythemia vera. About 20% of patients have thrombotic complications at diagnosis. Keeping hematocrit <45% and using aspirin dramatically reduces thrombosis risk. Age >60 and prior thrombosis are the strongest predictors of future thrombotic events (Marchioli et al., 2013).

Elevated counts in all three cell lines suggest a myeloproliferative neoplasm. When you see polycythemia plus leukocytosis plus thrombocytosis, think polycythemia vera (or less commonly, another myeloproliferative neoplasm). Secondary polycythemia typically elevates only red cells.

Splenomegaly is common in polycythemia vera. About 70% of patients have palpable splenomegaly at diagnosis. The spleen enlarges due to congestion and extramedullary hematopoiesis. Progressive splenomegaly may indicate transformation to myelofibrosis.

Symptoms may be subtle or attributed to other causes. Fatigue, headache, dizziness, and pruritus (especially after warm showers—"aquagenic pruritus") are common but nonspecific. Many patients are diagnosed incidentally when a CBC is ordered for another reason. Don't overlook elevated hemoglobin found on routine testing.

Related Cases

This case connects to:

- **Case 14: Myelodysplastic Syndrome** (another bone marrow disorder, but causing low counts rather than high counts)
- **Case 10: Acute Leukemia Presentation** (malignant proliferation, but of immature blast cells)
- **Case 13: Factor V Leiden Thrombophilia** (another disorder causing increased thrombosis risk)

Case 7: The Young Woman with Confusion and Fever

Clinical Presentation

A 29-year-old woman is brought to the emergency department by her boyfriend because of increasing confusion and odd behavior over the past two days. He reports that she's been unusually forgetful, repeating questions, and seeming "not herself." This morning she had difficulty getting dressed and couldn't remember how to make coffee.

She also has fever (temperature 38.9°C or 102°F), headache, and malaise. Her boyfriend initially thought she had the flu, but her mental status changes worried him enough to bring her to the ED.

Her past medical history is unremarkable. She takes oral contraceptives and no other medications. No recent travel, no sick contacts, no history of drug use. She works as a graphic designer. Last month she had what she thought was a stomach virus with diarrhea lasting several days.

Physical examination reveals a confused young woman who is oriented to person but not to place or time. She has fever, tachycardia (heart rate 115 beats per minute), and blood pressure of 128/82 mmHg. Neurologic examination shows confusion but no focal deficits. She has scattered petechiae on her legs and arms. No neck stiffness. The rest of the examination is unremarkable.

Initial Laboratory Findings

CBC:

- Hemoglobin: 7.8 g/dL (normal: 12.0-16.0 g/dL) - **VERY LOW**

- Hematocrit: 23% (normal: 36-46%) - **VERY LOW**

- MCV: 90 fL (normal) - NORMAL

- **Platelet count: 18,000/µL (normal: 150,000-400,000/µL) - VERY LOW**

- White blood cell count: 11,200/µL (normal) - slightly elevated

Chemistry Panel:

- Creatinine: 2.1 mg/dL (normal: 0.6-1.2 mg/dL) - **ELEVATED** (kidney dysfunction)

- BUN: 35 mg/dL (normal: 7-20 mg/dL) - elevated

- **LDH: 1,248 U/L (normal: 122-222 U/L) - MARKEDLY ELEVATED**

- **Indirect bilirubin: 3.2 mg/dL (normal: 0.2-0.8 mg/dL) - ELEVATED**

- Direct bilirubin: 0.3 mg/dL (normal) - NORMAL

Stop and Think

This case screams emergency. A young woman with fever, confusion, severe anemia, severe thrombocytopenia, and kidney injury—this is a medical crisis requiring immediate action.

The combination of findings suggests several life-threatening possibilities:

1. **Thrombotic thrombocytopenic purpura (TTP)** - Top consideration

2. Hemolytic uremic syndrome (HUS)

3. Disseminated intravascular coagulation (DIC)

4. Severe sepsis

5. Meningococcemia

The markedly elevated LDH and indirect bilirubin with normal direct bilirubin indicate **hemolysis** (red blood cell destruction). When red cells break apart, they release hemoglobin, which gets metabolized to indirect bilirubin. LDH, an enzyme inside red cells, spills into the bloodstream.

So we have:

- **Hemolytic anemia** (low hemoglobin, high LDH, high indirect bilirubin)
- **Thrombocytopenia** (low platelets)
- **Acute kidney injury** (elevated creatinine)
- **Neurologic symptoms** (confusion)
- **Fever**

This pentad of findings—anemia, thrombocytopenia, neurologic symptoms, kidney injury, and fever—is classic for **thrombotic thrombocytopenic purpura (TTP)**.

Diagnostic Reasoning Questions

What's the next most important test?

Peripheral blood smear immediately. You need to look for schistocytes (fragmented red blood cells).

In TTP, microthrombi (tiny blood clots) form in small blood vessels throughout the body. Red blood cells get sheared as they squeeze through vessels partially occluded by these clots, creating fragmented cells called schistocytes. The presence of schistocytes confirms microangiopathic hemolytic anemia (Joly et al., 2017).

What causes TTP?

TTP is caused by severe deficiency of **ADAMTS13**, an enzyme that cleaves von Willebrand factor (vWF) multimers. Without ADAMTS13:

- Ultra-large vWF multimers accumulate in plasma
- These giant vWF molecules cause platelets to aggregate spontaneously
- Microthrombi form throughout the microcirculation
- Red cells fragment as they pass through partially occluded vessels
- Organs (brain, kidneys) suffer ischemic damage

ADAMTS13 deficiency can be:

- **Acquired** (most common): Autoantibodies against ADAMTS13 develop
- **Hereditary** (rare): Genetic mutations in ADAMTS13 gene

How do you distinguish TTP from HUS?

Both cause microangiopathic hemolytic anemia and thrombocytopenia, making them hard to distinguish initially. Key differences:

TTP:

- Neurologic symptoms prominent
- ADAMTS13 severely deficient (<10% activity)
- Often triggered by infection, autoimmune disease, or idiopathic
- Treatment: Plasma exchange

HUS:

- Kidney injury more severe
- Often preceded by bloody diarrhea (E. coli O157:H7)
- ADAMTS13 normal or only mildly reduced
- More common in children
- Treatment: Supportive care (though atypical HUS may need complement inhibitors)

What about DIC?

DIC (disseminated intravascular coagulation) also causes:

- Anemia
- Thrombocytopenia
- Schistocytes
- Organ damage

But DIC shows abnormal coagulation studies (prolonged PT/aPTT, low fibrinogen, elevated D-dimer). In TTP, coagulation studies are typically normal because TTP doesn't consume clotting factors—it's a problem of platelet aggregation, not coagulation activation.

Sequential Test Results

Peripheral Blood Smear: Severe schistocytosis—numerous fragmented red blood cells visible on every field. Helmet cells, microspherocytes, and other RBC fragments present. Severely reduced platelet count confirmed. Polychromasia present (indicating increased reticulocyte production as bone marrow tries to compensate for hemolysis).

Coagulation Studies:

- PT: 12.8 seconds (normal) - NORMAL
- aPTT: 31 seconds (normal) - NORMAL
- Fibrinogen: 320 mg/dL (normal: 200-400 mg/dL) - NORMAL
- D-dimer: Mildly elevated

Additional Tests:

- Haptoglobin: <10 mg/dL (normal: 30-200 mg/dL) - **UNDETECTABLE** (confirms hemolysis)

- Reticulocyte count: 6.2% (normal: 0.5-1.5%) - ELEVATED (bone marrow responding to anemia)

- Direct antiglobulin test (Coombs): Negative (rules out immune-mediated hemolysis)

- **ADAMTS13 activity: <5%** (normal: >60%) - **SEVERELY DEFICIENT**

- **ADAMTS13 inhibitor: POSITIVE** (autoantibody detected)

The ADAMTS13 activity <5% confirms severe deficiency. The positive inhibitor indicates this is acquired (immune-mediated) TTP, not hereditary.

What's Happening Here?

This patient has **acquired thrombotic thrombocytopenic purpura (TTP)** due to autoantibodies against ADAMTS13.

The pathophysiology creates a cascade of problems:

1. Autoantibodies inhibit ADAMTS13 enzyme

2. Ultra-large vWF multimers accumulate

3. Platelets bind to vWF, forming microthrombi in capillaries and arterioles

4. Brain microthrombi → confusion, stroke-like symptoms

5. Kidney microthrombi → acute kidney injury

6. Widespread microthrombi → organ ischemia

7. Red cells shear through partially occluded vessels → schistocytes

8. Platelet consumption in clots → thrombocytopenia

9. Red cell destruction → hemolytic anemia

TTP is a hematologic emergency with >90% mortality if untreated. With prompt plasma exchange therapy, survival exceeds 80% (Joly et al., 2017).

Her recent diarrheal illness may have triggered the immune response that produced ADAMTS13 autoantibodies, though often no clear trigger is identified.

Final Diagnosis

Acquired thrombotic thrombocytopenic purpura (immune-mediated TTP) with ADAMTS13 deficiency

Treatment and Management

Immediate Treatment:

TTP is a medical emergency. Treatment must begin immediately—don't wait for ADAMTS13 results.

1. Plasma Exchange (Plasmapheresis): The cornerstone of TTP treatment. Plasma exchange:

- Removes autoantibodies against ADAMTS13

- Removes ultra-large vWF multimers

- Replaces ADAMTS13 enzyme

Performed daily until platelets normalize and hemolysis resolves. Usually requires 7-14 days of daily exchanges.

She's admitted to the ICU and urgent plasma exchange is arranged. A central venous catheter is placed for large-volume plasma exchange.

2. Corticosteroids: High-dose prednisone or methylprednisolone to suppress autoantibody production. Usually given alongside plasma exchange.

3. Rituximab: Anti-CD20 monoclonal antibody that depletes B cells (which produce autoantibodies). Now considered standard first-line therapy along with plasma exchange. Reduces relapse rates significantly (Scully et al., 2019).

4. Supportive Care:

- Avoid platelet transfusions unless life-threatening bleeding (platelets may worsen thrombosis)

- Folic acid supplementation (hemolysis increases folate needs)

- Avoid unnecessary procedures that could cause bleeding

- Monitor neurologic status closely

What NOT to do:

- Don't give platelets routinely (may worsen microthrombosis)

- Don't anticoagulate (bleeding risk is high, not clearly beneficial)

Follow-up

Day 1-3: Daily plasma exchange initiated. She receives rituximab and high-dose methylprednisolone.

Day 4: Her mental status begins improving. Confusion lessens. Platelet count rises to 35,000/µL.

Day 7: Platelet count reaches 95,000/µL. Hemoglobin stabilizes at 9.2 g/dL. LDH declining. Schistocytes decreasing on smear. She's alert and oriented. Creatinine improving to 1.4 mg/dL.

Day 10: Platelet count normalizes at 165,000/µL. No schistocytes on smear. LDH normal. She's discharged on oral prednisone taper and completes four weekly rituximab infusions.

3 months: Complete remission. ADAMTS13 activity has recovered to 48% (no longer severely deficient). She's off all medications. Regular monitoring for relapse continues.

Prognosis:

With modern treatment (plasma exchange + rituximab), about 80-90% of patients achieve remission. However, relapse occurs in 30-50% of patients at some point, requiring repeat treatment. Long-term monitoring of ADAMTS13 activity helps predict relapse risk (Scully et al., 2019).

Teaching Points

TTP is a medical emergency—recognize it fast and start treatment immediately. The classic pentad (fever, anemia, thrombocytopenia, neurologic symptoms, kidney injury) occurs in only about 40% of cases. Most patients present with just the triad of hemolytic anemia, thrombocytopenia, and neurologic or kidney abnormalities. Don't wait for all five features to make the diagnosis (Joly et al., 2017).

Schistocytes on blood smear are the key finding. If you see severe thrombocytopenia with hemolytic anemia (elevated LDH, elevated indirect bilirubin, low haptoglobin), immediately look at the peripheral smear. Abundant schistocytes indicate microangiopathic hemolytic anemia and should trigger immediate consideration of TTP, HUS, or DIC.

Normal coagulation studies help distinguish TTP from DIC. In TTP, PT, aPTT, and fibrinogen are typically normal because the problem is platelet aggregation in microvessels, not activation of the coagulation cascade. In DIC, clotting factors are consumed and coagulation studies are abnormal. This distinction is crucial because treatments differ.

Don't wait for ADAMTS13 results to start plasma exchange. ADAMTS13 testing takes days to result. If you strongly suspect TTP based on clinical and laboratory findings, start plasma exchange immediately. Delayed treatment increases mortality dramatically. You can always stop plasma exchange if ADAMTS13 comes back normal and an alternative diagnosis is confirmed.

ADAMTS13 activity <10% with inhibitor present confirms immune-mediated TTP. This distinguishes acquired TTP (autoantibodies) from hereditary TTP (genetic mutations) and from other microangiopathic hemolytic anemias where ADAMTS13 is normal or only mildly reduced.

Avoid platelet transfusions unless absolutely necessary. Giving platelets to a TTP patient can worsen microthrombosis by providing more "fuel" for clot formation. Platelet transfusions are reserved for life-threatening bleeding or before urgent neurosurgery—situations where bleeding risk outweighs thrombosis risk (Joly et al., 2017).

Rituximab has changed TTP outcomes. Adding rituximab to plasma exchange and steroids significantly reduces relapse rates from about 50% to 10-20%. It's now considered standard first-line therapy for acquired TTP (Scully et al., 2019).

Related Cases

This case connects to:

- **Case 2: Unexplained Bruising** (ITP—another cause of isolated thrombocytopenia but without hemolysis)

- **Case 12: Disseminated Intravascular Coagulation** (another microangiopathic hemolytic anemia but with abnormal coagulation studies)

- **Case 5: The Man Who Couldn't Stop Bleeding** (discusses von Willebrand factor, which is central to TTP pathophysiology)

Case 8: The Young Man with Joint Pain

Clinical Presentation

A 22-year-old African American man presents to the emergency department with severe pain in his right knee and left hip that began suddenly six hours ago. He describes the pain as throbbing and constant, rating it 9 out of 10. He has difficulty bearing weight and appears in obvious distress.

He reports a three-day history of fever, chills, and general malaise that he thought was the flu. The joint pain developed suddenly this afternoon and has progressively worsened. He also mentions chest pain with deep breathing and some shortness of breath.

His medical history is significant for multiple similar episodes since childhood—painful episodes involving his bones and joints that his mother called "crises." He was diagnosed with sickle cell disease at birth through newborn screening. He takes folic acid daily and received penicillin prophylaxis as a child but stopped several years ago. He missed his last hematology follow-up appointment six months ago.

Physical examination reveals a young man in severe pain, holding his right leg still. Temperature is 38.7°C (101.7°F), heart rate 108 beats per minute, blood pressure 128/75 mmHg, respiratory rate 22 breaths/minute, oxygen saturation 91% on room air (low). His right knee and left hip are swollen, warm, and exquisitely tender to palpation. He has decreased range of motion due to pain. Lung examination reveals decreased breath sounds at the left base. Abdominal examination shows splenomegaly was absent (the spleen has likely auto-infarcted from prior crises—common in sickle cell disease).

Initial Laboratory Findings

CBC:

- Hemoglobin: 7.8 g/dL (normal: 13.5-17.5 g/dL) - **LOW** (but his baseline)

- Hematocrit: 23% (normal: 41-53%)

- MCV: 85 fL (normal) - NORMAL

- **Reticulocyte count: 12% (normal: 0.5-1.5%) - MARKEDLY ELEVATED**

- White blood cell count: 18,500/μL (normal: 4,000-11,000/μL) - elevated

- Platelet count: 425,000/μL (normal) - elevated

Chemistry:

- **Total bilirubin: 4.2 mg/dL (normal: 0.3-1.2 mg/dL) - ELEVATED**

- **Indirect bilirubin: 3.8 mg/dL (normal: 0.2-0.8 mg/dL) - ELEVATED**

- Direct bilirubin: 0.4 mg/dL (normal)

- **LDH: 856 U/L (normal: 122-222 U/L) - ELEVATED**

- Creatinine: 1.1 mg/dL (normal)

Chest X-ray: Left lower lobe infiltrate consistent with pneumonia or acute chest syndrome.

Stop and Think

This patient with known sickle cell disease presents with a **vaso-occlusive crisis** (also called pain crisis) complicated by **acute chest syndrome**.

Let's understand what's happening. In sickle cell disease, abnormal hemoglobin (HbS) polymerizes when deoxygenated, causing red blood cells to become rigid and sickle-shaped. These sickled cells:

- Obstruct small blood vessels (vaso-occlusion)
- Cause tissue ischemia and severe pain
- Hemolyze (break apart) more easily than normal red cells
- Have shortened lifespan (10-20 days vs. 120 days for normal RBCs)

The laboratory findings reflect chronic hemolysis:

- Low hemoglobin (chronic anemia from shortened RBC lifespan)
- Elevated reticulocyte count (bone marrow working overtime to replace destroyed cells)
- Elevated indirect bilirubin (breakdown product of hemoglobin)
- Elevated LDH (released from damaged red cells)

The acute presentation suggests several sickle cell complications occurring simultaneously:

1. **Vaso-occlusive crisis**: Sickled cells blocking blood flow to bones/joints causing severe pain
2. **Acute chest syndrome**: Pulmonary complication with fever, chest pain, hypoxia, and infiltrate on chest X-ray
3. **Possible infection**: Fever and elevated WBC count (though these can occur in vaso-occlusive crisis without infection)

Diagnostic Reasoning Questions

What triggers sickle cell crises?

Common triggers include:

- **Infection** (most common—infections increase metabolic demand and stress on the body)
- Dehydration (concentrates red cells, promoting sickling)
- Cold exposure (causes vasoconstriction)
- Hypoxia (high altitude, lung disease)
- Physical or emotional stress
- Acidosis
- Often no identifiable trigger

What is acute chest syndrome, and why is it dangerous?

Acute chest syndrome is defined as new pulmonary infiltrate on chest X-ray plus one or more of:

- Fever

- Chest pain

- Respiratory symptoms

- Hypoxia

It's caused by:

- Vaso-occlusion in pulmonary vessels

- Infection (bacterial or viral)

- Fat embolism from bone marrow infarction

- Pulmonary infarction

Acute chest syndrome is the leading cause of death in adults with sickle cell disease and the second leading cause in children (after infection). It can rapidly progress to respiratory failure requiring mechanical ventilation (Gladwin & Vichinsky, 2008).

What additional tests are needed?

- **Blood cultures**: Before starting antibiotics (to identify bacterial infection)

- **Sputum culture**: If obtainable

- **Type and screen**: In case transfusion is needed

- **Hemoglobin electrophoresis or HPLC**: Confirms HbSS vs. other sickle syndromes (though this patient has known diagnosis)

- **Arterial blood gas**: Assess severity of hypoxia and acid-base status

- **Peripheral blood smear**: Visualize sickled cells

What's the difference between HbSS, HbSC, and sickle cell trait?

- **HbSS (sickle cell anemia)**: Two copies of sickle gene (homozygous). Most severe form. Hemoglobin mostly HbS.

- **HbSC disease**: One sickle gene, one hemoglobin C gene. Milder than HbSS but still causes complications.

- **HbS/β-thalassemia**: One sickle gene, one beta-thalassemia gene. Severity varies based on beta-thalassemia type.

- **Sickle cell trait (HbAS)**: One normal gene, one sickle gene (heterozygous carrier). Usually asymptomatic. About 8% of African Americans carry the trait.

Sequential Test Results

Peripheral Blood Smear: Numerous sickle-shaped red blood cells visible. Target cells present. Howell-Jolly bodies noted (indicating asplenia—absent or non-functioning spleen). Polychromasia present (reflecting elevated reticulocytes). Nucleated red blood cells occasionally seen (extreme marrow stress).

Blood Cultures: Pending (results take 24-48 hours)

Arterial Blood Gas:

- pH: 7.38 (normal: 7.35-7.45)

- pCO2: 35 mmHg (normal: 35-45 mmHg)

- pO2: 62 mmHg (normal: 80-100 mmHg) - **LOW** (hypoxemia)

- Oxygen saturation: 91%

Hemoglobin Analysis: (From previous records—electrophoresis done at diagnosis)

- HbS: 92%

- HbF: 6%

- HbA2: 2%

- HbA: 0%

This confirms homozygous sickle cell disease (HbSS). No normal adult hemoglobin (HbA) is present.

What's Happening Here?

This patient is experiencing a **vaso-occlusive crisis with acute chest syndrome** in the setting of possible infection.

The pathophysiology involves:

1. Triggering event (likely infection based on fever and respiratory symptoms): Infection increases metabolic demands and may cause local hypoxia in tissues. Inflammatory cytokines promote adhesion of sickled cells to blood vessel walls.

2. Sickling cascade: HbS polymerizes when deoxygenated → RBCs become rigid and sickle-shaped → sickled cells obstruct microvasculature → tissue ischemia → pain, organ damage.

3. Vaso-occlusion in bones: Bone marrow has slow blood flow and low oxygen tension, making it especially vulnerable. Vaso-occlusion in bone marrow causes severe pain in long bones and joints. This is the hallmark of vaso-occlusive crisis—excruciating pain that patients describe as worse than anything else they've experienced.

4. Acute chest syndrome: Pulmonary vessels become occluded by sickled cells. This can be triggered by:

- Primary pulmonary vaso-occlusion

- Fat embolism from bone marrow infarction (fat from infarcted marrow enters bloodstream)

- Infection (bacterial pneumonia)

- Hypoventilation from pain (leading to atelectasis)

The combination creates a dangerous cycle: hypoxia promotes more sickling → more vaso-occlusion → worsening hypoxia.

5. Chronic hemolysis: His baseline hemoglobin of 7.8 g/dL reflects chronic destruction of sickled red cells. The bone marrow compensates with reticulocyte count of 12% (massively increased production), but can't keep up with the shortened RBC lifespan.

Final Diagnosis

Sickle cell disease (HbSS) with acute vaso-occlusive crisis complicated by acute chest syndrome

Treatment and Management

This is a hematologic emergency requiring aggressive management.

Immediate Priorities:

1. Pain Control: Severe pain requires opioid analgesia. Under-treatment of pain is unfortunately common in sickle cell patients due to provider bias and concerns about addiction. Pain should be treated aggressively.

- IV morphine or hydromorphone on a scheduled basis (not just "as needed")
- Titrate to pain control
- Patient-controlled analgesia (PCA) pump often works well
- Add NSAIDs if not contraindicated

He receives IV hydromorphone 1 mg every 2 hours initially, then transitions to PCA.

2. Hydration: Aggressive IV hydration (1.5 times maintenance) to:

- Reduce blood viscosity
- Improve blood flow
- Prevent further sickling

D5 1/2 normal saline at 150 mL/hour is started.

3. Oxygen: Supplemental oxygen to maintain saturation >92% to prevent further sickling. He's placed on 4 liters nasal cannula, which improves his saturation to 94%.

4. Antibiotics: Broad-spectrum antibiotics to cover typical and atypical pneumonia organisms. Sickle cell patients have functional asplenia (from repeated splenic infarctions) making them susceptible to encapsulated organisms.

Ceftriaxone 1g IV daily plus azithromycin 500 mg IV daily is started.

5. Incentive Spirometry: Aggressive pulmonary toilet to prevent atelectasis. Every 2 hours while awake, he uses an incentive spirometer to take deep breaths. Atelectasis can worsen acute chest syndrome.

6. Exchange Transfusion (for severe acute chest syndrome): Simple transfusion or exchange transfusion may be needed if:

- Oxygen requirements increase

- Respiratory status deteriorates

- Hemoglobin drops significantly from baseline

- Patient fails to improve with supportive care

The goal is to reduce the percentage of HbS and improve oxygen-carrying capacity without causing hyperviscosity.

In this case, his oxygen requirements remain stable, so exchange transfusion is held in reserve but not immediately needed.

7. Monitor Closely:

- Oxygen saturation

- Respiratory rate and work of breathing

- Hemoglobin (watch for sudden drops indicating splenic sequestration or acute anemia)

- Intake and output (ensure adequate hydration)

- Pain scores

Follow-up

Day 1-2: He requires high-dose opioids around the clock. His pain gradually improves from 9/10 to 6/10. Fever resolves on antibiotics. Blood cultures show no growth (suggesting viral trigger or sterile vaso-occlusion rather than bacterial infection).

Day 3: Pain decreases to 4/10. He's able to ambulate with assistance. Oxygen saturation remains stable at 94% on 2 liters. Chest X-ray shows slight improvement in infiltrate.

Day 4: Pain controlled with oral opioids. Oxygen saturation 96% on room air. He's tolerating oral fluids and food.

Day 5: Discharged home with oral pain medications, instructions to stay well-hydrated, and follow-up with his hematologist in one week.

Long-term Management

Disease-Modifying Therapy:

Hydroxyurea is the cornerstone of chronic management. It:

- Increases fetal hemoglobin (HbF) production

- HbF inhibits HbS polymerization and sickling

- Reduces frequency of vaso-occlusive crises by 50%

- Reduces acute chest syndrome episodes

- Reduces need for transfusions

- Improves survival (Steinberg et al., 2003)

Hydroxyurea 500 mg daily is started with plan to titrate up based on response and blood counts.

Other Management Strategies:

- **Folic acid supplementation**: 1 mg daily (chronic hemolysis depletes folate)

- **Penicillin prophylaxis**: Recommended through age 5, but some continue lifelong due to functional asplenia

- **Vaccinations**: Pneumococcal, meningococcal, Haemophilus influenzae, annual influenza vaccine

- **Avoid triggers**: Stay hydrated, avoid temperature extremes, avoid high altitude

- **Regular hematology follow-up**: Monitor for complications, adjust hydroxyurea

- **Transcranial Doppler ultrasound**: Screen children for stroke risk

- **Retinal examination**: Screen for retinopathy

- **Renal function monitoring**: Sickle cell nephropathy is common

Newer Therapies:

- **L-glutamine** (Endari): Reduces oxidative stress, decreases crisis frequency

- **Crizanlizumab** (Adakveo): Monoclonal antibody that prevents cell adhesion, reduces crises

- **Voxelotor** (Oxbryta): Increases hemoglobin oxygen affinity, prevents sickling

Curative Options:

- **Bone marrow/stem cell transplant**: Only curative option. High risk. Usually reserved for severe cases with matched sibling donor.

- **Gene therapy**: Experimental but promising. Clinical trials ongoing.

Prognosis

With modern care, median survival for sickle cell disease (HbSS) has improved to about 45-50 years. However, quality of life is often impaired by recurrent painful crises, chronic organ damage, and disease complications.

Major causes of mortality include:

- Acute chest syndrome

- Infection (due to functional asplenia)

- Stroke

- Multi-organ failure

- Chronic kidney disease

- Pulmonary hypertension

Hydroxyurea and other disease-modifying therapies are improving outcomes significantly.

Teaching Points

Sickle cell crises require aggressive pain management. Under-treatment of pain is a major problem. Patients with sickle cell disease are often labeled as "drug-seeking" when they present in crisis, but studies show they actually receive inadequate analgesia. Trust the patient's pain report and treat aggressively with opioids, scheduled dosing, and multimodal pain management (Brandow & Panepinto, 2010).

Acute chest syndrome is a medical emergency. It's the leading cause of death in adults with sickle cell disease. New pulmonary infiltrate plus fever, chest pain, or respiratory symptoms in a sickle cell patient requires immediate aggressive management—hydration, oxygen, antibiotics, incentive spirometry, and low threshold for transfusion. Early recognition and treatment prevent progression to respiratory failure (Gladwin & Vichinsky, 2008).

Chronic hemolysis creates a characteristic laboratory pattern. Low hemoglobin, elevated reticulocyte count, elevated indirect bilirubin, and elevated LDH all reflect ongoing red cell destruction. This is the patient's baseline—not necessarily a crisis. During acute crises, hemoglobin may drop further if bone marrow becomes temporarily suppressed (aplastic crisis) or if sequestration occurs.

Howell-Jolly bodies indicate functional asplenia. These are nuclear remnants that normally get removed by the spleen. Their presence on blood smear indicates the spleen isn't functioning. In sickle cell disease, repeated splenic infarctions lead to "auto-splenectomy" by adolescence/adulthood. This increases infection risk, particularly from encapsulated bacteria (Streptococcus pneumoniae, Haemophilus influenzae, Neisseria meningitidis).

Hydroxyurea dramatically improves outcomes. All patients with HbSS should be offered hydroxyurea unless contraindicated. It reduces crisis frequency by about 50%, reduces acute chest syndrome, and improves survival. Despite clear benefits, it remains underutilized (Steinberg et al., 2003).

Sickle cell trait (HbAS) is usually benign. Carriers have one normal and one sickle gene. They're typically asymptomatic under normal conditions. However, extreme conditions (severe dehydration, high altitude, extreme exercise) can rarely cause complications. Genetic counseling is important—two carriers have a 25% chance with each pregnancy of having a child with sickle cell disease.

Infection is a major trigger for crises and a leading cause of death. Functional asplenia makes sickle cell patients vulnerable to overwhelming infection. Fever in a sickle cell patient requires blood cultures and empiric broad-spectrum antibiotics. Vaccination against encapsulated organisms is critical preventive care.

Related Cases

This case connects to:

- **Case 15: Hereditary Spherocytosis** (another inherited hemolytic anemia but with different pathophysiology)

- **Case 7: TTP** (another cause of hemolysis and schistocytes, but acquired rather than inherited)

- **Case 1: The Tired Graduate Student** (anemia, but due to iron deficiency rather than hemolysis)

Case 9: The Child with Lifelong Mild Anemia

Clinical Presentation

A 7-year-old boy is brought to his pediatrician for his annual well-child check. His mother mentions that he's always been "slightly anemic" since birth, but multiple doctors have told her not to worry. He's been taking iron supplements for two years without improvement in his hemoglobin. She's concerned that "the iron isn't working" and wonders if something more serious is wrong.

The child is active, plays soccer, does well in school, and has no significant symptoms. No fatigue, no jaundice, no bleeding or bruising. He eats a normal diet. Family history is significant—his father is from Greece and has "mild anemia that runs in the family."

Physical examination reveals a well-appearing child with normal growth and development. No pallor, no jaundice, no lymphadenopathy, no hepatosplenomegaly. Examination is completely normal.

Initial Laboratory Findings

CBC (current):

- Hemoglobin: 10.2 g/dL (normal for age: 11.5-15.5 g/dL) - LOW

- Hematocrit: 32% (normal: 34-40%) - LOW

- MCV: 64 fL (normal for age: 77-95 fL) - **VERY LOW**

- RBC count: 5.8 million/µL (normal: 4.0-5.2 million/µL) - **HIGH**

- RDW: 13.8% (normal: 11.5-14.5%) - NORMAL

- White blood cell count: 7,200/µL (normal)

- Platelet count: 305,000/µL (normal)

CBC from 2 years ago (before starting iron):

- Hemoglobin: 10.4 g/dL

- MCV: 65 fL

- RBC count: 5.7 million/µL

CBC from newborn screening (cord blood):

- Hemoglobin: 16.8 g/dL (normal for newborn)

- MCV: 96 fL (normal for newborn)

Stop and Think

This case immediately recalls Case 3 (the athletic young man with thalassemia trait). The pattern is similar—marked microcytosis (very low MCV) with elevated or high-normal RBC count and only mild anemia.

Key observations:

1. **Lifelong anemia since birth** suggests inherited condition

2. **No improvement with iron supplementation** for two years argues against iron deficiency

3. **MCV of 64 fL is severely low** for a 7-year-old

4. **RBC count is elevated** at 5.8 million (many small cells)

5. **Family history of similar anemia** in father of Mediterranean descent

6. **RDW is normal** (cells are uniformly small, unlike iron deficiency where RDW is usually elevated)

Calculate the Mentzer index: MCV ÷ RBC count = 64 ÷ 5.8 = **11.0**

A Mentzer index <13 strongly suggests thalassemia rather than iron deficiency.

The failure to respond to iron supplementation is a critical clue. Iron deficiency improves with supplementation. Thalassemia doesn't because the problem isn't iron—it's defective hemoglobin synthesis.

Diagnostic Reasoning Questions

Why didn't the anemia show up at birth?

Newborns have high levels of fetal hemoglobin (HbF), which doesn't contain beta globin chains. Beta thalassemia only becomes apparent after 3-6 months of age when HbF decreases and HbA (adult hemoglobin containing beta chains) becomes predominant. The newborn CBC showed normal hemoglobin and MCV because HbF was still predominant.

Alpha thalassemia, by contrast, can affect newborns because alpha chains are needed for both fetal and adult hemoglobin.

What tests confirm thalassemia?

- **Hemoglobin electrophoresis or HPLC** (high-performance liquid chromatography): Shows elevated HbA2 in beta thalassemia trait

- **Iron studies**: Normal in thalassemia, abnormal in iron deficiency

- **Peripheral blood smear**: Characteristic findings

- **Genetic testing**: Can identify specific mutations if needed

Could this be both iron deficiency AND thalassemia?

Yes, it's possible to have both conditions simultaneously. In Mediterranean populations with high thalassemia prevalence, some individuals have thalassemia trait plus coexisting iron deficiency. However, this child's iron studies are normal (see below), ruling out iron deficiency.

Sequential Test Results

Iron Studies:

- Serum iron: 88 µg/dL (normal: 50-120 µg/dL) - NORMAL

- TIBC: 280 µg/dL (normal: 250-400 µg/dL) - NORMAL

- Ferritin: 45 ng/mL (normal: 7-140 ng/mL for children) - NORMAL

- Transferrin saturation: 31% (normal: 20-50%) - NORMAL

These normal iron studies confirm he's not iron deficient. The iron supplementation he's been taking was unnecessary and ineffective.

Peripheral Blood Smear: Microcytic, hypochromic red blood cells with remarkable uniformity in size. Numerous target cells present. Occasional basophilic stippling noted. No anisocytosis (variation in size) or poikilocytosis (variation in shape). Contrast this with iron deficiency, which shows marked variation in cell size and shape.

Hemoglobin Analysis (HPLC):

- HbA: 92.8% (normal: 96-98%)

- **HbA2: 5.8%** (normal: 2.5-3.5%) - **ELEVATED** (diagnostic)

- HbF: 1.4% (normal: <1%)

The elevated HbA2 at 5.8% confirms the diagnosis.

What's Happening Here?

This child has **beta thalassemia minor** (beta thalassemia trait), inherited from his Greek father. He has one normal beta globin gene and one defective beta globin gene.

Beta thalassemia results from decreased or absent production of beta globin chains. In beta thalassemia trait:

- One gene produces normal beta globin

- One gene produces little or no beta globin

- Overall beta globin production is reduced (but not absent)

- The body compensates by producing more HbA2 (which uses delta chains instead of beta chains)

- Red cells are microcytic because they contain less hemoglobin

- RBC count increases to partially compensate for low hemoglobin per cell

- Mild anemia results (hemoglobin typically 10-13 g/dL)

The condition is **clinically benign**. Children and adults with beta thalassemia trait are typically asymptomatic. The mild anemia doesn't cause problems. This boy playing soccer without limitation confirms he's not functionally impaired.

The **major issue is misdiagnosis and inappropriate treatment**. Many people with thalassemia trait are mistakenly diagnosed with iron deficiency and given years of unnecessary iron supplementation. This child has been taking iron for two years with no benefit because iron deficiency was never his problem.

Final Diagnosis

Beta thalassemia minor (beta thalassemia trait)

Management and Counseling

Discontinue Iron Supplementation: The first step is stopping the unnecessary iron. Continued iron supplementation in someone without iron deficiency can lead to iron overload over many years. His ferritin is normal now, but continued supplementation could eventually cause problems.

Education: The pediatrician explains to his mother:

- This is a genetic condition, not a nutritional deficiency
- It's lifelong but benign (not a disease requiring treatment)
- His mild anemia is his normal baseline
- He can participate in all normal activities without restriction
- Iron supplements don't help and should be stopped

Inform Future Healthcare Providers: He should wear a medical alert bracelet or carry a card stating "Beta thalassemia trait - not iron deficient" to prevent future misdiagnosis and inappropriate iron supplementation.

Avoid Unnecessary Testing: He doesn't need repeat CBCs unless clinically indicated. His hemoglobin will always be mildly low—that's expected and normal for him.

Genetic Counseling: His parents should understand the inheritance pattern:

- His father has beta thalassemia trait
- His mother presumably has normal hemoglobin genes (based on family history)
- Each child has a 50% chance of inheriting the trait
- If both parents had trait, each child would have a 25% chance of thalassemia major (severe disease requiring lifelong transfusions)

His mother is offered hemoglobin electrophoresis to confirm she's not a carrier. Results show normal hemoglobin pattern (she's not a carrier), so future children have no risk of thalassemia major.

Implications for Future: If this child has children in the future, genetic counseling with his partner will be important. If his partner also carries a thalassemia gene, prenatal genetic counseling and testing would be recommended.

Distinguishing Thalassemia Trait from Iron Deficiency

This case highlights a critical clinical challenge. The table below compares these two common causes of microcytic anemia:

Feature	Thalassemia Trait	Iron Deficiency
MCV	Very low (<75 fL)	Low but less severe initially

Feature	Thalassemia Trait	Iron Deficiency
RBC count	High or high-normal	Low or normal
RDW	Normal	Elevated (>15%)
Mentzer index	<13	>13
Iron studies	Normal	Low iron, high TIBC, low ferritin
HbA2	Elevated (>3.5%) in beta thal	Normal
Family history	Often positive	Usually negative
Response to iron	None	Hemoglobin increases

Peripheral smear Uniform microcytosis, target cells Varied cell sizes, pencil cells

The Mentzer index (MCV ÷ RBC count) is a useful screening tool but not definitive. When in doubt, check iron studies and hemoglobin electrophoresis.

Follow-up

His mother is relieved to learn this isn't a serious condition and that stopping iron is appropriate. She's given written information about thalassemia trait to share with future healthcare providers.

At follow-up one year later, his hemoglobin remains stable at 10.3 g/dL. He continues to do well in school and sports. No further intervention is needed.

Teaching Points

Always check iron studies before assuming microcytic anemia is iron deficiency. Millions of people worldwide have thalassemia trait and are mistakenly given iron supplements for years. Iron studies distinguish these conditions quickly and cheaply. Hemoglobin electrophoresis confirms the diagnosis.

Lack of response to iron supplementation should prompt reconsideration of the diagnosis. If a patient takes iron supplements for 2-3 months with no improvement in hemoglobin, they either don't have iron deficiency, or have ongoing blood loss, or have malabsorption. Investigate further rather than continuing ineffective treatment.

Thalassemia trait is clinically benign but genetically significant. Individuals with trait don't need treatment and have normal life expectancy. However, they can pass the gene to children. Two parents with trait have a 25% chance with each pregnancy of having a child with thalassemia major, which requires lifelong transfusions and chelation therapy. Genetic counseling is essential.

Ethnicity provides important clues. Thalassemia trait is common in people of Mediterranean (Italian, Greek, Turkish), Middle Eastern, Asian (especially Southeast Asian), African, and Caribbean descent. Always ask about ethnic background when evaluating microcytic anemia. However, thalassemia can occur in any ethnicity.

The Mentzer index and other discriminating indices help but aren't perfect. Mentzer index <13 suggests thalassemia; >13 suggests iron deficiency. Other indices exist (Shine and Lal, Ehsani, etc.). These are screening tools—definitive diagnosis requires iron studies and hemoglobin electrophoresis (Urrechaga et al., 2015).

Don't miss coexisting iron deficiency in thalassemia trait patients. While this child didn't have iron deficiency, it's possible to have both conditions. If a known thalassemia trait patient's hemoglobin drops below their usual baseline, check iron studies. Coexisting iron deficiency should be treated.

Target cells and basophilic stippling on smear are characteristic of thalassemia. These findings, along with uniformly small red cells, point toward thalassemia rather than iron deficiency. However, smear interpretation requires expertise, and some features overlap between conditions.

Related Cases

This case connects to:

- **Case 1: The Tired Graduate Student** (iron deficiency—the condition this is most often confused with)

- **Case 3: The Athletic Young Man** (another beta thalassemia trait case in an adult)

- **Case 15: Hereditary Spherocytosis** (another inherited red cell disorder)

Case 10: The Teenager with Fatigue and Easy Bruising

Clinical Presentation

A 16-year-old girl presents to her pediatrician with complaints of increasing fatigue, weakness, and easy bruising over the past three weeks. She's also noticed frequent nosebleeds and gum bleeding when brushing her teeth. Her mother reports that she's been sleeping more than usual and seems "pale and tired all the time."

She denies fever initially, but her mother mentions low-grade fevers off and on for the past week. She's lost about 8 pounds without trying. Her appetite has decreased. She reports vague bone pain, especially in her legs.

Her past medical history is unremarkable. No chronic illnesses, no medications. She's a good student, doesn't use drugs or alcohol, and is active in her school's theater program. Family history is negative for blood disorders or cancers.

Physical examination reveals a pale, ill-appearing adolescent. Temperature is 37.8°C (100°F). Scattered petechiae are present on her lower extremities. Multiple ecchymoses in various stages of healing are noted on her arms and legs. Oral examination reveals gingival bleeding and pallor. Lymph nodes are not enlarged. She has mild hepatomegaly (liver edge palpable 2 cm below costal margin) and splenomegaly (spleen tip palpable 3 cm below left costal margin). Sternal tenderness is present on palpation.

Initial Laboratory Findings

CBC:

- **Hemoglobin: 6.9 g/dL** (normal: 12.0-16.0 g/dL) - **SEVERELY LOW**

- Hematocrit: 21% (normal: 36-46%) - SEVERELY LOW

- MCV: 92 fL (normal) - NORMAL

- **White blood cell count: 68,000/µL** (normal: 4,000-11,000/µL) - **MARKEDLY ELEVATED**

- **Platelet count: 28,000/µL** (normal: 150,000-400,000/µL) - **VERY LOW**

WBC Differential:

- Neutrophils: 5%

- Lymphocytes: 3%

- Monocytes: 2%

- **Blasts: 90%** - **ABNORMAL** (blasts should be 0% in peripheral blood)

Stop and Think

This case is dramatically different from anything we've seen so far. The presence of **90% blasts** in the peripheral blood is alarming and diagnostic.

Blasts are immature, undifferentiated blood cells that normally reside only in the bone marrow, where they mature into functional blood cells. Blasts should never appear in significant numbers in peripheral blood. Their presence indicates:

1. **Acute leukemia** (most likely given the high percentage)

2. Blastic phase of chronic myeloid leukemia (rare in teenagers)

3. Severe bone marrow stress (rare to see this many blasts)

The clinical picture fits acute leukemia perfectly:

- **Anemia** → fatigue, pallor, weakness (bone marrow replaced by leukemia cells, can't produce normal RBCs)

- **Thrombocytopenia** → easy bruising, petechiae, nosebleeds, gum bleeding (can't produce normal platelets)

- **Neutropenia** (only 5% neutrophils of 68,000 = 3,400 absolute neutrophils) → infection risk (can't produce normal functional white cells)

- **Bone pain** → leukemia cells expanding in bone marrow

- **Hepatosplenomegaly** → leukemia cells infiltrating organs

- **Weight loss, low-grade fever** → systemic effects of malignancy

This is a hematologic emergency. This teenager has acute leukemia and needs immediate referral to a pediatric oncology center.

Diagnostic Reasoning Questions

What types of acute leukemia exist?

Acute Lymphoblastic Leukemia (ALL):

- Malignant proliferation of lymphoid precursor cells

- Most common childhood cancer (75% of childhood leukemia)

- Peak incidence age 2-5 years, but can occur in adolescents and adults

- Better prognosis than AML, especially in children

- Subtypes: B-ALL (most common) and T-ALL

Acute Myeloid Leukemia (AML):

- Malignant proliferation of myeloid precursor cells

- Less common in children (25% of childhood leukemia)

- More common in adults

- Generally worse prognosis than ALL

- Multiple subtypes based on FAB classification

How do you distinguish ALL from AML?

Morphology alone isn't sufficient. You need:

Flow cytometry (immunophenotyping):

- ALL blasts express lymphoid markers: CD19, CD10 (B-ALL) or CD3, CD7 (T-ALL)

- AML blasts express myeloid markers: CD13, CD33, CD117, MPO

Cytochemistry:

- Myeloperoxidase (MPO) positive → AML

- MPO negative → ALL

Cytogenetics and molecular studies:

- Identify specific chromosomal abnormalities

- Determine prognosis

- Guide treatment decisions

What other tests are needed urgently?

- **Peripheral blood smear**: Examine blast morphology

- **Bone marrow aspiration and biopsy**: Confirm diagnosis, determine blast percentage, perform flow cytometry and cytogenetics

- **Comprehensive metabolic panel**: Check for tumor lysis syndrome (elevated uric acid, potassium, phosphorus, creatinine)

- **Coagulation studies**: Check for DIC (can occur in acute promyelocytic leukemia, a subtype of AML)

- **Blood type and screen**: Transfusions will be needed

- **Chest X-ray**: Look for mediastinal mass (common in T-ALL)

- **Lumbar puncture**: Check for CNS involvement (done after platelet transfusion if platelets very low)

Sequential Test Results

Peripheral Blood Smear: Numerous large blast cells with high nuclear-to-cytoplasmic ratio, fine chromatin, and prominent nucleoli. Blasts comprise the vast majority of white blood cells. Severe anemia and thrombocytopenia confirmed. Occasional smudge cells present.

Chemistry Panel:

- Potassium: 5.8 mEq/L (normal: 3.5-5.0) - **ELEVATED**

- **Uric acid: 11.2 mg/dL (normal: 2.5-5.5 mg/dL) - MARKEDLY ELEVATED**

- **LDH: 2,450 U/L (normal: 122-222 U/L) - MARKEDLY ELEVATED**

- Phosphorus: 6.2 mg/dL (normal: 2.5-4.5 mg/dL) - ELEVATED

- Calcium: 8.1 mg/dL (normal: 8.5-10.5 mg/dL) - slightly low

- Creatinine: 1.1 mg/dL (normal) - NORMAL (for now)

These findings suggest **early tumor lysis syndrome**—metabolic derangements from rapid breakdown of cancer cells releasing intracellular contents.

Coagulation Studies:

- PT: 13.2 seconds (normal)

- aPTT: 32 seconds (normal)

- Fibrinogen: 285 mg/dL (normal)

No evidence of DIC.

Chest X-ray: No mediastinal mass. Heart size normal. Lungs clear.

Bone Marrow Aspiration and Biopsy:

Performed urgently. Bone marrow is hypercellular (>90% cellularity) with near-complete replacement by blast cells. **Blasts comprise 92% of marrow cells** (normal: <5%). Normal hematopoiesis is nearly absent.

Flow Cytometry (Immunophenotyping):

Blasts are positive for:

- **CD19** (B-cell marker)

- **CD10** (CALLA—common ALL antigen)

- **CD34** (immature cell marker)

- **TdT** (terminal deoxynucleotidyl transferase—marker of lymphoid precursors)

Blasts are negative for:

- Myeloid markers (CD13, CD33, MPO)

- T-cell markers (CD3, CD7)

This immunophenotype confirms **B-cell acute lymphoblastic leukemia (B-ALL)**.

Cytogenetics:

Conventional chromosome analysis and FISH (fluorescence in situ hybridization) are performed. Results show:

- **Philadelphia chromosome negative** (good—Philadelphia positive ALL has worse prognosis)

- Hyperdiploidy (>50 chromosomes) - **FAVORABLE PROGNOSTIC FACTOR**

- No high-risk translocations identified

Molecular Studies:

- BCR-ABL fusion: Negative (confirms Philadelphia chromosome negative)

- MLL rearrangement: Negative

What's Happening Here?

This teenager has **B-cell acute lymphoblastic leukemia (B-ALL)**, the most common form of leukemia in children and adolescents.

ALL results from malignant transformation of lymphoid precursor cells. These leukemic blasts:

- Proliferate rapidly in the bone marrow

- Crowd out normal hematopoiesis (causing cytopenias)

- Spill into peripheral blood (causing elevated WBC with blasts)

- Infiltrate organs (liver, spleen, lymph nodes, CNS)

- Can infiltrate any organ if untreated

The pathophysiology explains her symptoms:

- **Bone marrow failure** → anemia (fatigue), thrombocytopenia (bleeding), neutropenia (infection risk)

- **Bone marrow expansion** → bone pain, sternal tenderness

- **Organ infiltration** → hepatosplenomegaly

- **Systemic effects** → fever, weight loss, malaise

- **High cell turnover** → elevated LDH, elevated uric acid (tumor lysis)

The hyperdiploidy (>50 chromosomes) in her leukemia cells is actually a **favorable prognostic factor**. Hyperdiploid ALL has better treatment response and survival compared to other cytogenetic patterns (Pui & Evans, 2006).

Final Diagnosis

B-cell acute lymphoblastic leukemia (B-ALL) with hyperdiploid karyotype

Treatment and Management

She is immediately admitted to the pediatric oncology unit at a tertiary care center. ALL treatment is complex, intensive, and prolonged.

Immediate Priorities:

1. Prevent/Treat Tumor Lysis Syndrome: High leukemia cell burden means massive cell death will occur once chemotherapy starts. Cell contents (potassium, phosphorus, uric acid, nucleic acids) flood the bloodstream, potentially causing:

- Hyperkalemia → cardiac arrhythmias

- Hyperphosphatemia and hypocalcemia → seizures, cardiac issues

- Hyperuricemia → acute kidney injury from uric acid crystals

Management:

- **Aggressive IV hydration** (200 mL/m²/hour)

- **Allopurinol** or **rasburicase** (lowers uric acid)

- Monitor electrolytes every 4-6 hours

- Avoid potassium and phosphorus in IV fluids

- Daily weights, strict intake/output

2. Transfusion Support:

- **Packed red blood cells**: For hemoglobin <7 g/dL or symptomatic anemia

- **Platelets**: For platelet count <10,000/µL (prophylactic) or <50,000/µL before procedures

She receives 1 unit of packed RBCs and 1 unit of platelets.

3. Infection Prophylaxis: Severe neutropenia plus chemotherapy-induced immunosuppression creates extreme infection risk.

- Broad-spectrum antibiotics for any fever

- Antifungal prophylaxis

- Pneumocystis jirovecii prophylaxis (trimethoprim-sulfamethoxazole)

- Protective precautions (handwashing, avoiding sick contacts, no fresh flowers or raw foods)

Chemotherapy Treatment Phases:

ALL treatment follows a multi-phase approach lasting 2-3 years:

1. Induction (4-6 weeks): Goal: Achieve complete remission (no detectable leukemia cells)

Medications:

- Vincristine (IV weekly)

- Daunorubicin or doxorubicin (IV)

- PEG-asparaginase (IM)

- Prednisone or dexamethasone (oral daily)

- Intrathecal chemotherapy (methotrexate or cytarabine into spinal fluid to prevent CNS leukemia)

About 95% of children achieve complete remission after induction.

2. Consolidation (2-4 months): Goal: Eliminate residual leukemia cells

High-dose methotrexate, 6-mercaptopurine, continued intrathecal chemotherapy

3. Maintenance (2-3 years): Goal: Prevent relapse

Daily oral 6-mercaptopurine and weekly oral methotrexate, with periodic vincristine and steroid pulses. Continued intrathecal chemotherapy every 2-3 months.

CNS Prophylaxis: ALL commonly spreads to the central nervous system. Intrathecal chemotherapy (injecting chemotherapy directly into spinal fluid via lumbar puncture) is given throughout treatment to prevent CNS leukemia. Some high-risk patients receive cranial radiation.

Monitoring:

- Bone marrow assessments at end of induction, during consolidation, and periodically during maintenance

- **Minimal residual disease (MRD) testing**: Highly sensitive flow cytometry or PCR detects 1 leukemia cell among 10,000-100,000 normal cells. MRD negativity is the strongest predictor of cure (Pui & Evans, 2006).

- Blood counts (frequently during intensive phases)

- Infection surveillance

- Growth and development monitoring

- Late effects screening (cardiac function, endocrine function, learning)

Follow-up and Prognosis

End of Induction (Week 5): Bone marrow shows complete remission—blasts <5%, recovery of normal hematopoiesis. MRD testing shows no detectable leukemia (MRD-negative). This is excellent prognostic sign.

Her blood counts recover:

- Hemoglobin: 11.2 g/dL

- White blood cells: 4,800/μL

- Platelets: 185,000/μL

6 Months: She's midway through consolidation therapy. Tolerating treatment with manageable side effects (nausea, fatigue, hair loss). Continues attending school part-time. MRD remains negative.

1 Year: She's transitioned to maintenance chemotherapy. Takes daily oral chemotherapy at home. Returns to clinic monthly. Hair has regrown. She's back in school full-time and involved in drama club again. Energy improving.

2.5 Years: Completes maintenance therapy. Final bone marrow shows continued complete remission, MRD-negative. She's declared in remission and off all chemotherapy.

5 Years: She's now 21 years old, attending college, and thriving. No evidence of leukemia. She's considered cured. Long-term follow-up continues to monitor for late effects of treatment.

Prognosis for B-ALL:

Modern treatment has transformed ALL from uniformly fatal to one of the most curable cancers:

- **Children (ages 1-10):** 90% long-term survival

- **Adolescents (ages 10-18):** 75-80% long-term survival

- **Adults (>18):** 40-50% long-term survival

Prognostic factors affecting survival:

- **Favorable:** Age 1-10, low initial WBC count (<50,000), hyperdiploid cytogenetics, rapid treatment response, MRD negativity

- **Unfavorable:** Infant or adult age, very high WBC (>50,000), certain cytogenetic abnormalities (Philadelphia chromosome, MLL rearrangement), slow treatment response, MRD positivity

This patient has mostly favorable factors (adolescent age, hyperdiploid karyotype, excellent treatment response), predicting high cure probability.

Teaching Points

Blasts in peripheral blood indicate acute leukemia until proven otherwise. Normal peripheral blood contains 0% blasts. Any significant number of blasts (>5%) requires urgent evaluation. High blast percentages (>20%) are diagnostic of acute leukemia. This is a hematologic emergency requiring same-day referral to hematology/oncology.

The combination of cytopenias plus elevated WBC is classic for leukemia. Leukemia causes low hemoglobin, low platelets, often low functional WBCs (despite high total WBC from blasts). This pattern—pancytopenia with leukocytosis—should immediately raise concern for leukemia. Order a peripheral smear urgently.

Flow cytometry distinguishes ALL from AML. You cannot reliably distinguish these by morphology alone. Immunophenotyping (flow cytometry) identifies whether blasts are lymphoid (ALL) or myeloid (AML) based on surface markers. This distinction is critical because treatments differ dramatically.

Tumor lysis syndrome is a life-threatening emergency. High leukemia burden means billions of cancer cells will die once treatment starts, releasing intracellular contents. Aggressive hydration and uric acid-lowering therapy (allopurinol or rasburicase) are essential preventive measures. Hyperkalemia and acute kidney injury can be fatal without proper management.

ALL treatment is prolonged but highly successful. Unlike most cancers treated with surgery or short chemotherapy courses, ALL requires 2-3 years of continuous chemotherapy. Compliance is critical—stopping treatment early dramatically increases relapse risk. Despite the long duration, cure rates in children approach 90% (Pui & Evans, 2006).

Minimal residual disease (MRD) is the strongest prognostic factor. MRD testing after induction chemotherapy detects leukemia cells that are invisible by standard microscopy (which only detects 1 in 20 malignant cells, while MRD detects 1 in 10,000-100,000). MRD-negative patients have >90% cure rates, while MRD-positive patients need treatment intensification (Conter et al., 2010).

Adolescents have worse outcomes than younger children. Survival for adolescents with ALL (75-80%) is significantly lower than young children (90%). Reasons include biological differences in leukemia subtypes, poorer tolerance of chemotherapy, and compliance issues with prolonged treatment. Adolescents treated on pediatric protocols fare better than those treated on adult protocols.

Related Cases

This case connects to:

- **Case 4: The Teenager with Night Sweats** (Hodgkin lymphoma—another hematologic malignancy in an adolescent but with different presentation)
- **Case 14: Myelodysplastic Syndrome** (another bone marrow disorder causing cytopenias)
- **Case 6: The Older Man with Increasing Fatigue** (polycythemia vera—opposite problem, too many cells, but also a bone marrow disorder)

Case 11: The College Student with Sore Throat

Clinical Presentation

A 19-year-old college freshman presents to student health services complaining of severe sore throat, fever, and extreme fatigue for the past week. He initially thought he had strep throat, but an earlier rapid strep test was negative. His symptoms have progressively worsened. He reports difficulty swallowing, headache, body aches, and profound tiredness that makes it hard to stay awake in classes.

He mentions that several of his dormmates have been sick with similar symptoms. He denies cough, chest pain, or shortness of breath. No nausea, vomiting, or diarrhea. He's taking ibuprofen for fever and pain with minimal relief.

His past medical history is unremarkable. He takes no regular medications. He socially drinks alcohol at parties and doesn't smoke or use drugs. He recently started dating someone new about a month ago.

Physical examination reveals an ill-appearing young man with temperature of 39.2°C (102.6°F), heart rate 98 beats per minute, blood pressure 122/76 mmHg. His pharynx is markedly erythematous with tonsillar hypertrophy and white exudates covering both tonsils. **Bilateral cervical lymphadenopathy** is prominent—multiple enlarged, tender lymph nodes palpable along both sides of his neck, some measuring 2-3 cm. He has **splenomegaly**—spleen tip palpable 4 cm below the left costal margin. No hepatomegaly. A faint maculopapular rash is noted on his trunk.

Initial Laboratory Findings

CBC:

- Hemoglobin: 14.2 g/dL (normal) - NORMAL

- Hematocrit: 42% (normal) - NORMAL

- MCV: 88 fL (normal) - NORMAL

- **White blood cell count: 18,500/µL** (normal: 4,000-11,000/µL) - **ELEVATED**

- Platelet count: 165,000/µL (normal) - NORMAL

WBC Differential:

- Neutrophils: 35%

- **Lymphocytes: 58%** (normal: 20-40%) - **ELEVATED**

- **Atypical lymphocytes: 18% - ABNORMAL**

- Monocytes: 7%

- Eosinophils: 2%

Stop and Think

This case presents the classic triad of infectious mononucleosis ("mono"):

1. **Pharyngitis** with tonsillar exudates

2. **Lymphadenopathy** (especially posterior cervical)

3. **Splenomegaly**

The CBC shows lymphocytosis (elevated lymphocyte count) with atypical lymphocytes—the hallmark laboratory finding of infectious mononucleosis.

But let's think carefully. We saw atypical lymphocytes in Case 4 (the teenager with lymphoma). How do we distinguish infectious mononucleosis from lymphoma and other serious causes of atypical lymphocytes?

Clinical context is critical:

Infectious mononucleosis:

- Acute onset (days to weeks)
- Pharyngitis prominent
- Fever, malaise, lymphadenopathy
- Splenomegaly common
- Young adults (college-age peak incidence)
- Self-limited course

Lymphoma:

- Insidious onset (weeks to months)
- Painless lymphadenopathy
- B symptoms (fever, night sweats, weight loss)
- Splenomegaly sometimes
- Usually no pharyngitis
- Progressive without treatment

This patient's presentation—acute severe pharyngitis, fever, fatigue, lymphocytosis with atypical lymphocytes—screams infectious mononucleosis.

Diagnostic Reasoning Questions

What causes infectious mononucleosis?

Epstein-Barr virus (EBV) causes about 90% of infectious mononucleosis cases. Other causes include:

- Cytomegalovirus (CMV)
- HIV (acute retroviral syndrome)
- Toxoplasmosis
- Adenovirus
- HHV-6

EBV is a herpesvirus transmitted primarily through saliva (hence "kissing disease"). The virus infects B lymphocytes, which triggers a massive T lymphocyte response. The "atypical lymphocytes" seen on blood smear are actually activated T lymphocytes responding to EBV-infected B cells.

How do you confirm the diagnosis?

Monospot test (heterophile antibody test):

- Detects heterophile antibodies produced in response to EBV

- Positive in 70-90% of cases by the first week of illness

- False negatives occur early in illness and in young children

- Quick, inexpensive, point-of-care test

EBV-specific antibody testing (more sensitive and specific):

- **VCA IgM** (viral capsid antigen IgM): Positive in acute infection

- **VCA IgG**: Appears during acute infection, persists for life

- **EBNA** (Epstein-Barr nuclear antigen): Appears later (weeks to months after infection), persists for life

- **EA** (early antigen): Sometimes positive in acute infection

Antibody patterns distinguish:

- **Acute infection**: VCA IgM positive, VCA IgG positive, EBNA negative

- **Past infection**: VCA IgM negative, VCA IgG positive, EBNA positive

- **Never infected**: All negative

What complications should you watch for?

Most cases resolve uneventfully, but potential complications include:

- **Splenic rupture** (rare but life-threatening—occurs in 0.1-0.5% of cases)

- Airway obstruction from massive tonsillar hypertrophy

- Secondary bacterial pharyngitis (strep throat)

- Hepatitis (mild liver enzyme elevations common)

- Neurologic complications (Guillain-Barré syndrome, encephalitis—rare)

- Hemolytic anemia or thrombocytopenia (immune-mediated)

- Chronic active EBV infection (very rare)

Sequential Test Results

Monospot Test: POSITIVE - This confirms the diagnosis of infectious mononucleosis.

EBV Antibody Panel:

- VCA IgM: **Positive** (acute infection marker)

- VCA IgG: **Positive** (acute infection marker)

- EBNA IgG: **Negative** (not yet developed—confirms acute, not past, infection)

This serologic pattern confirms **acute EBV infection**.

Liver Function Tests:

- AST: 95 U/L (normal: 10-40 U/L) - elevated

- ALT: 112 U/L (normal: 7-56 U/L) - elevated

- Total bilirubin: 1.8 mg/dL (normal: 0.3-1.2 mg/dL) - slightly elevated

- Alkaline phosphatase: 145 U/L (normal: 44-147 U/L) - high normal

Mild hepatitis is common in infectious mononucleosis. About 80-90% of patients have some liver enzyme elevation, though clinically significant hepatitis is uncommon (Ebell, 2004).

Peripheral Blood Smear: Numerous atypical lymphocytes present. These are large lymphocytes with abundant cytoplasm, irregular nuclear contours, and darkly staining cytoplasm that "molds" around adjacent red blood cells—classic features of reactive lymphocytes (Downey cells) in infectious mononucleosis.

What's Happening Here?

This patient has **infectious mononucleosis** caused by acute Epstein-Barr virus infection.

The pathophysiology explains his symptoms:

1. EBV infection: EBV enters through oropharyngeal epithelium, infects B lymphocytes, and establishes lifelong latent infection in memory B cells.

2. Massive immune response: T lymphocytes (especially CD8+ cytotoxic T cells) mount vigorous response against EBV-infected B cells. These activated T cells are the "atypical lymphocytes" seen on blood smear. The lymphocytosis reflects the massive lymphocyte proliferation.

3. Lymphoid tissue hypertrophy: Lymph nodes enlarge (lymphadenopathy) as immune cells proliferate. Tonsils enlarge, sometimes causing airway compromise. Spleen enlarges (splenomegaly) from lymphoid proliferation and congestion.

4. Systemic symptoms: Cytokines released during the immune response cause fever, malaise, fatigue, and body aches. The profound fatigue is a hallmark of EBV infectious mononucleosis and can persist for weeks to months.

5. Pharyngitis: Tonsillar inflammation and exudates result from viral infection and immune response. This can mimic streptococcal pharyngitis.

About 90% of adults have been infected with EBV at some point (evidenced by positive VCA IgG antibodies). Infection in early childhood is usually asymptomatic or mild. Infection in adolescence or young adulthood more commonly causes symptomatic infectious mononucleosis. The classic college-age patient reflects this pattern—many students encounter EBV for the first time in the college setting (Ebell, 2004).

Final Diagnosis

Infectious mononucleosis due to acute Epstein-Barr virus infection

Treatment and Management

There's no specific antiviral treatment for EBV. Management is supportive:

Symptomatic Treatment:

- **Rest**: Important, especially during the acute phase (first 2-3 weeks)
- **Hydration**: Oral fluids to maintain hydration
- **Acetaminophen or ibuprofen**: For fever and pain (he's already taking ibuprofen)
- **Throat lozenges or sprays**: For sore throat
- **Salt water gargles**: May provide some relief

What NOT to do:

- **Avoid ampicillin and amoxicillin**: These antibiotics cause a distinctive maculopapular rash in 80-100% of patients with infectious mononucleosis. The mechanism isn't fully understood but isn't a true penicillin allergy. He already has a faint rash, which could be from EBV itself or from any antibiotics given before the diagnosis was made.
- **Avoid corticosteroids (usually)**: Not routinely indicated. Reserved for severe complications like impending airway obstruction from massive tonsillar hypertrophy, severe thrombocytopenia, or hemolytic anemia.

Activity Restrictions:

- **Avoid contact sports and strenuous activity for at least 3-4 weeks** due to splenomegaly. Splenic rupture is rare (0.1-0.5% of cases) but can be fatal. The enlarged spleen is vulnerable to trauma. Most ruptures occur in the second or third week of illness.
- Athletes should get clearance from their physician before returning to contact sports. Some experts recommend waiting until splenomegaly has resolved (confirmed by physical exam or ultrasound).

When to Seek Urgent Care: He's instructed to return immediately for:

- Severe abdominal pain (especially left upper quadrant) - could indicate splenic rupture
- Difficulty breathing or swallowing - airway obstruction
- Severe headache, confusion, weakness - neurologic complications
- Worsening symptoms or no improvement after 2-3 weeks

Follow-up

Week 2: His fever has resolved. Sore throat is much improved. Lymphadenopathy is decreasing. He still feels tired but can attend classes. He's following activity restrictions and resting when needed.

Week 4: He's feeling much better, though still tires more easily than before illness. Physical examination shows resolution of pharyngitis, significant reduction in lymphadenopathy, and spleen no longer palpable.

He's cleared to gradually resume normal activities but continue avoiding contact sports for another 2-3 weeks.

Week 8: He's back to baseline energy levels and has returned to all normal activities including recreational sports. Repeat examination shows complete resolution of splenomegaly. He's cleared for full activity without restrictions.

Long-term: About 10-20% of patients experience prolonged fatigue lasting several months after acute infectious mononucleosis. This doesn't represent ongoing acute infection but rather post-viral fatigue syndrome. Most eventually recover completely.

He remains EBV VCA IgG positive and EBNA positive for life—markers of past infection and immunity. He won't get infectious mononucleosis again, though EBV remains latent in his B cells permanently.

Teaching Points

Infectious mononucleosis presents with the classic triad of pharyngitis, lymphadenopathy, and splenomegaly. This combination in an adolescent or young adult should immediately suggest mono. The posterior cervical lymphadenopathy is particularly characteristic—more prominent than in typical pharyngitis.

Atypical lymphocytes are reactive T cells, not malignant cells. The "atypical" appearance reflects activation and enlargement of normal T lymphocytes responding to viral infection. These are different from the abnormal lymphocytes in lymphoma. Infectious mononucleosis typically shows 10-20% atypical lymphocytes (sometimes up to 50%), while other cell lines remain normal. In lymphoma, you'd expect progressive lymphadenopathy, B symptoms, and abnormal findings on flow cytometry.

The monospot test is quick but can be falsely negative early in illness. Heterophile antibodies may not develop until the second week of symptoms. If clinical suspicion is high and monospot is negative in the first week, repeat testing in 7-10 days or order EBV-specific antibodies. The monospot can also be falsely negative in young children (<4 years) and in CMV-associated mononucleosis (Ebell, 2004).

Avoid ampicillin and amoxicillin in suspected infectious mononucleosis. These antibiotics cause a distinctive rash in most patients with mono—not a true allergy but an interaction between the antibiotic and the acute EBV infection. Unfortunately, mono is often initially misdiagnosed as strep throat, leading to unnecessary antibiotic prescriptions. Always consider mono in the differential for severe pharyngitis, especially if accompanied by prominent lymphadenopathy and splenomegaly.

Splenic rupture is rare but potentially fatal. It occurs in 0.1-0.5% of cases, usually in the second or third week of illness. Most ruptures follow trauma (sports injury, motor vehicle accident), though spontaneous rupture can occur. This is why activity restriction is critical—the risk may seem small, but the consequences are severe. Patients with suspected rupture (severe abdominal pain, hypotension, referred shoulder pain) need emergent surgical evaluation (Asgari & Begos, 1997).

Most adults have been infected with EBV at some point. About 90-95% of adults worldwide have serologic evidence of past EBV infection (VCA IgG and EBNA positive). Primary infection in childhood is often asymptomatic or mild. Adolescents and young adults are more likely to develop classic infectious mononucleosis when first infected. This explains why mono is common in college settings—students from different geographic areas (some previously exposed, some not) mix together (Ebell, 2004).

CMV can cause a mononucleosis-like syndrome. Cytomegalovirus causes about 5-7% of mononucleosis cases. The clinical presentation is similar to EBV mono but typically with less severe pharyngitis and more prominent hepatitis. The monospot test is negative in CMV mono. CMV-specific antibody testing distinguishes it from EBV. Treatment is still supportive.

Fatigue can persist for months after acute illness. While most symptoms resolve within 2-4 weeks, profound fatigue lasting several months affects 10-20% of patients. This doesn't represent ongoing infection—EBV becomes latent once acute illness resolves. Post-viral fatigue syndrome is poorly understood but eventually resolves. Pushing too hard too soon may prolong recovery. Gradual return to activities as tolerated works better than forced rest or aggressive exercise.

Related Cases

This case connects to:

- **Case 4: The Teenager with Night Sweats** (Hodgkin lymphoma—another cause of lymphadenopathy and atypical lymphocytes, but with different clinical course)

- **Case 10: The Teenager with Fatigue and Easy Bruising** (acute leukemia—another cause of cytopenias in a young person)

- **Case 2: Unexplained Bruising** (discusses immune thrombocytopenia, which rarely complicates infectious mononucleosis)

-

Case 12: The Postoperative Patient with Bleeding

Clinical Presentation

A 58-year-old woman is hospitalized on the surgical ward three days after undergoing emergency surgery for a ruptured appendix with peritonitis. She initially did well postoperatively, but over the past 12 hours she's developed concerning symptoms.

The nurse calls the physician because the patient is bleeding from her IV sites and surgical incision. Blood is oozing around the surgical drain. She has multiple new bruises on her arms. Her vital signs show temperature 38.9°C (102°F), heart rate 115 beats per minute, blood pressure 92/58 mmHg (low), respiratory rate 24 breaths/minute, oxygen saturation 92% on 2 liters nasal cannula.

She appears acutely ill and confused. Her surgical incision is oozing blood despite pressure. Multiple ecchymoses are present on her arms and trunk. Petechiae are noted on her chest and legs. Abdominal examination reveals diffuse tenderness. She has decreased urine output over the past 6 hours.

Her past medical history includes hypertension and type 2 diabetes. Home medications include metformin and lisinopril. The surgical team is concerned about sepsis from intra-abdominal infection.

Initial Laboratory Findings

CBC:

- Hemoglobin: 8.2 g/dL (baseline pre-surgery was 13.5 g/dL) - **SIGNIFICANTLY DECREASED**

- Hematocrit: 25% (was 40% pre-surgery)

- MCV: 88 fL (normal)

- **Platelet count: 45,000/μL** (was 280,000/μL pre-surgery) - **VERY LOW**

- White blood cell count: 18,500/μL (elevated—consistent with infection)

Coagulation Studies:

- **PT: 22 seconds** (normal: 11-13 seconds) - **PROLONGED**

- **INR: 2.8** (normal: 0.8-1.2) - **ELEVATED**

- **aPTT: 68 seconds** (normal: 25-35 seconds) - **PROLONGED**

- **Fibrinogen: 85 mg/dL** (normal: 200-400 mg/dL) - **VERY LOW**

- **D-dimer: >20,000 ng/mL** (normal: <500 ng/mL) - **MARKEDLY ELEVATED**

Chemistry:

- Creatinine: 2.4 mg/dL (baseline 0.9 mg/dL) - ELEVATED (acute kidney injury)

- Lactate: 4.2 mmol/L (normal: 0.5-2.0 mmol/L) - ELEVATED (tissue hypoxia)

Stop and Think

This case presents a dramatically different bleeding disorder than we've seen before. Let's analyze the pattern:

What's abnormal?

1. Bleeding from multiple sites (IV sites, surgical incision, diffuse bruising, petechiae)

2. Severe thrombocytopenia (platelet count dropped from 280,000 to 45,000)

3. Prolonged PT and aPTT (both coagulation pathways affected)

4. Low fibrinogen (consumption of clotting factors)

5. Very high D-dimer (fibrin breakdown products)

6. Clinical sepsis (fever, hypotension, confusion, acute organ dysfunction)

This constellation—bleeding, thrombocytopenia, prolonged coagulation times, low fibrinogen, elevated D-dimer, and underlying sepsis—is pathognomonic for **disseminated intravascular coagulation (DIC)**.

DIC is not a primary disease but a **consumptive coagulopathy** that occurs secondary to severe underlying conditions. In this case, the trigger is sepsis from intra-abdominal infection after ruptured appendix.

Think about the paradox: inappropriate clotting (intravascular) leads to bleeding (consumption of platelets and clotting factors). Let's understand the mechanism.

Diagnostic Reasoning Questions

What is disseminated intravascular coagulation?

DIC is a syndrome of pathologic activation of coagulation throughout the microvasculature, characterized by:

1. Widespread microthrombi formation:

- Excessive thrombin generation activates coagulation

- Small clots form throughout small blood vessels

- These microthrombi can cause organ dysfunction (kidney, liver, brain, lungs)

2. Consumption of platelets and clotting factors:

- Platelets get used up making all these clots → thrombocytopenia

- Clotting factors (fibrinogen, factors V, VIII, II) get consumed → prolonged PT/aPTT

- This consumption leads to bleeding despite ongoing clotting

3. Fibrinolysis activation:

- The body tries to break down all the clots

- Plasmin degrades fibrin → elevated fibrin degradation products (D-dimer)

- Excessive fibrinolysis contributes to bleeding

The result is simultaneous thrombosis (causing organ damage) and bleeding (from consumption of hemostatic components).

What triggers DIC?

Common triggers include:

- **Sepsis** (most common—especially gram-negative bacteria)

- Trauma with tissue injury

- Malignancy (especially acute promyelocytic leukemia, adenocarcinomas)

- Obstetric complications (placental abruption, amniotic fluid embolism, retained dead fetus)

- Severe tissue injury (burns, heat stroke)

- Vascular disorders (giant hemangiomas)

- Severe transfusion reactions

This patient's DIC is triggered by **sepsis** from intra-abdominal infection following ruptured appendix with peritonitis.

How do you distinguish DIC from other coagulopathies?

Finding	DIC	Liver Disease	Vitamin K Deficiency	TTP/HUS
Platelet count	Low	Low or normal	Normal	Very low
PT	Prolonged	Prolonged	Prolonged	Normal
aPTT	Prolonged	Prolonged	Prolonged	Normal
Fibrinogen	Low	Low or normal	Normal	Normal
D-dimer	Very high	Elevated	Normal	Elevated
Schistocytes	Sometimes	No	No	Yes, many
Clinical context	Sepsis, trauma	Chronic liver disease	Malnutrition, antibiotics	Hemolysis, thrombocytopenia

The combination of low platelets, prolonged PT/aPTT, **low fibrinogen**, and **very high D-dimer** in the setting of sepsis is diagnostic for DIC.

What about the peripheral blood smear?

In DIC, you may see schistocytes (fragmented red cells) from mechanical damage as red cells pass through vessels partially occluded by microthrombi. This creates microangiopathic hemolytic anemia similar to TTP, though typically less severe.

Sequential Test Results

Peripheral Blood Smear: Thrombocytopenia confirmed. Occasional schistocytes present (about 1-2% of red cells), indicating mild microangiopathic hemolysis. Some large platelets present (megathrombocytes—young platelets released from bone marrow trying to compensate).

Additional Studies:

- Haptoglobin: 15 mg/dL (normal: 30-200 mg/dL) - LOW (indicates hemolysis)
- LDH: 485 U/L (normal: 122-222 U/L) - ELEVATED (indicates hemolysis and tissue damage)
- Indirect bilirubin: 2.1 mg/dL (elevated—from hemolysis)

Blood Cultures: Positive for **Escherichia coli** (gram-negative bacteria) and **Bacteroides fragilis** (anaerobic bacteria)—organisms typical of intra-abdominal infections.

Imaging: CT scan of abdomen shows intra-abdominal abscess and fluid collections consistent with ongoing infection.

What's Happening Here?

This patient has **acute disseminated intravascular coagulation (DIC) secondary to sepsis** from intra-abdominal infection.

The pathophysiology creates a vicious cycle:

1. Sepsis triggers systemic inflammation: Bacterial endotoxin and inflammatory cytokines activate the coagulation cascade. Tissue factor is expressed on monocytes and endothelial cells, initiating widespread thrombin generation.

2. Uncontrolled coagulation activation: Massive thrombin generation leads to:

- Fibrinogen → fibrin (forming microthrombi throughout microvasculature)
- Platelet activation and aggregation
- Consumption of clotting factors V, VIII, XIII, and prothrombin
- Depletion of natural anticoagulants (protein C, protein S, antithrombin)

3. Fibrinolysis activation: The fibrinolytic system activates to break down clots, producing massive amounts of fibrin degradation products (D-dimer).

4. Consumption coagulopathy: Depletion of platelets and clotting factors leads to:

- Thrombocytopenia (platelets consumed in clots)
- Prolonged PT/aPTT (clotting factors consumed)
- Low fibrinogen (converted to fibrin, then degraded)
- Paradoxical bleeding despite ongoing clotting

5. Organ dysfunction: Microthrombi in small vessels cause:

- Acute kidney injury (from renal microthrombi)
- Respiratory failure (pulmonary microthrombi)
- Confusion (cerebral microthrombi)
- Liver dysfunction
- Skin necrosis

6. Microangiopathic hemolysis: Red blood cells are sheared as they pass through vessels partially occluded by fibrin strands, producing schistocytes and contributing to anemia.

The combination of bleeding (from consumption) and thrombosis (from ongoing coagulation) creates the complex clinical picture of DIC.

Final Diagnosis

Acute disseminated intravascular coagulation (DIC) secondary to septic shock from intra-abdominal infection (E. coli and Bacteroides fragilis bacteremia)

Treatment and Management

DIC treatment focuses on two priorities:

1. Treat the underlying condition (most important) **2. Supportive care for coagulopathy**

Treating the Underlying Sepsis:

This is the MOST IMPORTANT intervention. DIC won't resolve until the underlying trigger is addressed.

- **Broad-spectrum antibiotics**: Already started (piperacillin-tazobactam and metronidazole for intra-abdominal infection)

- **Source control**: Surgical drainage of intra-abdominal abscess is planned

- **Hemodynamic support**: IV fluids for hypotension, vasopressors if needed (norepinephrine)

- **Supportive care**: Oxygen, monitoring, ICU-level care

Supportive Care for Coagulopathy:

Platelet transfusion:

- Indicated if platelet count <10,000-20,000/μL (spontaneous bleeding risk) or <50,000/μL with active bleeding or before procedures

- She receives 1 unit of platelets to support hemostasis during abscess drainage

Fresh Frozen Plasma (FFP):

- Replaces clotting factors (including fibrinogen)

- Indicated for active bleeding with prolonged PT/aPTT or before procedures

- She receives 4 units of FFP

Cryoprecipitate:

- Concentrated source of fibrinogen, factor VIII, vWF, factor XIII

- Indicated if fibrinogen <100 mg/dL

- She receives 10 units of cryoprecipitate to raise fibrinogen

Packed Red Blood Cells:

- For symptomatic anemia or hemoglobin <7 g/dL

- She receives 2 units PRBCs

What about anticoagulation?

Anticoagulation (heparin) is **controversial and usually not given**. While ongoing coagulation drives DIC, giving anticoagulants to a bleeding patient seems counterintuitive and dangerous. Anticoagulation may be considered in specific situations:

- Severe thrombotic complications (venous thromboembolism, acral ischemia)

- Chronic DIC with predominant thrombosis

- Under hematology guidance

In this case, with active bleeding, anticoagulation is **not given**.

Follow-up

Day 1 (Day 4 post-surgery): She undergoes CT-guided drainage of intra-abdominal abscess. Large volume of purulent material is drained. She's admitted to the ICU for close monitoring. She receives antibiotics, blood products, and vasopressor support.

Day 2-3: With abscess drainage and antibiotics, her clinical status begins improving. Fever decreases. Blood pressure stabilizes. Mental status clears. Bleeding from IV sites and incision slows.

Laboratory improvement:

- Platelet count: 78,000/μL (rising)

- PT: 16 seconds (improving)

- aPTT: 42 seconds (improving)

- Fibrinogen: 165 mg/dL (rising)

- D-dimer: 8,500 ng/mL (decreasing but still very elevated)

Day 7: She's transferred out of ICU to regular medical floor. Infection is resolving. Coagulation studies are near-normal:

- Platelet count: 145,000/μL

- PT: 13 seconds

- aPTT: 34 seconds

- Fibrinogen: 280 mg/dL

- D-dimer: 1,200 ng/mL (still elevated but much improved)

Day 14: She's discharged home on oral antibiotics to complete treatment course. Follow-up coagulation studies two weeks later are completely normal. She's recovered fully from both the surgical complication and the DIC.

Teaching Points

DIC is always secondary to an underlying condition—identify and treat the trigger. DIC doesn't occur in isolation. Common triggers include sepsis, trauma, malignancy, and obstetric complications. Treatment of the underlying condition is the most important intervention. Without addressing the trigger, DIC won't resolve despite supportive transfusions (Levi & Ten Cate, 1999).

The combination of low platelets, prolonged PT/aPTT, low fibrinogen, and high D-dimer in the right clinical context is diagnostic. No single test diagnoses DIC. The pattern of abnormalities combined with clinical presentation (sepsis, trauma, etc.) makes the diagnosis. Some scoring systems (like the ISTH DIC score) use these parameters to diagnose DIC objectively.

DIC causes both bleeding and thrombosis simultaneously. This seems paradoxical but makes sense with the pathophysiology. Widespread activation of coagulation forms microthrombi (causing organ damage), while consumption of platelets and clotting factors leads to bleeding. Some patients present primarily with bleeding, others with thrombotic complications, many with both (Levi & Ten Cate, 1999).

Schistocytes may be present but are usually less prominent than in TTP. Both DIC and TTP cause microangiopathic hemolytic anemia with schistocytes. In TTP, schistocytes are numerous and hemolysis is severe. In DIC, schistocytes may be present but are usually less prominent, and hemolysis is milder. The coagulation studies distinguish them—normal in TTP, markedly abnormal in DIC.

Blood product transfusion is supportive, not curative. Platelets, FFP, and cryoprecipitate replace consumed components temporarily but don't stop the underlying consumptive process. They're indicated for active bleeding or before procedures, but shouldn't be given "to correct numbers" in stable patients without bleeding. Treating the underlying condition is what actually resolves DIC.

Fibrinogen is a key marker. In DIC, fibrinogen is typically <100 mg/dL due to consumption. In contrast, most other coagulopathies (liver disease, vitamin K deficiency) show normal or only mildly reduced fibrinogen. Very low fibrinogen with prolonged coagulation times points toward DIC. Cryoprecipitate (which concentrates fibrinogen) is the blood product of choice when fibrinogen is critically low.

D-dimer is extremely elevated in DIC. D-dimer reflects fibrin breakdown. In DIC, massive fibrin formation followed by lysis produces very high D-dimer levels (often >10,000-20,000 ng/mL or even >50,000 ng/mL). While D-dimer is also elevated in other conditions (pulmonary embolism, recent surgery), the extreme elevation in DIC is characteristic. However, D-dimer alone doesn't diagnose DIC—it's part of the overall pattern.

Related Cases

This case connects to:

- **Case 7: TTP** (another cause of thrombocytopenia with microangiopathic hemolysis, but with normal coagulation studies)

- **Case 5: The Man Who Couldn't Stop Bleeding** (von Willebrand disease—inherited bleeding disorder with prolonged aPTT)

- **Case 2: Unexplained Bruising** (ITP—isolated thrombocytopenia without coagulation abnormalities)

Case 13: The Woman with Recurrent Miscarriages

Clinical Presentation

A 32-year-old woman is referred to hematology clinic by her obstetrician for evaluation of possible thrombophilia. She has a concerning history of pregnancy complications and now presents with a new deep vein thrombosis.

Three days ago, she developed left leg pain and swelling. Ultrasound confirmed deep vein thrombosis (DVT) in her left femoral vein. She was started on anticoagulation with low molecular weight heparin and is transitioning to warfarin.

Her obstetric history is troubling:

- **Three pregnancy losses**: Two first-trimester miscarriages and one second-trimester fetal demise at 22 weeks

- One successful pregnancy resulting in a healthy child (now age 5)

- Current pregnancy: 8 weeks pregnant when DVT diagnosed

She has no personal history of prior blood clots before this DVT. However, her father had a pulmonary embolism at age 45, and her paternal aunt had multiple DVTs. She doesn't smoke, isn't obese, and has no other significant medical history. She takes prenatal vitamins and no other medications.

Physical examination reveals left leg edema with 3 cm greater circumference than the right leg. The left leg is mildly tender but without erythema or warmth. The rest of her examination is unremarkable.

Initial Laboratory Findings

CBC:

- Hemoglobin: 12.8 g/dL (normal)

- Hematocrit: 38% (normal)

- MCV: 88 fL (normal)

- White blood cell count: 8,500/μL (normal)

- Platelet count: 245,000/μL (normal)

Coagulation Studies:

- PT: 12.5 seconds (normal)

- INR: 1.0 (normal)

- aPTT: 28 seconds (normal)

Chemistry:

- Normal renal and liver function

Stop and Think

This case presents a very different type of hematologic problem. Rather than bleeding (like previous cases), this patient has **thrombosis** (inappropriate clot formation).

The key features raising concern for inherited thrombophilia:

1. **Venous thromboembolism (VTE) at young age** (age 32)

2. **Strong family history** of VTE (father and paternal aunt)

3. **Recurrent pregnancy losses** (three miscarriages/fetal demise)

4. **No obvious provoking factors** (not obese, doesn't smoke, wasn't immobilized)

Pregnancy itself is a hypercoagulable state due to increased clotting factors and decreased protein S. However, DVT in early pregnancy plus recurrent pregnancy losses suggests an underlying thrombophilia.

What is thrombophilia?

Thrombophilia refers to conditions that increase risk of abnormal blood clot formation. Thrombophilias can be:

Inherited (genetic):

- Factor V Leiden (most common)
- Prothrombin G20210A mutation
- Protein C deficiency
- Protein S deficiency
- Antithrombin deficiency

Acquired:

- Antiphospholipid syndrome
- Pregnancy
- Malignancy
- Immobility
- Oral contraceptives/hormone replacement

The family history (father and aunt with clots) strongly suggests an **inherited thrombophilia**, likely **autosomal dominant** (affecting multiple generations).

Diagnostic Reasoning Questions

What is Factor V Leiden?

Factor V Leiden is the **most common inherited thrombophilia**, affecting about 5% of Caucasians (less common in other ethnicities). It's caused by a mutation in the Factor V gene that makes Factor V resistant to degradation by activated protein C.

Normal hemostasis involves both clotting and anticoagulation. Activated protein C (APC) is a natural anticoagulant that inactivates Factors Va and VIIIa, limiting clot formation. In Factor V Leiden, the mutated Factor V can't be inactivated efficiently by APC, leading to:

- Prolonged clotting activity
- Increased thrombin generation
- Increased risk of venous thrombosis

Inheritance:

- Autosomal dominant
- Heterozygotes (one mutation): 5-7 fold increased VTE risk
- Homozygotes (two mutations): 50-80 fold increased VTE risk

What about pregnancy complications?

Factor V Leiden and other thrombophilias are associated with:

- **Recurrent pregnancy loss** (placental thrombosis impairs blood flow to fetus)

- **Late pregnancy complications** (preeclampsia, placental abruption, fetal growth restriction, stillbirth)

- **Increased VTE risk during pregnancy** (pregnancy is already hypercoagulable; thrombophilia adds additional risk)

The mechanism involves placental thrombosis—tiny clots in placental vessels compromise blood flow, oxygen delivery, and nutrient transfer to the fetus.

When should you test for thrombophilia?

Testing is appropriate for:

- First VTE at age <50 without provocation

- Recurrent VTE

- VTE in unusual location (cerebral, mesenteric, portal veins)

- VTE with strong family history

- Women with recurrent pregnancy loss (≥3 losses) or unexplained late pregnancy complications

Testing is **NOT recommended** for:

- VTE with clear provocation (surgery, trauma, prolonged immobilization)

- Older patients with first VTE

- Screening asymptomatic family members (controversial)

- Routine screening before oral contraceptive use

This patient meets criteria: young age, family history, recurrent pregnancy losses, and now VTE.

What tests should be ordered?

Genetic testing:

- **Factor V Leiden mutation** (PCR-based genetic test)

- **Prothrombin G20210A mutation** (PCR-based genetic test)

Functional assays:

- Protein C activity

- Protein S activity (total and free)

- Antithrombin activity

Antiphospholipid antibodies (acquired thrombophilia):

- Lupus anticoagulant

- Anticardiolipin antibodies (IgG and IgM)

- Anti-beta-2-glycoprotein I antibodies (IgG and IgM)

Timing matters: Some tests are affected by acute thrombosis, pregnancy, and anticoagulation. Ideally, test when:

- Not acutely ill with thrombosis (wait 2-4 weeks)

- Not pregnant (protein S is falsely low in pregnancy)

- Off anticoagulation (if possible)

However, genetic tests (Factor V Leiden, prothrombin mutation) are **not affected** by these factors and can be done anytime. Functional assays should ideally be delayed.

Given she's pregnant and on anticoagulation, the hematologist proceeds with genetic testing now and defers functional assays until after pregnancy and anticoagulation are completed.

Sequential Test Results

Thrombophilia Genetic Testing:

- **Factor V Leiden mutation: Heterozygous - POSITIVE**

- Prothrombin G20210A mutation: Negative

She's heterozygous for Factor V Leiden—she has one normal Factor V gene and one mutated Factor V Leiden gene.

Antiphospholipid Antibody Panel:

- Lupus anticoagulant: Negative

- Anticardiolipin antibodies: Negative

- Anti-beta-2-glycoprotein I antibodies: Negative

No evidence of antiphospholipid syndrome.

Family Testing:

Her father (who had pulmonary embolism at age 45) is tested and found to be **heterozygous for Factor V Leiden** as well. This confirms the inherited nature—she inherited the mutation from her father.

What's Happening Here?

This patient has **Factor V Leiden thrombophilia (heterozygous)**, which explains both her venous thromboembolism and her recurrent pregnancy losses.

The pathophysiology:

1. Resistance to activated protein C: The Factor V Leiden mutation (G1691A) changes amino acid 506 from arginine to glutamine. This is the site where activated protein C normally cleaves and inactivates Factor Va. The mutation prevents efficient inactivation, so Factor Va remains active longer than normal.

2. Increased thrombin generation: Prolonged Factor Va activity leads to more thrombin generation and increased clot formation. This shifts the hemostatic balance toward thrombosis.

3. Pregnancy amplifies risk: Pregnancy is naturally hypercoagulable (increased fibrinogen, increased Factors VII, VIII, X, decreased protein S). Adding Factor V Leiden creates a "perfect storm" for thrombosis—both systemic (DVT/PE) and placental (pregnancy complications).

4. Placental thrombosis: Microthrombi in placental vessels compromise uteroplacental blood flow, leading to:

- Early pregnancy loss (impaired implantation or early placental insufficiency)

- Late pregnancy complications (fetal growth restriction, stillbirth, preeclampsia)

Her history of three pregnancy losses likely resulted from placental insufficiency due to thrombosis. Her one successful pregnancy occurred despite Factor V Leiden—many women with thrombophilia have successful pregnancies, especially with proper management.

Final Diagnosis

Factor V Leiden thrombophilia (heterozygous) with deep vein thrombosis in pregnancy and history of recurrent pregnancy loss

Treatment and Management

Acute DVT Management:

She's already appropriately started on anticoagulation. For pregnant women with acute VTE:

- **Low molecular weight heparin (LMWH):** Drug of choice in pregnancy

- Examples: enoxaparin, dalteparin

- Advantages: doesn't cross placenta, predictable pharmacokinetics, once or twice daily dosing

- Continue throughout pregnancy and 6-12 weeks postpartum (minimum 3 months total treatment)

Warfarin is contraindicated in pregnancy (teratogenic in first trimester, risks fetal bleeding). She should NOT transition to warfarin as initially planned.

Preventing Recurrent VTE:

Lifelong considerations:

- Avoid estrogen-containing contraceptives (significantly increase VTE risk in Factor V Leiden)

- Use prophylactic anticoagulation for high-risk situations (surgery, hospitalization, long flights)

- Maintain healthy weight and stay active

- Consider prophylactic anticoagulation during future pregnancies

Managing Future Pregnancies:

For women with Factor V Leiden and history of pregnancy complications or VTE:

Option 1: Prophylactic anticoagulation throughout pregnancy

- LMWH at prophylactic doses (lower than treatment doses)

- Reduces VTE risk

- May improve pregnancy outcomes (though data are mixed)

Option 2: Clinical surveillance without prophylaxis

- Reserve anticoagulation for VTE if it occurs

- Appropriate for women with thrombophilia but no VTE history

Given her history of both VTE and recurrent pregnancy losses, **prophylactic anticoagulation in future pregnancies is recommended**.

Low-dose aspirin (81 mg daily) starting in first trimester may also help prevent pregnancy complications by inhibiting platelet aggregation in placental vessels.

Current Pregnancy Management:

She continues therapeutic LMWH throughout this pregnancy (since she has acute DVT). Close obstetric monitoring includes:

- Serial ultrasounds to assess fetal growth

- Surveillance for preeclampsia

- Fetal testing in third trimester

Postpartum:

Continue anticoagulation for at least 6 weeks postpartum (postpartum period has highest VTE risk). Some experts recommend 12 weeks postpartum or 3 months total from DVT diagnosis.

After completing acute treatment, discuss long-term thromboprophylaxis strategy for future high-risk situations.

Family Counseling and Genetic Implications

Her children's risk:

- Each child has 50% chance of inheriting Factor V Leiden

- Her 5-year-old son can be tested if desired (controversial—some test, others defer until adulthood)

- Future children will have 50% risk

Her siblings:

- 50% chance of having Factor V Leiden

- Should be informed so they can make decisions about testing
- Female siblings should avoid estrogen contraceptives if positive

Genetic counseling:

- Autosomal dominant inheritance explained
- Testing implications discussed
- Reproductive options reviewed

Follow-up

Pregnancy outcome: With therapeutic anticoagulation throughout pregnancy, she delivers a healthy baby at 38 weeks via scheduled induction. No pregnancy complications occur. Baby is healthy.

Postpartum: She continues LMWH for 6 weeks postpartum, then stops. No further VTE episodes occur.

Long-term: She's counseled about VTE prevention strategies. She chooses an IUD for contraception (avoiding estrogen). She takes prophylactic LMWH during a future pregnancy two years later and delivers another healthy baby. No further pregnancy losses occur.

Teaching Points

Factor V Leiden is the most common inherited thrombophilia. About 5% of Caucasians carry the mutation (less common in African Americans, Hispanics, and Asians). It increases VTE risk 5-7 fold in heterozygotes and 50-80 fold in homozygotes. Most carriers never experience thrombosis, but risk increases with additional factors (pregnancy, oral contraceptives, surgery) (Kujovich, 2011).

Thrombophilia testing should be targeted, not universal. Test patients with unprovoked VTE at young age, recurrent VTE, strong family history, or VTE in unusual locations. Don't screen low-risk populations or test for thrombophilia when results won't change management. Testing asymptomatic family members is controversial—positive results may cause anxiety and insurance discrimination without proven benefit.

Estrogen-containing contraceptives are contraindicated in Factor V Leiden. Oral contraceptives increase VTE risk 3-4 fold in normal women. In women with Factor V Leiden, the combined risk is 30-40 fold increased. Progestin-only methods (IUD, implant, progestin-only pill) and non-hormonal methods are safer alternatives (Kujovich, 2011).

Pregnancy management in thrombophilia is individualized. Not all women with thrombophilia need anticoagulation during pregnancy. Those with VTE history definitely need it. Those with thrombophilia but no VTE history may or may not need it, depending on specific thrombophilia type and obstetric history. Decisions are made case-by-case balancing VTE risk against bleeding risk.

Thrombophilia contributes to recurrent pregnancy loss but isn't the only cause. About 10-15% of recurrent pregnancy loss is attributable to thrombophilia. Other causes include anatomic abnormalities, chromosomal abnormalities, endocrine disorders, and immunologic factors. Antiphospholipid syndrome (acquired thrombophilia) is strongly associated with pregnancy loss and should be tested in women with recurrent losses.

Genetic test results aren't affected by anticoagulation or acute thrombosis. Factor V Leiden and prothrombin G20210A mutations are detected by DNA testing, which doesn't change with anticoagulation, pregnancy, or acute illness. Functional assays (protein C, protein S, antithrombin) ARE affected by these factors and should ideally be performed when patient is well, not pregnant, and off anticoagulation for at least 2-4 weeks.

Family history is a critical clue. Multiple family members with VTE, especially at young ages, suggests inherited thrombophilia. Always obtain detailed family history including VTE in parents, siblings, and extended family. Autosomal dominant thrombophilias (Factor V Leiden, prothrombin mutation) often show vertical transmission (multiple generations affected).

Related Cases

This case connects to:

- **Case 6: The Older Man with Increasing Fatigue** (polycythemia vera—another condition causing increased thrombosis risk)

- **Case 5: The Man Who Couldn't Stop Bleeding** (von Willebrand disease—opposite problem, bleeding rather than clotting)

- **Case 12: The Postoperative Patient with Bleeding** (DIC—paradoxical thrombosis and bleeding)

Case 14: The Elderly Man with Persistent Cytopenias

Clinical Presentation

A 72-year-old retired teacher presents to his primary care physician for follow-up of abnormal blood counts first noted three months ago during routine screening. At that time, his hemoglobin was mildly low at 11.2 g/dL, and his white blood cell count was at the low end of normal. His doctor attributed it to "getting older" and recommended repeat testing.

The repeat CBC today shows worsening:

- Progressive fatigue and weakness

- Increasing shortness of breath with minimal exertion

- Occasional bruising

- Two nosebleeds in the past month (unusual for him)

He denies fever, night sweats, or weight loss. His appetite is normal. He's had no recent infections. No bone pain. Medical history includes hypertension and benign prostatic hypertrophy. Medications include lisinopril and tamsulosin. He's a lifelong nonsmoker and drinks alcohol only occasionally.

Physical examination reveals a pale elderly man in no acute distress. No lymphadenopathy. No hepatosplenomegaly. Scattered ecchymoses on his arms. The rest of the examination is unremarkable—specifically, no sternal tenderness, no petechiae.

Initial Laboratory Findings

CBC (current):

- **Hemoglobin: 9.8 g/dL** (normal: 13.5-17.5 g/dL) - **LOW**

- Hematocrit: 30% (normal: 41-53%) - LOW

- MCV: 102 fL (normal: 80-100 fL) - **SLIGHTLY ELEVATED** (macrocytic)

- **White blood cell count: 3,200/μL** (normal: 4,000-11,000/μL) - **LOW**

- **Platelet count: 88,000/μL** (normal: 150,000-400,000/μL) - **LOW**

WBC Differential:

- Neutrophils: 52% (absolute neutrophil count = 1,664/μL) - slightly low

- Lymphocytes: 38%

- Monocytes: 8%

- Eosinophils: 2%

- Basophils: 0%

- No blasts seen

CBC from 3 months ago:

- Hemoglobin: 11.2 g/dL

- WBC: 4,100/μL

- Platelets: 125,000/μL

All three cell lines have progressively declined.

Stop and Think

This case presents **pancytopenia**—decreased counts in all three cell lines (red cells, white cells, platelets). The progressive worsening over three months is concerning.

Pancytopenia indicates bone marrow is not producing adequate numbers of blood cells. Causes include:

1. Bone marrow failure syndromes:

- Aplastic anemia

- Myelodysplastic syndrome (MDS)

- Myelofibrosis

- Bone marrow infiltration (leukemia, lymphoma, metastatic cancer)

2. Peripheral destruction:

- Hypersplenism (enlarged spleen sequestering and destroying cells)

- Autoimmune cytopenias

3. Nutritional deficiencies:

- Vitamin B12 or folate deficiency (though usually causes isolated anemia, not full pancytopenia)

4. Medications/toxins:

- Chemotherapy
- Certain antibiotics, anticonvulsants
- Alcohol (chronic heavy use)

Key features in this case:

- **Elderly patient** (MDS is a disease of the elderly—median age 70-75)
- **Progressive pancytopenia** (worsening over months)
- **Macrocytic anemia** (MCV 102—slightly elevated)
- **No splenomegaly** (rules out hypersplenism)
- **No obvious toxic exposure**

Myelodysplastic syndrome (MDS) is high on the differential for an elderly patient with progressive pancytopenia and macrocytosis.

Diagnostic Reasoning Questions

What is myelodysplastic syndrome?

MDS is a group of clonal bone marrow disorders characterized by:

- **Ineffective hematopoiesis** (bone marrow makes abnormal cells that die before maturing)
- **Cytopenias** (low blood counts despite cellular bone marrow)
- **Dysplasia** (abnormal-appearing cells in bone marrow and sometimes peripheral blood)
- **Risk of transformation to acute myeloid leukemia** (10-30% progress to AML)

MDS is called a "clonal" disorder because it arises from a single abnormal hematopoietic stem cell that acquires mutations. This clone produces dysplastic (abnormal) progeny that undergo apoptosis (programmed cell death) before fully maturing, resulting in low peripheral blood counts despite a cellular (or even hypercellular) bone marrow—a phenomenon called "ineffective hematopoiesis."

Who gets MDS?

- Median age: 70-75 years
- More common in men
- Incidence increases dramatically with age
- Risk factors: prior chemotherapy or radiation (therapy-related MDS), benzene exposure, smoking

What tests are needed?

Peripheral blood smear: May show dysplastic features:

- Macrocytic red cells

- Hypo granular or pseudo-Pelger-Huët neutrophils (neutrophils with hyposegmented nuclei)

- Giant platelets or hypogranular platelets

Bone marrow aspiration and biopsy: Essential for diagnosis. Shows:

- Cellularity (often normal or increased despite cytopenias)

- Dysplasia in one or more cell lines (>10% dysplastic cells)

- Blast percentage (must be <20% to diagnose MDS; ≥20% is AML)

- Iron staining (may show ring sideroblasts)

Cytogenetics: Chromosomal abnormalities are common in MDS and help with prognosis. Common findings:

- Deletion 5q [del(5q)]

- Trisomy 8

- Deletion 7q or monosomy 7

- Complex karyotype (multiple abnormalities—poor prognosis)

Molecular testing: Next-generation sequencing can identify gene mutations (SF3B1, TET2, ASXL1, TP53, etc.) that help with diagnosis and prognosis.

How do you distinguish MDS from other causes of pancytopenia?

- **Vitamin B12/folate deficiency**: Check levels. Macrocytic anemia common, but cytopenias usually less severe. Bone marrow shows megaloblastic changes, not dysplasia.

- **Aplastic anemia**: Bone marrow is hypocellular (empty), not cellular with dysplasia.

- **AML**: Blasts ≥20% in marrow or blood. MDS has <20% blasts by definition.

- **Medications**: Detailed medication and exposure history. Stop offending agent if identified.

Sequential Test Results

Peripheral Blood Smear: Macrocytic red blood cells with moderate anisocytosis. Occasional teardrop cells. Neutrophils show decreased granulation and some hyposegmentation (pseudo-Pelger-Huët anomaly). Platelets are decreased in number and show variation in size. No blasts seen.

The findings—macrocytosis, hypogranular neutrophils, and dysmorphic features—suggest MDS.

Vitamin B12 and Folate:

- Vitamin B12: 425 pg/mL (normal: 200-900 pg/mL) - NORMAL

- Folate: 12 ng/mL (normal: >4 ng/mL) - NORMAL

Nutritional deficiencies are ruled out.

Bone Marrow Aspiration and Biopsy:

Aspirate smears: Bone marrow is normocellular to hypercellular (50-60% cellularity for age). Significant dysplasia noted in multiple cell lines:

- **Erythroid dysplasia**: Multinucleated erythroid precursors, nuclear budding, irregular nuclear contours

- **Myeloid dysplasia**: Hypogranular neutrophils, hyposegmented nuclei (pseudo-Pelger-Huët)

- **Megakaryocytic dysplasia**: Small hypolobated megakaryocytes (normally megakaryocytes are large with multiple nuclear lobes)

Blasts comprise 6% of marrow cells (normal: <5%, elevated but below the 20% threshold for AML).

Iron stain (Prussian blue): Increased iron stores. **Ring sideroblasts present** (erythroid precursors with iron-laden mitochondria forming a ring around the nucleus) comprising 18% of erythroid precursors.

The presence of ≥15% ring sideroblasts is diagnostic of a specific MDS subtype called **MDS with ring sideroblasts**.

Biopsy: Confirms normocellular marrow with trilineage dysplasia. No evidence of fibrosis. No lymphoma or metastatic disease.

Cytogenetics (Karyotype): Normal male karyotype, 46,XY. No chromosomal abnormalities detected.

Normal cytogenetics actually occur in about 50% of MDS cases. Some chromosomal abnormalities confer better prognosis (isolated del(5q)), while others are worse (monosomy 7, complex karyotype). Normal cytogenetics are intermediate risk.

Molecular Studies: Next-generation sequencing panel shows mutation in **SF3B1 gene**.

SF3B1 mutations are strongly associated with MDS with ring sideroblasts and generally confer a favorable prognosis with lower risk of progression to AML.

What's Happening Here?

This patient has **myelodysplastic syndrome with ring sideroblasts (MDS-RS)**, specifically MDS with multilineage dysplasia and ring sideroblasts.

The pathophysiology:

1. Clonal stem cell disorder: A hematopoietic stem cell acquires mutations (in this case, SF3B1 mutation). This abnormal clone proliferates but produces dysplastic progeny.

2. Ineffective hematopoiesis: The dysplastic cells undergo premature apoptosis in the bone marrow before fully maturing. This creates the paradox of MDS:

- Cellular bone marrow (actively producing cells)

- But peripheral cytopenias (cells dying before release into bloodstream)

3. Ring sideroblasts: SF3B1 mutations affect RNA splicing and lead to mitochondrial iron overload in erythroid precursors. Iron-laden mitochondria encircle the nucleus, creating the characteristic "ring sideroblast" appearance on iron staining.

4. Progressive cytopenias: Over time, ineffective hematopoiesis worsens, and cytopenias deepen. This causes:

- Anemia → fatigue, weakness, dyspnea

- Thrombocytopenia → bruising, bleeding

- Neutropenia → infection risk (though often mild)

5. Risk of AML transformation: MDS can progress to acute myeloid leukemia in 10-30% of patients over time. The blast percentage increases, and eventually crosses the 20% threshold defining AML. Patients with MDS-RS and SF3B1 mutations have relatively low risk of AML transformation compared to other MDS subtypes (Malcovati et al., 2020).

Final Diagnosis

Myelodysplastic syndrome with ring sideroblasts and multilineage dysplasia, associated with SF3B1 mutation

Prognosis and Risk Stratification

MDS prognosis varies widely from relatively indolent disease with years of survival to aggressive disease rapidly progressing to AML. Risk stratification guides treatment decisions.

IPSS-R (Revised International Prognostic Scoring System):

Scores based on:

- Cytogenetics (chromosomal abnormalities)

- Bone marrow blast percentage

- Hemoglobin level

- Platelet count

- Absolute neutrophil count

His IPSS-R score calculation:

- Cytogenetics: Normal (0 points—intermediate risk)

- Blasts 6%: (1 point)

- Hemoglobin 9.8 g/dL: (1.5 points)

- Platelets 88,000/μL: (0.5 points)

- ANC 1,664/μL: (0 points)

Total: 3 points = Intermediate risk

Median survival for intermediate-risk MDS is approximately 3-5 years. Risk of AML transformation is moderate (10-20% at 5 years).

However, the presence of SF3B1 mutation and ring sideroblasts is a **favorable prognostic factor** that improves his outlook compared to other intermediate-risk MDS patients.

Treatment and Management

MDS treatment is individualized based on:

- Risk stratification (IPSS-R score)
- Patient age and comorbidities
- Severity of cytopenias
- Patient goals and preferences

For this patient (intermediate risk, elderly, symptomatic anemia):

1. Supportive Care:

Red blood cell transfusions:

- For symptomatic anemia (fatigue, dyspnea)
- Typically transfuse when hemoglobin <8 g/dL or symptomatic at higher levels
- Goal: maintain hemoglobin where patient feels functional

Erythropoiesis-stimulating agents (ESAs):

- Epoetin alfa or darbepoetin
- May reduce transfusion needs in some patients
- Best response in patients with lower transfusion burden and lower baseline EPO levels

Iron chelation:

- Patients receiving chronic transfusions develop iron overload
- Chelation (deferasirox, deferoxamine) removes excess iron and prevents organ damage
- Considered after 20-30 units of blood transfused

Platelet transfusions:

- For significant thrombocytopenia (<10,000-20,000/μL) or bleeding

Antibiotics:

- For infections (neutropenia increases infection risk)

2. Disease-Modifying Therapy:

Luspatercept:

- New agent approved for MDS with ring sideroblasts and SF3B1 mutation

- Promotes late-stage red blood cell maturation

- Reduces transfusion needs in about 50-60% of patients

- Well-tolerated

- Ideal for this patient given his MDS subtype

He's started on luspatercept with good response—transfusion needs decrease, and hemoglobin improves to 10.5-11 g/dL.

Hypomethylating agents (azacitidine, decitabine):

- For higher-risk MDS

- Can improve cytopenias and delay AML progression

- Not typically first-line for lower/intermediate risk with ring sideroblasts

Lenalidomide:

- Specifically for MDS with isolated del(5q) chromosomal abnormality

- Not applicable to this patient (he has normal cytogenetics)

3. Potentially Curative Therapy:

Allogeneic stem cell transplant:

- Only curative option for MDS

- High risk (mortality 20-40%)

- Generally reserved for younger patients (<65-70) or higher-risk disease

- Not pursued in this 72-year-old with intermediate-risk disease

Follow-up

Month 3 on luspatercept: Hemoglobin improves to 10.8 g/dL. He feels less fatigued and no longer requires transfusions. Platelets and white count remain stable.

Year 1: He continues luspatercept with maintained hemoglobin around 10-11 g/dL. Quality of life is good. He's able to continue his hobbies (gardening, reading). Repeat bone marrow at 1 year shows persistent dysplasia but stable blast percentage (5%). No progression to AML.

Year 3: He remains transfusion-independent on luspatercept. Occasional monitoring shows stable disease. No AML transformation.

Prognosis: With MDS-RS and SF3B1 mutation (favorable features) and good response to luspatercept, he has a relatively good prognosis for MDS. Median survival may exceed 5-7 years with low risk of AML transformation. Quality of life is maintained with treatment.

Teaching Points

MDS is primarily a disease of the elderly. Median age at diagnosis is 70-75 years. Always consider MDS in elderly patients with unexplained, progressive cytopenias. The incidence of MDS increases dramatically after age 60, affecting about 1 in 500 people over age 70 (Malcovati et al., 2020).

Ineffective hematopoiesis explains the paradox of cellular marrow with peripheral cytopenias. In MDS, the bone marrow is often normal or even hypercellular, yet blood counts are low. The dysplastic cells die prematurely in the marrow before maturing and entering the bloodstream. This distinguishes MDS from aplastic anemia (where the marrow is empty).

Bone marrow examination is essential for diagnosis. You cannot diagnose MDS from peripheral blood alone, though certain findings (macrocytosis, hypogranular neutrophils, giant platelets) raise suspicion. Bone marrow shows the characteristic dysplasia in ≥10% of cells in one or more lineages, which is the diagnostic criterion for MDS.

Ring sideroblasts are pathognomonic for certain MDS subtypes. These erythroblasts with perinuclear iron-laden mitochondria are seen on iron staining of bone marrow. The presence of ≥15% ring sideroblasts defines MDS with ring sideroblasts (MDS-RS), which is often associated with SF3B1 mutations and has relatively favorable prognosis compared to other MDS subtypes (Malcovati et al., 2020).

MDS can transform to acute myeloid leukemia. About 10-30% of MDS cases progress to AML over time. The blast percentage gradually increases from <5% (normal) to 5-19% (MDS) to ≥20% (AML). Risk of transformation varies by MDS subtype, cytogenetics, and molecular features. MDS-RS with SF3B1 mutations has lower transformation risk.

Prognosis varies widely and requires risk stratification. The IPSS-R score incorporates cytogenetics, blast percentage, and severity of cytopenias to categorize patients as very low, low, intermediate, high, or very high risk. This guides treatment decisions—lower-risk patients receive supportive care and mild therapies, while higher-risk patients need aggressive treatment or transplant consideration.

Treatment is individualized and often supportive. Most elderly patients with lower/intermediate-risk MDS are managed with supportive care (transfusions) and mild disease-modifying agents (ESAs, luspatercept). Aggressive chemotherapy and stem cell transplant are reserved for younger patients or higher-risk disease. The goal is often quality of life rather than cure in elderly patients.

Related Cases

This case connects to:

- **Case 10: The Teenager with Fatigue and Easy Bruising** (acute leukemia—MDS can transform to AML)

- **Case 6: The Older Man with Increasing Fatigue** (polycythemia vera—another myeloproliferative disorder, but causing too many cells rather than too few)

- **Case 1: The Tired Graduate Student** (anemia, but due to iron deficiency rather than bone marrow failure)

Case 15: The Child with Anemia and Jaundice

Clinical Presentation

A 4-year-old boy is brought to the pediatrician by his parents for evaluation of persistent pallor and yellowish discoloration of his eyes noticed over the past few weeks. His mother reports that he seems more tired than usual and has been less interested in playing.

She also mentions that his urine has been darker than normal, sometimes appearing cola-colored, especially in the morning. He's had several similar episodes over the past year, usually lasting a few days before improving spontaneously.

His past medical history includes neonatal jaundice requiring phototherapy and mild anemia noted on previous well-child visits. His father had similar problems as a child and underwent splenectomy at age 10. Family history is otherwise notable for a paternal grandfather who had "gallstones at a young age."

Physical examination reveals a pale child with noticeable scleral icterus (yellow discoloration of the whites of the eyes). His spleen is enlarged, palpable 3 cm below the left costal margin. No hepatomegaly. No lymphadenopathy. The rest of the examination is unremarkable.

Initial Laboratory Findings

CBC:

- **Hemoglobin: 8.9 g/dL** (normal for age: 11.5-15.5 g/dL) - **LOW**
- Hematocrit: 27% (normal: 34-40%) - LOW
- **MCV: 76 fL** (normal for age: 77-95 fL) - **SLIGHTLY LOW**
- **MCHC: 37 g/dL** (normal: 32-36 g/dL) - **ELEVATED**
- **RDW: 18%** (normal: 11.5-14.5%) - **ELEVATED**
- **Reticulocyte count: 12%** (normal: 0.5-1.5%) - **MARKEDLY ELEVATED**
- White blood cell count: 9,200/μL (normal)
- Platelet count: 385,000/μL (normal)

Chemistry:

- **Total bilirubin: 4.8 mg/dL** (normal: 0.3-1.2 mg/dL) - **ELEVATED**
- **Indirect bilirubin: 4.2 mg/dL** (normal: 0.2-0.8 mg/dL) - **MARKEDLY ELEVATED**
- Direct bilirubin: 0.6 mg/dL (normal)
- **LDH: 645 U/L** (normal: 122-222 U/L) - **ELEVATED**
- Haptoglobin: <10 mg/dL (normal: 30-200 mg/dL) - **UNDETECTABLE**

Stop and Think

This case presents a young child with:

1. **Anemia** (low hemoglobin)

2. **Jaundice** (elevated indirect bilirubin, scleral icterus)

3. **Dark urine** (hemoglobinuria from hemolysis)

4. **Splenomegaly**

5. **Markedly elevated reticulocyte count** (12%)

6. **Strong family history** (father with similar condition requiring splenectomy, grandfather with early gallstones)

The laboratory pattern screams **hemolytic anemia**:

- Low hemoglobin (anemia)

- High reticulocyte count (bone marrow responding to anemia)

- Elevated indirect bilirubin (hemoglobin breakdown product)

- Elevated LDH (released from lysed red cells)

- Undetectable haptoglobin (consumed binding free hemoglobin)

This is chronic hemolysis—the reticulocyte count of 12% indicates massive red cell turnover. The bone marrow is working overtime to replace destroyed red cells.

The **elevated MCHC** (mean corpuscular hemoglobin concentration) is an unusual and important clue. MCHC is rarely elevated in most anemias. When it is elevated, think **hereditary spherocytosis**.

The **family history** (father with same condition, grandfather with early gallstones) strongly suggests an **inherited hemolytic anemia**. Hereditary spherocytosis is autosomal dominant—the father likely has it, the son inherited it, and the grandfather probably had it too (gallstones are common in chronic hemolysis due to increased bilirubin).

Diagnostic Reasoning Questions

What is hereditary spherocytosis?

Hereditary spherocytosis (HS) is the most common inherited hemolytic anemia in people of Northern European descent, affecting about 1 in 2,000 people. It's caused by mutations in genes encoding red blood cell membrane proteins (spectrin, ankyrin, band 3, protein 4.2).

These membrane protein defects lead to:

- Loss of red cell membrane

- Red cells become spherical rather than biconcave disc-shaped

- Spherical cells are less deformable

- Spherocytes get trapped and destroyed in the spleen

- Chronic hemolysis results

Inheritance:

- Usually autosomal dominant (75% of cases)
- Affected parent passes it to 50% of children
- Sometimes autosomal recessive or new mutations

Clinical features:

- Anemia (variable severity—mild to severe)
- Jaundice (from indirect hyperbilirubinemia)
- Splenomegaly (the spleen destroys spherocytes)
- Gallstones (common—from chronic hyperbilirubinemia)
- Aplastic crises (temporary bone marrow shutdown during viral infections, especially parvovirus B19)

Why is MCHC elevated?

Spherocytes have decreased surface area relative to volume (spheres have the lowest surface-to-volume ratio). They appear densely packed with hemoglobin, creating elevated MCHC. This is a characteristic finding in hereditary spherocytosis, though not 100% sensitive (Bolton-Maggs et al., 2012).

What tests confirm the diagnosis?

Peripheral blood smear:

- Spherocytes visible (small, round red cells without central pallor)
- Polychromasia (blue-tinged cells representing reticulocytes)

Osmotic fragility test:

- Spherocytes are more fragile than normal red cells
- When placed in hypotonic (low salt) solution, spherocytes lyse more readily than normal cells
- Classic test but being replaced by newer methods

Eosin-5-maleimide (EMA) binding test:

- Flow cytometry-based test
- Measures binding of fluorescent dye to red cell membrane proteins
- Reduced binding in hereditary spherocytosis
- More sensitive and specific than osmotic fragility

Molecular genetic testing:

- Can identify specific mutations
- Not always necessary if clinical and laboratory features are diagnostic

Sequential Test Results

Peripheral Blood Smear: Numerous spherocytes present—small, round red blood cells lacking central pallor. Marked polychromasia (reflecting the elevated reticulocyte count). No schistocytes, no target cells, no sickle cells.

The presence of abundant spherocytes confirms the suspected diagnosis.

Direct Antiglobulin Test (Coombs test): Negative

This rules out immune-mediated hemolysis (autoimmune hemolytic anemia), which can also cause spherocytes. In immune hemolytic anemia, antibodies coat red cells and the Coombs test is positive. In hereditary spherocytosis, there are no antibodies—the problem is intrinsic to the red cell membrane.

Osmotic Fragility Test: Increased osmotic fragility. Spherocytes begin lysing at higher salt concentrations than normal red cells, confirming they're more fragile.

EMA Binding Test: Reduced EMA binding (68% of normal control mean). This supports hereditary spherocytosis.

Abdominal Ultrasound: Splenomegaly confirmed (spleen 12 cm in longest dimension; normal for age is <8 cm). No gallstones noted yet (though he's at high risk for developing them over time). Liver is normal size.

What's Happening Here?

This child has **hereditary spherocytosis**, inherited from his father (who had the same condition and underwent splenectomy).

The pathophysiology:

1. Membrane protein deficiency: Mutations in genes encoding membrane skeleton proteins (most commonly spectrin or ankyrin) weaken the red cell membrane's structural integrity.

2. Membrane loss: The weakened membrane sheds small vesicles over the red cell's lifespan. With each pass through the spleen, a bit more membrane is lost.

3. Spherocyte formation: As membrane is lost, the surface-to-volume ratio decreases. The cell becomes spherical (spheres have the minimum surface area for a given volume).

4. Decreased deformability: Normal red cells are highly deformable biconcave discs that can squeeze through narrow splenic sinusoids. Spherocytes are rigid and less deformable.

5. Splenic sequestration and destruction: The spleen's narrow sinusoids (5-8 micrometers) trap the rigid spherocytes. Splenic macrophages recognize and destroy these abnormal cells. This is called **extravascular hemolysis** (hemolysis outside blood vessels, in the spleen).

6. Chronic hemolysis: Continuous red cell destruction in the spleen leads to:

- Anemia (hemoglobin drops because destruction exceeds production)

- Elevated reticulocyte count (bone marrow compensates by producing new cells rapidly)

- Indirect hyperbilirubinemia (hemoglobin breakdown releases unconjugated bilirubin)

- Jaundice (visible when bilirubin >2-3 mg/dL)

- Splenomegaly (chronic workload enlarges the spleen)

- Dark urine during hemolytic crises (hemoglobinuria and urobilinogen)

7. Long-term complications:

- **Gallstones** (pigment stones from chronic hyperbilirubinemia—develop in 50-85% of patients by adulthood)

- **Aplastic crises** (parvovirus B19 infection temporarily shuts down red cell production, causing severe anemia)

- **Hemolytic crises** (infections or other stressors worsen hemolysis temporarily)

- **Folate deficiency** (chronic hemolysis increases folate requirements)

His father's splenectomy at age 10 makes sense—splenectomy removes the site of red cell destruction and dramatically improves or eliminates anemia in hereditary spherocytosis, though it doesn't cure the underlying membrane defect.

Final Diagnosis

Hereditary spherocytosis

Treatment and Management

Treatment depends on severity of hemolysis and symptoms.

Current Management:

1. Folic Acid Supplementation:

- 1 mg daily

- Chronic hemolysis depletes folate stores

- Prevents megaloblastic anemia superimposed on hemolytic anemia

2. Monitoring:

- Regular CBC to track hemoglobin

- Monitor for complications (gallstones, aplastic crises)

- Annual ultrasound to check for gallstone development

3. Vaccinations (in preparation for potential splenectomy): If splenectomy is being considered, vaccinate **before** surgery:

- Pneumococcal (Prevnar 13 and Pneumovax 23)

- Meningococcal (Menactra or Menveo)

- Haemophilus influenzae type b

- Annual influenza vaccine

4. Education: Parents are educated about:

- **Aplastic crisis warning signs**: Sudden worsening of anemia, fatigue, pallor without jaundice (because reticulocytes disappear, bilirubin may actually drop)

- **Hemolytic crisis**: Increased jaundice, dark urine, abdominal pain

- **When to seek urgent care**: Severe fatigue, pallor, dizziness, fever with severe symptoms

Splenectomy Considerations:

Splenectomy is **curative** for the hematologic manifestations of hereditary spherocytosis. After splenectomy:

- Hemoglobin normalizes

- Reticulocyte count drops (but remains slightly elevated)

- Jaundice resolves

- Quality of life improves

However, splenectomy has risks:

- **Lifelong infection risk** from encapsulated bacteria (overwhelming post-splenectomy infection/OPSI)

- **Thrombosis risk** (platelets often rise post-splenectomy)

- **Surgical risks**

Guidelines for splenectomy timing:

- **Defer until age 5-6 years** (allows immune system maturation, reduces infection risk)

- Consider earlier if severe symptomatic anemia

- Consider later or never if mild disease

Indications for splenectomy:

- Moderate to severe anemia requiring transfusions

- Significant symptoms (fatigue, growth delay, exercise intolerance)

- Complications (recurrent gallstones, aplastic crises)

Not indicated if:

- Mild disease with minimal symptoms

- Can maintain adequate hemoglobin without transfusions

This child has moderate disease—hemoglobin 8.9 g/dL is symptomatic (fatigue, pallor) but not transfusion-dependent. The family will monitor him over the next 1-2 years. If symptoms worsen or complications develop, splenectomy will be considered around age 5-6.

Follow-up

Age 5: His anemia has remained stable (hemoglobin 8.5-9.5 g/dL range). He's experiencing more fatigue and difficulty keeping up with peers during physical activities. His parents opt for splenectomy.

Pre-operative: He receives all recommended vaccinations 2-4 weeks before surgery. Pneumococcal, meningococcal, and Haemophilus vaccines are administered.

Surgery: Laparoscopic splenectomy is performed successfully. The spleen weighed 180 grams (normal for age is 40-80 grams), confirming splenomegaly.

Post-operative: Within 2 weeks, his hemoglobin rises to 12.8 g/dL. Reticulocyte count drops to 4% (still elevated but much improved from 12%). Jaundice completely resolves. His energy level dramatically improves.

3 Months Post-splenectomy: He's thriving. Hemoglobin stable at 13.2 g/dL. He's active, playing sports, and has no limitations. Peripheral blood smear still shows spherocytes (the membrane defect remains), but they're no longer being destroyed because the spleen is absent.

Platelet count is elevated at 520,000/μL (thrombocytosis is common after splenectomy). He's started on daily aspirin 81 mg to reduce thrombosis risk until platelet count stabilizes.

Long-term Management Post-splenectomy:

- **Lifelong penicillin prophylaxis** (or amoxicillin) until at least age 18-21

- **Immediate antibiotics for fever** (any fever >101°F warrants urgent evaluation and empiric antibiotics)

- **Medical alert bracelet** indicating asplenia

- **Annual influenza vaccination**

- **Re-vaccination** with pneumococcal vaccine every 5 years

- **Malaria prophylaxis** if traveling to endemic areas

- **Monitor for gallstones** (risk remains even after splenectomy)

Age 16: Develops gallstones (common even after splenectomy due to years of chronic hyperbilirubinemia before splenectomy). Undergoes laparoscopic cholecystectomy. Recovers well.

Adulthood: He lives a normal life with no activity restrictions. His hemoglobin remains stable at 13-14 g/dL. He understands his infection risk and takes appropriate precautions. He receives genetic counseling before having children—each child will have a 50% chance of inheriting hereditary spherocytosis.

Teaching Points

Hereditary spherocytosis presents with the triad of anemia, jaundice, and splenomegaly. Symptoms range from mild (incidental finding) to severe (requiring transfusions). Most patients have moderate disease with compensated hemolysis—chronic anemia but adequate reticulocyte response. The severity often correlates with the specific genetic mutation (Bolton-Maggs et al., 2012).

Elevated MCHC is a valuable clue. MCHC is rarely elevated in most conditions (it's usually normal or low). When MCHC is >36 g/dL, think hereditary spherocytosis or autoimmune hemolytic anemia. Spherocytes have high hemoglobin concentration per unit volume because of their decreased surface-to-volume ratio, creating the elevated MCHC.

Family history is critical. About 75% of cases show autosomal dominant inheritance with affected parents. Always ask about family members with anemia, jaundice, splenomegaly, splenectomy, or gallstones at young age. However, 25% are de novo mutations or recessive inheritance, so negative family history doesn't exclude hereditary spherocytosis.

Distinguish hereditary spherocytosis from autoimmune hemolytic anemia. Both cause hemolysis with spherocytes on smear. The Direct Antiglobulin Test (Coombs test) distinguishes them—negative in hereditary spherocytosis (intrinsic red cell defect), positive in autoimmune hemolytic anemia (antibodies coating red cells). This is a critical distinction because treatments differ completely.

Aplastic crisis is a life-threatening complication. Parvovirus B19 infection specifically targets red blood cell precursors in the bone marrow, temporarily shutting down red cell production. In healthy people, this causes minimal problems because red cells live 120 days. In hereditary spherocytosis, red cells only live 10-20 days, so stopping production for even one week causes severe anemia. Aplastic crisis presents with sudden worsening of anemia, fatigue, and pallor WITHOUT jaundice (because reticulocytes disappear, bilirubin actually drops). Treatment is supportive—transfusions if needed until bone marrow recovers (Bolton-Maggs et al., 2012).

Splenectomy is curative for the hematologic manifestations but creates lifelong infection risk. After splenectomy, hemoglobin normalizes and symptoms resolve. However, the spleen plays a critical role in fighting encapsulated bacteria (Streptococcus pneumoniae, Haemophilus influenzae, Neisseria meningitidis). Without a spleen, patients are at lifelong risk of overwhelming post-splenectomy infection (OPSI), which has 50% mortality even with treatment. This is why vaccination before splenectomy and lifelong vigilance for fever are essential.

Defer splenectomy until age 5-6 if possible. Younger children have higher infection risk after splenectomy. Waiting until age 5-6 allows immune system maturation and reduces OPSI risk. However, if severe symptomatic anemia or complications occur, earlier splenectomy may be necessary. Partial splenectomy is being explored as an alternative that preserves some immune function while reducing hemolysis.

Gallstones develop in most patients by adulthood. Chronic hyperbilirubinemia leads to pigment gallstone formation in 50-85% of hereditary spherocytosis patients. They often develop in childhood or young adulthood (much younger than typical cholesterol gallstones). Some centers recommend concurrent cholecystectomy at the time of splenectomy if gallstones are present or advocate for prophylactic cholecystectomy to prevent future symptomatic gallstones.

Related Cases

This case connects to:

- **Case 8: The Young Man with Joint Pain** (sickle cell disease—another inherited hemolytic anemia but with different pathophysiology)

- **Case 3: The Athletic Young Man** (thalassemia trait—another inherited red cell disorder but causing microcytic anemia without hemolysis)

- **Case 7: TTP** (acquired hemolytic anemia with thrombocytopenia, but microangiopathic rather than extravascular hemolysis)

Key Lessons from These Hematology Cases

After working through these 15 hematology cases, several overarching principles emerge:

Pattern recognition accelerates diagnosis. Microcytic anemia → think iron deficiency or thalassemia. Isolated thrombocytopenia with normal other counts → think ITP. Schistocytes plus thrombocytopenia → think TTP or DIC. Blasts in blood → think leukemia. Learning these patterns makes you faster and more accurate.

Context matters enormously. The same finding means different things in different patients. Anemia in a menstruating vegan woman likely means iron deficiency. Anemia in a Mediterranean man with elevated RBC count likely means thalassemia. Anemia in an elderly patient with cytopenias suggests MDS or malignancy. Always consider age, gender, ethnicity, family history, and clinical presentation.

The peripheral blood smear is your friend. Automated analyzers provide numbers, but the smear shows morphology. Schistocytes, spherocytes, target cells, blasts, atypical lymphocytes—these findings guide diagnosis in ways numbers alone cannot. When results don't make sense or serious pathology is suspected, look at the smear.

Follow-up matters. Many diagnoses require observing trends over time. Stable mild anemia in thalassemia trait versus progressive anemia in MDS. Single episode of thrombocytopenia versus recurrent episodes in ITP. Response to treatment confirms or refutes diagnoses. Always reassess and adjust your thinking based on clinical course.

Inherited disorders often present in childhood but sometimes in adulthood. Hereditary spherocytosis, sickle cell disease, and severe thalassemias usually present early. But Factor V Leiden, mild thalassemia trait, and von Willebrand disease may not become apparent until adulthood when triggers occur. Don't assume adult-onset means acquired—ask about family history.

Treatment addresses both the underlying condition and its complications. Iron deficiency needs iron supplementation AND identification of the bleeding source. Sickle cell needs pain management AND treatment of infection AND prevention strategies. TTP needs plasma exchange for the acute crisis AND immunosuppression for the autoimmune process. DIC needs treatment of sepsis AND blood product support. Always address the root cause, not just the symptoms.

Hematology integrates with all of medicine. These cases involved infectious disease (EBV, sepsis triggering DIC), obstetrics (pregnancy complications in thrombophilia), oncology (lymphoma, leukemia), and many other specialties. Blood touches every organ system, so hematologic disorders have wide-ranging effects. Think broadly and integrate information across systems.

You've now worked through diverse hematology presentations—from simple iron deficiency to life-threatening TTP, from inherited spherocytosis to acquired MDS. These cases provide a foundation for approaching real patients with blood disorders. The diagnostic reasoning skills you've practiced—generating differentials, ordering appropriate tests, interpreting results in context, considering complications—transfer directly to clinical practice.

Moving Forward

You've completed the hematology cases in Chapter 2. These 15 cases covered the major categories of hematologic disorders—anemia (iron deficiency, thalassemia, hemolysis), thrombocytopenia (ITP, TTP, DIC), thrombophilia (Factor V Leiden), coagulation disorders (von Willebrand disease), proliferative disorders (polycythemia vera, leukemia, lymphoma), and bone marrow failure (MDS).

In Chapter 3, you'll encounter clinical chemistry and metabolic disorder cases covering electrolyte abnormalities, acid-base disturbances, endocrine disorders, liver and kidney disease, and more. The same diagnostic reasoning framework applies—careful history, pattern recognition, systematic workup, and thoughtful interpretation in clinical context.

The skills you've developed working through these hematology cases—generating differential diagnoses, selecting appropriate tests, interpreting results, recognizing patterns, considering complications—transfer directly to chemistry cases and to clinical practice. Keep practicing, keep thinking systematically, and keep learning from each case.

You're building expertise one case at a time.

Chapter 3: Clinical Chemistry and Metabolic Disorders

Chemistry panels tell stories about metabolism, hormones, electrolytes, and organ function. A sodium level isn't just a number—it reflects fluid balance, kidney function, and hormonal regulation. An elevated glucose doesn't just mean "high sugar"—it tells you about insulin production, cellular metabolism, and potentially life-threatening metabolic crises.

Clinical chemistry encompasses a huge territory: electrolytes that keep your heart beating regularly, hormones that regulate everything from metabolism to mood, enzymes that reveal organ damage, and metabolic byproducts that signal disease. Learning to interpret these values in context—not just identifying what's abnormal, but understanding what it means for this specific patient—separates competent laboratory professionals from exceptional ones.

These 15 cases will take you through common and critical chemistry presentations. You'll work through diabetic emergencies, electrolyte disasters, hormone imbalances, and metabolic syndromes. Some cases unfold quickly with clear answers. Others twist through multiple possibilities before revealing the diagnosis. All reflect real clinical scenarios you'll encounter.

Why Chemistry Cases Challenge Even Experienced Clinicians

Chemistry results rarely exist in isolation. A low sodium could mean too little sodium, too much water, or hormonal problems affecting both. High calcium might reflect parathyroid disease, cancer, vitamin D toxicity, or kidney failure. The same potassium level that's acceptable in a healthy person could be deadly in someone taking certain medications.

Context matters enormously in chemistry. Lab values interact with each other, with medications, with underlying diseases. You can't interpret a chemistry panel by looking at each value independently and checking if it's flagged high or low. You need to see patterns, understand physiology, and integrate clinical information.

Research shows that about 30-40% of electrolyte and metabolic abnormalities are initially misinterpreted, leading to delayed or incorrect treatment (Weisberg, 2008). The consequences range from minor (unnecessary testing) to catastrophic (death from untreated hyperkalemia or diabetic ketoacidosis). Getting chemistry interpretation right matters.

The Chemistry Diagnostic Framework

Before starting these cases, here's a systematic approach that works for most chemistry problems:

Identify the primary abnormality. Don't try to solve everything at once. Is the main problem hyperglycemia? Hyponatremia? Elevated liver enzymes? Start with the most abnormal or clinically significant finding.

Determine the mechanism. Most chemistry abnormalities have three possible mechanisms: too much intake, too little excretion, or abnormal distribution. For electrolytes, consider whether the problem is renal (kidneys), endocrine (hormones), or extrarenal (GI losses, medications).

Look for patterns and relationships. Chemistry values interact. High glucose with high ketones suggests diabetic ketoacidosis. Low sodium with low potassium and high bicarbonate suggests vomiting or diuretic use. These patterns accelerate diagnosis.

Consider the clinical context always. A glucose of 180 mg/dL in a non-diabetic person is concerning. The same glucose in a type 1 diabetic is routine. A potassium of 5.5 mEq/L in a healthy person is borderline. In someone on ACE inhibitors with kidney disease, it's dangerous.

Follow the cascade. One abnormality often causes others. Severe hyperglycemia causes osmotic diuresis, which causes dehydration and electrolyte losses, which causes kidney injury. Understanding these cascades helps you anticipate complications and order appropriate follow-up tests.

Now, let's meet your first patient.

Case 1: The Confused Diabetic

Clinical Presentation

A 28-year-old woman with type 1 diabetes is brought to the emergency department by her roommate after being found confused and lethargic in her apartment. The roommate reports the patient has been sick with what seemed like the flu for the past three days—fever, vomiting, poor appetite. She hasn't been eating much and apparently stopped taking her insulin because she "didn't think she needed it if she wasn't eating."

The patient is drowsy and difficult to arouse. She's oriented to person but not to place or time. She complains of severe abdominal pain, nausea, and extreme thirst. She admits she hasn't urinated much today despite drinking water constantly yesterday.

Her past medical history includes type 1 diabetes diagnosed at age 14, generally well-controlled on an insulin pump. She takes no other medications. She doesn't smoke, drink alcohol occasionally, and works as a graphic designer.

Physical examination reveals a lethargic young woman in obvious distress. Vital signs show temperature 37.2°C (99°F), heart rate 118 beats per minute, blood pressure 98/62 mmHg (low), respiratory rate 28 breaths per minute (rapid and deep—Kussmaul breathing), oxygen saturation 98% on room air. She has dry mucous membranes and poor skin turgor (signs of dehydration). Her breath has a fruity odor. Abdominal examination reveals diffuse tenderness without guarding or rebound. The rest of the examination is unremarkable.

Initial Laboratory Findings

Chemistry Panel (Basic Metabolic Panel):

- **Glucose: 485 mg/dL** (normal: 70-100 mg/dL) - **SEVERELY ELEVATED**
- Sodium: 132 mEq/L (normal: 136-145 mEq/L) - slightly low
- **Potassium: 5.8 mEq/L** (normal: 3.5-5.0 mEq/L) - **ELEVATED**

- Chloride: 98 mEq/L (normal: 98-107 mEq/L) - normal
- **Bicarbonate: 8 mEq/L** (normal: 22-28 mEq/L) - **VERY LOW**
- BUN: 28 mg/dL (normal: 7-20 mg/dL) - elevated
- **Creatinine: 1.4 mg/dL** (normal: 0.6-1.2 mg/dL) - elevated
- **Anion gap: 26 mEq/L** (normal: 8-12 mEq/L) - **MARKEDLY ELEVATED**

Arterial Blood Gas:

- pH: **6.98** (normal: 7.35-7.45) - **SEVERELY LOW** (severe acidosis)
- pCO2: 18 mmHg (normal: 35-45 mmHg) - LOW (respiratory compensation)
- pO2: 102 mmHg (normal: 80-100 mmHg) - normal
- HCO3: 8 mEq/L - LOW (matches serum bicarbonate)

Urinalysis:

- **Glucose: 4+ (large amount)**
- **Ketones: 4+ (large amount)**
- Specific gravity: 1.030 (elevated—concentrated urine)
- No blood, protein, or white blood cells

Stop and Think

This case screams medical emergency. Let's break down what we're seeing:

Severe hyperglycemia (485 mg/dL) plus **severe metabolic acidosis (pH 6.98, bicarbonate 8 mEq/L)** plus **positive urine ketones** equals **diabetic ketoacidosis (DKA)**.

The pathophysiology makes sense when you understand insulin's role. Insulin allows glucose to enter cells for energy. Without insulin:

1. Glucose can't enter cells despite high blood glucose
2. Cells are "starving" despite abundant glucose in blood
3. The body breaks down fat for energy
4. Fat breakdown produces ketone bodies (acetoacetate, beta-hydroxybutyrate, acetone)
5. Ketones are acids, causing metabolic acidosis
6. High glucose causes osmotic diuresis (glucose in urine pulls water) → dehydration
7. Dehydration → prerenal kidney injury (elevated BUN and creatinine)

Her **rapid, deep breathing (Kussmaul respirations)** is the body trying to compensate for metabolic acidosis by blowing off CO2 (respiratory alkalosis to counteract metabolic acidosis). That's why pCO2 is low at 18 mmHg.

The **fruity breath odor** comes from acetone (a ketone) being exhaled.

The **elevated anion gap** indicates the presence of unmeasured anions (in this case, ketones). Calculate anion gap: Sodium - (Chloride + Bicarbonate) = 132 - (98 + 8) = 26. Normal is 8-12. An anion gap >20 strongly suggests metabolic acidosis from ketones, lactic acid, toxins, or kidney failure.

The **elevated potassium (5.8 mEq/L)** seems paradoxical because total body potassium is actually low in DKA. Acidosis causes potassium to shift out of cells into the bloodstream (hydrogen ions move into cells, potassium moves out to maintain electrical neutrality). Once insulin treatment starts and acidosis corrects, potassium will drop—sometimes dramatically and dangerously. This is a critical management issue.

The **abdominal pain** is common in DKA, though the mechanism isn't fully understood. It can mimic acute abdomen, leading to unnecessary surgical consultations.

Diagnostic Reasoning Questions

What triggered this DKA episode?

Common DKA triggers include:

- **Infection** (most common—30-40% of cases)

- **Insulin omission** (10-20% of cases, especially in young patients)

- New diagnosis of diabetes

- Medications (steroids, antipsychotics)

- Myocardial infarction or stroke

- Pregnancy

- Pancreatitis

In this case, she had flu-like symptoms (possible viral infection) AND stopped taking insulin because she wasn't eating. Both factors contributed. The misconception that "no food = no insulin needed" is dangerous and common. The body always needs basal insulin, even when not eating.

How do you distinguish DKA from other causes of high anion gap metabolic acidosis?

The mnemonic **MUDPILES** lists causes of elevated anion gap metabolic acidosis:

- **M**ethanol

- **U**remia (kidney failure)

- **D**iabetic ketoacidosis

- **P**araldehyde (rarely used sedative)

- **I**soniazid or Iron

- **L**actic acidosis

- **E**thylene glycol

- Salicylates (aspirin overdose)

In this patient, the clinical context (known type 1 diabetes, stopped insulin) plus positive urine ketones confirms DKA. If urine ketones were negative, you'd need to consider other causes like lactic acidosis or toxic ingestions.

What additional tests are needed?

- **Beta-hydroxybutyrate level** (most abundant ketone in DKA—more specific than urine ketones)

- **Complete blood count** (to look for infection—white blood cells are often elevated in DKA even without infection due to stress response)

- **Lipase** (to rule out pancreatitis as cause or complication)

- **Troponin** (if chest pain—MI can trigger DKA)

- **Hemoglobin A1c** (reflects average glucose over past 2-3 months—tells you if diabetes was poorly controlled before this crisis)

- **Blood and urine cultures** (if infection suspected)

- **Chest X-ray** (to look for pneumonia)

- **ECG** (hyperkalemia can cause dangerous arrhythmias)

Sequential Test Results

Additional Laboratory Tests:

- **Beta-hydroxybutyrate: 8.2 mmol/L** (normal: <0.5 mmol/L) - **MARKEDLY ELEVATED** (confirms ketosis)

- White blood cell count: 18,500/µL (elevated—could be stress response or infection)

- Hemoglobin A1c: 9.8% (normal: <5.7%) - ELEVATED (indicates poor long-term glucose control)

- Lipase: 68 U/L (normal: 13-60 U/L) - slightly elevated (mild pancreatitis can occur in DKA)

- Troponin: <0.01 ng/mL - normal

- Blood cultures: Pending

- Chest X-ray: Clear, no pneumonia

ECG: Sinus tachycardia at 118 bpm. Peaked T waves (sign of hyperkalemia) noted. No ST segment changes. No life-threatening arrhythmias.

The peaked T waves are concerning—they indicate that hyperkalemia is affecting cardiac conduction. While her potassium of 5.8 mEq/L isn't immediately life-threatening, it needs monitoring because further elevation could cause cardiac arrest.

What's Happening Here?

This patient has **severe diabetic ketoacidosis** triggered by inadequate insulin administration in the setting of likely viral illness.

The complete pathophysiology:

1. Insulin deficiency: She stopped her insulin pump, creating absolute insulin deficiency. Her illness increased stress hormones (cortisol, catecholamines, glucagon, growth hormone), which further antagonize insulin action and increase glucose production.

2. Hyperglycemia: Without insulin:

- Hepatic glucose production increases (gluconeogenesis and glycogenolysis)

- Peripheral glucose utilization decreases

- Blood glucose rises to 485 mg/dL

3. Ketogenesis: Without glucose entering cells, the body thinks it's starving and breaks down fat for energy. Free fatty acids convert to ketone bodies in the liver. Ketones accumulate faster than tissues can use them.

4. Metabolic acidosis: Ketones are organic acids. Accumulation lowers blood pH from normal 7.40 to 6.98 (severe acidosis). The bicarbonate buffer system is overwhelmed (bicarbonate drops from normal 24 to 8 mEq/L).

5. Respiratory compensation: Chemoreceptors detect acidosis and stimulate hyperventilation. Rapid deep breathing (Kussmaul respirations) blows off CO_2, creating respiratory alkalosis to partially compensate for metabolic acidosis. This is why pCO_2 is 18 mmHg (low).

6. Osmotic diuresis: Glucose >180 mg/dL exceeds the kidney's reabsorption capacity. Glucose spills into urine, pulling water with it (osmotic diuresis). This causes:

- Polyuria (frequent urination)

- Dehydration (low blood pressure, dry mucous membranes, poor skin turgor)

- Electrolyte losses (sodium, potassium, magnesium, phosphorus)

7. Electrolyte abnormalities:

- **Potassium:** Total body potassium is depleted (lost in urine), but serum potassium is elevated due to acidosis-induced shift from cells. This will reverse with treatment, potentially causing dangerous hypokalemia.

- **Sodium:** Appears low (132 mEq/L) but this is partly dilutional from hyperglycemia. For every 100 mg/dL glucose elevation above 100, sodium decreases by about 1.6 mEq/L. Corrected sodium = 132 + [(485-100)/100 × 1.6] = 132 + 6.2 = 138.2 mEq/L (nearly normal).

8. Prerenal azotemia: Dehydration reduces kidney perfusion, causing BUN and creatinine to rise (prerenal acute kidney injury).

9. Abdominal pain: Mechanism unclear, but common in DKA. May relate to gastric distention, ileus, or metabolic effects on gut motility.

Final Diagnosis

Severe diabetic ketoacidosis (DKA) in a patient with type 1 diabetes due to insulin omission in the setting of intercurrent illness

Severity classification:

- Mild DKA: pH 7.25-7.30, bicarbonate 15-18 mEq/L

- Moderate DKA: pH 7.00-7.24, bicarbonate 10-15 mEq/L

- Severe DKA: pH <7.00, bicarbonate <10 mEq/L

She has **severe DKA** with pH 6.98 and bicarbonate 8 mEq/L.

Treatment and Management

DKA is a medical emergency requiring ICU-level care. The four pillars of treatment are: fluids, insulin, potassium replacement, and treating the underlying trigger.

1. Fluid Resuscitation (MOST IMPORTANT initial step):

Patients with DKA are severely dehydrated (typically 5-10 liters fluid deficit). Fluid resuscitation:

- Improves perfusion

- Dilutes glucose and ketones

- Enhances insulin sensitivity

- Begins lowering glucose even before insulin

Protocol:

- **Normal saline (0.9% NaCl) 1-2 liters in first 1-2 hours** (rapid initial bolus)

- Then 250-500 mL/hour guided by blood pressure, urine output, and clinical assessment

- Switch to 0.45% saline when sodium normalizes

- Add dextrose (D5 or D10) when glucose drops to 200-250 mg/dL (to prevent hypoglycemia while continuing insulin to clear ketones)

She receives 2 liters normal saline over the first hour, then 500 mL/hour.

2. Insulin Therapy:

Do NOT start insulin before fluid resuscitation. Starting insulin before fluids can cause cardiovascular collapse (insulin causes water to shift into cells, worsening intravascular depletion).

Protocol:

- **Regular insulin IV continuous infusion** at 0.1 units/kg/hour (typically 5-10 units/hour)

- **Goal:** Glucose decrease of 50-75 mg/dL per hour (not faster—rapid drops can cause cerebral edema)

- Once glucose reaches 200-250 mg/dL, reduce insulin to 0.05 units/kg/hour and add dextrose to IV fluids

- Continue insulin until ketones clear (anion gap normalizes, pH >7.30, bicarbonate >15 mEq/L)

She receives regular insulin infusion at 0.14 units/kg/hour (8 units/hour for her weight).

3. Potassium Replacement (CRITICAL):

This is the most dangerous aspect of DKA treatment. Patients are total body potassium depleted, but serum potassium is elevated initially. Insulin therapy causes potassium to shift back into cells, and serum potassium can drop precipitously.

Hypokalemia is the leading cause of death in DKA treatment (Kitabchi et al., 2009).

Protocol:

- **Check potassium every 2 hours initially**

- If K+ <3.3 mEq/L: HOLD insulin, give aggressive potassium replacement

- If K+ 3.3-5.0 mEq/L: Add 20-30 mEq potassium to each liter of IV fluid

- If K+ >5.0 mEq/L: Withhold potassium initially, but monitor closely

Her initial potassium is 5.8 mEq/L, so no potassium is added initially. Two hours after starting treatment, potassium drops to 4.2 mEq/L. Potassium chloride 30 mEq/L is added to IV fluids.

4. Treat Underlying Cause:

Search for and treat infection, discontinue offending medications, address MI if present, etc. In her case, supportive care for viral illness and patient education about never stopping insulin.

5. Monitor Closely:

- Blood glucose hourly (fingerstick)

- Electrolytes (sodium, potassium, chloride, bicarbonate) every 2-4 hours

- Anion gap calculation each time

- Mental status and vital signs continuously

- Urine output hourly

- Cardiac monitoring (for hyperkalemia-induced arrhythmias)

What NOT to do:

- **Don't give bicarbonate** (except in extreme acidosis pH <6.9 with cardiovascular instability). Bicarbonate doesn't improve outcomes and may cause paradoxical CNS acidosis, hypokalemia, and cerebral edema (Kitabchi et al., 2009).

- **Don't correct glucose too rapidly** (risk of cerebral edema, especially in children)

- **Don't stop insulin too soon** (glucose normalizes before ketones clear—continue insulin until ketones resolve)

Follow-up

Hour 4:

- Glucose: 280 mg/dL (improved)

- Potassium: 4.0 mEq/L (stable on replacement)

- Bicarbonate: 12 mEq/L (improving)

- pH: 7.15 (improving)

- Mental status significantly improved—alert and oriented

Hour 12:

- Glucose: 180 mg/dL (dextrose added to IV fluids, insulin rate reduced)

- Potassium: 4.2 mEq/L

- Bicarbonate: 18 mEq/L

- pH: 7.32

- Anion gap: 14 mEq/L (nearly normal)

- She's feeling much better, eating small amounts

Hour 24:

- Anion gap normalized

- Bicarbonate 22 mEq/L

- pH 7.38

- Transitioned to subcutaneous insulin (overlap IV insulin for 1-2 hours to prevent gap in insulin coverage)

- Tolerating regular diet

Day 2: Transferred out of ICU to medical floor. Insulin pump restarted with diabetes educator consultation. Extensive education provided:

- **Never stop basal insulin, even when not eating**

- Sick day management (continue insulin, check glucose and ketones frequently, stay hydrated)

- When to go to ER (persistent vomiting, high ketones, confusion)

Discharge (Day 3): She's discharged home on her usual insulin pump regimen with close endocrinology follow-up. Blood cultures showed no growth—the trigger was likely viral gastroenteritis.

Prognosis and Prevention

DKA mortality is 1-5% overall, higher in elderly patients and those with severe comorbidities. Causes of death include:

- Hypokalemia-induced cardiac arrhythmias
- Cerebral edema (rare in adults, more common in children)
- Severe infection
- Cardiovascular collapse

With proper treatment, most patients recover completely within 24-48 hours. However, recurrent DKA episodes damage organs over time and indicate poor diabetes management.

Prevention strategies:

- Patient education on sick day management
- Never omit insulin
- Check ketones during illness (home ketone meters available)
- Early intervention at first sign of ketones
- Address barriers to insulin adherence (cost, psychological factors, needle phobia)

About 30-40% of DKA cases are preventable through better patient education and access to care (Benoit et al., 2018).

Teaching Points

DKA is characterized by the triad of hyperglycemia, ketosis, and metabolic acidosis. All three must be present. Diabetics can have high glucose without ketoacidosis (hyperosmolar hyperglycemic state), or ketosis without severe acidosis (starvation ketosis). The combination with severe acidosis (pH <7.30) defines DKA.

Never stop basal insulin, even when not eating. This is a critical teaching point. Type 1 diabetics need basal insulin 24/7 regardless of food intake. Their bodies produce NO insulin endogenously. Stopping insulin invites DKA. Adjust meal-time insulin based on food, but continue basal insulin always.

The anion gap is your friend in DKA. Calculate it: Na - (Cl + HCO3). Normal is 8-12 mEq/L. In DKA, it's typically >20 due to ketoacids. The anion gap helps distinguish DKA from other acidoses and tracks treatment response. As ketones are cleared, the anion gap normalizes—this is your signal that DKA is resolving.

Potassium management is the most dangerous aspect of DKA treatment. Serum potassium is falsely elevated initially due to acidosis. With insulin treatment and acidosis correction, potassium shifts back into cells and serum potassium can drop precipitously. Aggressive monitoring and replacement prevent fatal hypokalemia. Check potassium every 2 hours initially (Kitabchi et al., 2009).

Fluid resuscitation comes before insulin. This may seem counterintuitive since insulin deficiency caused DKA, but fluids address the immediate life-threat (shock from severe dehydration). Starting insulin before adequate fluid resuscitation can worsen cardiovascular status. Give 1-2 liters normal saline first, then start insulin.

Don't stop insulin when glucose normalizes. Glucose corrects faster than ketones. If you stop insulin when glucose reaches 200 mg/dL, ketoacidosis will persist. Continue insulin until ketones clear (anion gap normal, bicarbonate >15, pH >7.30), and add dextrose to IV fluids to prevent hypoglycemia.

Bicarbonate therapy is rarely needed and potentially harmful. Despite severe acidosis, bicarbonate administration doesn't improve outcomes in most cases. It's reserved for pH <6.9 with cardiovascular instability. Bicarbonate can cause paradoxical CNS acidosis, cerebral edema, and hypokalemia (Kitabchi et al., 2009).

DKA can occur with "normal" glucose levels. Euglycemic DKA (glucose <250 mg/dL) occurs in 5-10% of cases, especially with SGLT2 inhibitor use (newer diabetes drugs). Don't rule out DKA just because glucose isn't severely elevated—check ketones if clinical picture fits.

Related Cases

This case connects to:

- **Case 8: Acid-Base Disturbances** (explores metabolic acidosis mechanisms in depth)
- **Case 14: Adrenal Insufficiency** (another endocrine emergency with electrolyte abnormalities)
- **Case 4: Acute Kidney Injury** (DKA causes prerenal AKI from dehydration)

Case 2: The Man with Kidney Stones and Fatigue

Clinical Presentation

A 58-year-old man presents to his primary care physician complaining of persistent fatigue, weakness, and difficulty concentrating over the past four months. He mentions that he's had to urinate frequently, both day and night, and feels constantly thirsty. He's also experienced vague abdominal discomfort and constipation.

Two months ago, he passed a kidney stone—his third stone in five years. His urologist recommended metabolic stone evaluation but he never followed up.

His past medical history includes hypertension treated with lisinopril and osteoarthritis. He takes ibuprofen occasionally for joint pain. He doesn't smoke but drinks 2-3 beers daily. No family history of kidney stones or endocrine disorders.

Physical examination reveals a mildly overweight man who appears somewhat depressed or fatigued. Vital signs are blood pressure 142/88 mmHg, heart rate 72 beats per minute, temperature normal. His mood seems flat. Deep tendon reflexes are somewhat sluggish. The rest of the examination is unremarkable—no thyroid enlargement, no neck masses, no abdominal tenderness.

Initial Laboratory Findings

Chemistry Panel (Comprehensive Metabolic Panel):

- Glucose: 102 mg/dL (normal: 70-100 mg/dL) - slightly elevated (impaired fasting glucose)

- Sodium: 142 mEq/L (normal: 136-145 mEq/L) - normal

- Potassium: 4.1 mEq/L (normal: 3.5-5.0 mEq/L) - normal

- Chloride: 105 mEq/L (normal: 98-107 mEq/L) - normal

- Bicarbonate: 26 mEq/L (normal: 22-28 mEq/L) - normal

- BUN: 22 mg/dL (normal: 7-20 mg/dL) - slightly elevated

- Creatinine: 1.3 mg/dL (normal: 0.7-1.3 mg/dL) - high normal

- **Calcium: 12.2 mg/dL** (normal: 8.5-10.5 mg/dL) - **ELEVATED**

- **Albumin: 4.2 g/dL** (normal: 3.5-5.0 g/dL) - normal

Stop and Think

The key finding here is **hypercalcemia**—calcium of 12.2 mg/dL when normal is 8.5-10.5 mg/dL. This isn't mild hypercalcemia—it's moderate and symptomatic.

But wait—before we jump to conclusions, we need to calculate the **corrected calcium**. About 40% of serum calcium is bound to albumin. If albumin is abnormal (low in liver disease, malnutrition, or nephrotic syndrome), the measured total calcium will be misleadingly low. We correct for this:

Corrected Calcium = Measured Calcium + 0.8 × (4.0 - Patient's Albumin)

For this patient: Corrected Calcium = 12.2 + 0.8 × (4.0 - 4.2) = 12.2 + 0.8 × (-0.2) = 12.2 - 0.16 = 12.04 mg/dL

His albumin is normal, so the correction doesn't change much. He truly has hypercalcemia.

Now look at his symptoms through the lens of hypercalcemia:

- **Fatigue and weakness** → classic hypercalcemia symptoms

- **Polyuria and polydipsia** (frequent urination, excessive thirst) → hypercalcemia impairs kidney concentrating ability

- **Constipation** → hypercalcemia decreases GI motility

- **Difficulty concentrating** → hypercalcemia affects mental function

- **Depression/flat affect** → neuropsychiatric effects of hypercalcemia

- **Recurrent kidney stones** → hypercalcemia causes calcium stone formation

- **Sluggish reflexes** → hypercalcemia dampens neuromuscular function

The classic mnemonic for hypercalcemia symptoms is "**stones, bones, groans, and psychiatric overtones**":

- **Stones** = kidney stones

- **Bones** = bone pain (from underlying bone disease)

118

- **Groans** = abdominal pain, constipation, nausea
- **Psychiatric overtones** = depression, confusion, lethargy

This patient has stones, groans, and psychiatric overtones. The question is: why is his calcium elevated?

Diagnostic Reasoning Questions

What causes hypercalcemia?

The differential for hypercalcemia is actually pretty short. About 90% of cases are due to just two causes:

1. Primary hyperparathyroidism (most common in outpatients—40-50% of cases)

- Parathyroid adenoma (single overactive gland—80% of cases)
- Parathyroid hyperplasia (all four glands enlarged—15-20%)
- Parathyroid carcinoma (rare—<1%)

2. Malignancy (most common in hospitalized patients—30-40% of cases)

- Solid tumors with bone metastases (breast, lung, kidney, multiple myeloma)
- Tumors secreting PTH-related peptide (PTHrP)—lung, kidney, breast cancers
- Hematologic malignancies producing local osteolytic factors

3. Other causes (collectively 10-20%):

- Vitamin D excess (supplements, granulomatous diseases like sarcoidosis)
- Thiazide diuretics
- Hyperthyroidism
- Immobilization
- Familial hypocalciuric hypercalcemia (genetic condition)
- Milk-alkali syndrome (excessive calcium and antacid ingestion)
- Adrenal insufficiency (rare)

How do you narrow the differential?

The single most important next test is **parathyroid hormone (PTH) level**. PTH should be suppressed in hypercalcemia (negative feedback). If PTH is elevated or even inappropriately normal despite high calcium, it indicates **primary hyperparathyroidism**.

If PTH is appropriately suppressed (low), then you look for other causes:

- Malignancy (check PTHrP, look for cancer)
- Vitamin D excess (check 25-OH vitamin D level)
- Thyrotoxicosis (check TSH)

- Medications (review drug list)

Sequential Test Results

Additional Laboratory Tests:

- **PTH (intact parathyroid hormone): 78 pg/mL** (normal: 10-65 pg/mL) - **ELEVATED**

- Phosphorus: 2.1 mg/dL (normal: 2.5-4.5 mg/dL) - LOW

- 25-OH Vitamin D: 28 ng/mL (normal: 30-80 ng/mL) - low-normal

- TSH: 2.1 mIU/L (normal: 0.4-4.0 mIU/L) - normal

- Alkaline phosphatase: 142 U/L (normal: 44-147 U/L) - high normal

Urinalysis:

- Calcium: Elevated (>250 mg/24 hours on 24-hour urine collection)

- No blood, protein, or infection

Interpretation:

The PTH level of 78 pg/mL is **inappropriately elevated** given the calcium of 12.2 mg/dL. In a healthy person with calcium of 12.2, PTH should be suppressed to near-zero. A PTH of 78 (above the normal range) indicates **autonomous PTH secretion** despite hypercalcemia—this is the hallmark of **primary hyperparathyroidism**.

The **low phosphorus** supports this diagnosis. PTH causes renal phosphate wasting, so primary hyperparathyroidism typically shows hypercalcemia with hypophosphatemia.

The elevated 24-hour urine calcium confirms that calcium is being excreted (ruling out familial hypocalciuric hypercalcemia, where urine calcium is inappropriately low).

The slightly elevated alkaline phosphatase may indicate increased bone turnover from PTH effects on bone.

What's Happening Here?

This patient has **primary hyperparathyroidism**, most likely from a parathyroid adenoma (single enlarged parathyroid gland).

The pathophysiology:

1. Autonomous PTH secretion: One or more parathyroid glands becomes autonomous, secreting PTH regardless of calcium levels. The normal negative feedback (high calcium suppresses PTH) is lost.

2. Calcium elevation: Excess PTH increases serum calcium through three mechanisms:

- **Bone resorption**: PTH activates osteoclasts, breaking down bone and releasing calcium

- **Renal calcium reabsorption**: PTH increases calcium reabsorption in kidney tubules

- **Renal phosphate excretion**: PTH causes phosphorus wasting

- **Intestinal calcium absorption**: PTH stimulates 1,25-vitamin D production, increasing gut calcium absorption

3. Clinical manifestations: Chronic hypercalcemia from hyperparathyroidism causes:

- Kidney stones (calcium supersaturation in urine)

- Bone disease (osteopenia, osteoporosis, rarely osteitis fibrosa cystica)

- Neuromuscular symptoms (weakness, fatigue, sluggish reflexes)

- Neuropsychiatric symptoms (depression, cognitive impairment, lethargy)

- GI symptoms (constipation, nausea, peptic ulcers)

- Cardiovascular (hypertension, shortened QT interval on ECG)

- Polyuria/polydipsia (hypercalcemia impairs kidney concentrating ability, causing nephrogenic diabetes insipidus)

4. "Asymptomatic" hyperparathyroidism: Many patients with mild hyperparathyroidism are asymptomatic or have subtle symptoms they don't recognize. It's often found incidentally on routine lab work. However, this patient has multiple symptoms—he's far from asymptomatic.

Primary hyperparathyroidism affects about 1 in 1,000 people, with peak incidence in the 50s-60s. It's 2-3 times more common in women than men (Bilezikian et al., 2018).

Final Diagnosis

Primary hyperparathyroidism, symptomatic, likely due to parathyroid adenoma

Further Workup and Treatment

Imaging Studies:

To locate the abnormal parathyroid gland(s) before surgery:

Sestamibi scan (parathyroid scintigraphy):

- Nuclear medicine scan using technetium-99m sestamibi

- Abnormal parathyroid tissue takes up and retains the tracer

- Helps localize adenomas pre-operatively

- His scan shows increased uptake in the left inferior parathyroid region, consistent with adenoma

Neck ultrasound:

- Non-invasive imaging

- Can identify enlarged parathyroid glands

- Less sensitive than sestamibi but useful for surgical planning

- His ultrasound shows a 1.2 cm hypoechoic mass posterior to the left thyroid lobe, consistent with parathyroid adenoma

Bone Density Scan (DEXA):

- Assess for osteoporosis (complication of chronic hyperparathyroidism)

- His T-score shows osteopenia (bone density lower than normal but not yet osteoporosis)

Treatment Options:

1. Surgical Parathyroidectomy (definitive treatment):

Indications for surgery in primary hyperparathyroidism (per guidelines):

- Symptomatic hypercalcemia

- Calcium >1 mg/dL above upper limit of normal (>11.5 mg/dL)

- Age <50

- Reduced creatinine clearance (<60 mL/min)

- Osteoporosis (T-score <-2.5)

- History of kidney stones

- Complications (fractures, nephrolithiasis)

This patient meets multiple criteria (symptomatic, calcium 12.2, kidney stones, osteopenia, borderline renal function). **Surgery is indicated.**

Surgical approach:

- **Minimally invasive parathyroidectomy**: Remove identified adenoma

- Intraoperative PTH monitoring (PTH should drop >50% within 10-15 minutes after removing the correct gland)

- Success rate >95% in experienced hands

- Low complication rate (<2% permanent hypoparathyroidism, <1% recurrent laryngeal nerve injury)

2. Medical Management (for patients who can't/won't have surgery):

- **Calcimimetics** (cinacalcet): Activates calcium-sensing receptors, reducing PTH secretion

- **Bisphosphonates**: Reduce bone resorption, preserve bone density

- **Adequate hydration**: Prevents kidney stones

- **Avoid thiazide diuretics**: Can worsen hypercalcemia

- **Monitor calcium and bone density**: Regular follow-up

Medical management is less effective than surgery and doesn't cure the underlying problem. Reserved for patients with mild asymptomatic disease or surgical contraindications.

Follow-up

Surgery: He undergoes minimally invasive left inferior parathyroidectomy. A 1.5 cm parathyroid adenoma is removed. Intraoperative PTH drops from 82 to 22 pg/mL within 15 minutes (confirming successful removal of the hyperfunctioning gland). No complications.

Postoperative:

- Day 1: Calcium 9.2 mg/dL, PTH 18 pg/mL - **normalized**

- Symptoms dramatically improve within days—energy returns, polyuria resolves, mood lifts

- Risk of "hungry bone syndrome" (rapid calcium uptake into bones causing hypocalcemia) is monitored but doesn't occur since his bone disease was mild

3 Months Post-Surgery:

- Calcium: 9.4 mg/dL (normal)

- PTH: 32 pg/mL (normal)

- Phosphorus: 3.2 mg/dL (normalized)

- He feels "like a new person"—fatigue resolved, mental clarity improved

- No further kidney stones

1 Year Post-Surgery:

- Repeat DEXA scan shows improved bone density (osteopenia improving with treatment)

- He's started on calcium and vitamin D supplementation to rebuild bone

- No recurrence of hypercalcemia

Cure rate: >95% with experienced surgeons. Recurrence is rare (<5%) and usually from missed multi-gland disease or parathyroid carcinoma (Bilezikian et al., 2018).

Teaching Points

Primary hyperparathyroidism is the most common cause of hypercalcemia in outpatients. If you find hypercalcemia on routine lab work in an otherwise stable outpatient, think hyperparathyroidism first. Malignancy is more common in hospitalized patients with acute severe hypercalcemia.

PTH is the key test. An elevated or inappropriately normal PTH in the setting of hypercalcemia confirms primary hyperparathyroidism. PTH should be suppressed (near-zero) if calcium is elevated from other causes like malignancy or vitamin D toxicity. Any PTH >20 pg/mL with calcium >10.5 mg/dL is "inappropriate" and suggests hyperparathyroidism.

Correct calcium for albumin before interpretation. Low albumin (malnutrition, liver disease, nephrotic syndrome) causes falsely low total calcium. Use the formula: Corrected Ca = Measured Ca + 0.8 × (4.0 - Patient's Albumin). Alternatively, measure ionized calcium directly (not affected by albumin), though this is less commonly done.

Hyperparathyroidism causes stones, bones, groans, and psychiatric overtones. This classic mnemonic captures the multisystem effects: kidney stones (most common), bone disease (osteoporosis), GI symptoms (constipation, ulcers), and neuropsychiatric symptoms (depression, fatigue, cognitive impairment). However, many patients today are diagnosed before severe symptoms develop (Bilezikian et al., 2018).

Low phosphorus supports the diagnosis of hyperparathyroidism. PTH causes renal phosphate wasting, so primary hyperparathyroidism typically shows hypercalcemia with hypophosphatemia. This pattern distinguishes it from malignancy (where phosphorus is often normal or high) and vitamin D toxicity (where phosphorus may be high).

Surgery is curative for most patients. Parathyroidectomy has high success rate (>95%), low complication rate, and dramatically improves symptoms and prevents complications like kidney stones and fractures. Medical management is less effective and doesn't cure the disease. Surgery is indicated for symptomatic patients, those with complications, and those meeting guideline criteria even if "asymptomatic."

Not all hypercalcemia needs urgent treatment. Mild chronic hypercalcemia (calcium 10.5-12 mg/dL) in a stable patient can be worked up outpatient. Severe hypercalcemia (calcium >14 mg/dL) or symptomatic hypercalcemia with altered mental status, severe dehydration, or cardiac arrhythmias requires urgent hospitalization and aggressive treatment with IV fluids, calcitonin, and bisphosphonates.

Familial hypocalciuric hypercalcemia (FHH) mimics hyperparathyroidism. FHH is a benign genetic condition causing mild hypercalcemia with normal or slightly elevated PTH. The key distinguishing feature is low 24-hour urine calcium (<100 mg/24 hours or calcium-to-creatinine clearance ratio <0.01). FHH doesn't require treatment and surgery doesn't help. Always check urine calcium before recommending parathyroidectomy.

Related Cases

This case connects to:

- **Case 13: Parathyroid Hormone Disorders** (explores hypoparathyroidism and secondary hyperparathyroidism)
- **Case 4: Acute Kidney Injury** (chronic hypercalcemia can cause kidney damage)
- **Case 7: Hypokalemia and Cardiac Arrhythmia** (other electrolyte disturbances)

Case 3: The Marathon Runner Who Can't Stop Drinking Water

Clinical Presentation

A 32-year-old avid marathon runner is brought to the emergency department by her training partner after collapsing during a long training run. She completed a 20-mile run on a hot summer day, drinking large amounts of water throughout. About 30 minutes after finishing, she complained of a severe headache, nausea, and confusion. Within minutes, she became disoriented and collapsed.

In the ED, she's lethargic and confused. She doesn't know where she is or what day it is. She's nauseated and has vomited twice. She complains of severe headache. Her training partner reports that she drank "tons of water" during and after the run, probably 3-4 liters, because she was worried about dehydration after reading about heat-related illness online.

Her past medical history is unremarkable. She takes no medications. She doesn't smoke or use drugs. She's training for her fifth marathon and typically runs 50-60 miles per week.

Physical examination reveals a confused, disoriented woman in distress. Vital signs show temperature 37.8°C (100°F), heart rate 88 beats per minute, blood pressure 138/82 mmHg, respiratory rate 16 breaths per minute. She has no focal neurologic deficits but is globally confused with impaired memory. No signs of dehydration—mucous membranes are moist, skin turgor is normal. No edema. The rest of the examination is unremarkable.

Initial Laboratory Findings

Chemistry Panel:

- Glucose: 96 mg/dL (normal)

- **Sodium: 118 mEq/L** (normal: 136-145 mEq/L) - **SEVERELY LOW**

- Potassium: 3.9 mEq/L (normal)

- Chloride: 88 mEq/L (normal: 98-107 mEq/L) - LOW

- Bicarbonate: 24 mEq/L (normal)

- BUN: 8 mg/dL (normal: 7-20 mg/dL) - low-normal

- Creatinine: 0.9 mg/dL (normal)

- **Serum osmolality: 242 mOsm/kg** (normal: 275-295 mOsm/kg) - **LOW**

Urine Studies:

- **Urine sodium: 32 mEq/L** - inappropriately high given low serum sodium

- **Urine osmolality: 278 mOsm/kg** - inappropriately concentrated given low serum osmolality

Stop and Think

This patient has **severe symptomatic hyponatremia**—sodium of 118 mEq/L when normal is 136-145 mEq/L. This is a neurologic emergency. Sodium <120 mEq/L with neurologic symptoms (confusion, seizures, altered mental status) can be fatal without immediate treatment.

The clinical context is classic: **exercise-associated hyponatremia (EAH)**, also called **exercise-induced hyponatremia**. This occurs in endurance athletes who drink excessive amounts of water or hypotonic fluids during prolonged exercise, diluting their serum sodium.

The pathophysiology involves:

1. Excessive free water intake: She drank 3-4 liters of water during a 20-mile run (probably lasting 3-4 hours). That's excessive for most runners and overwhelms the kidney's ability to excrete free water, especially during exercise.

2. Non-osmotic ADH (vasopressin) release: During strenuous exercise, antidiuretic hormone (ADH) is released due to:

- Exercise stress

- Pain and nausea (potent ADH stimulators)

- Volume depletion from insensible losses (despite drinking water)

ADH causes the kidneys to retain water, preventing excretion of the excess water she drank.

3. Water intoxication: Excessive water intake plus impaired water excretion = dilutional hyponatremia. Water moves into cells (including brain cells) due to osmotic forces, causing cerebral edema.

4. Cerebral edema and symptoms: As brain cells swell, intracranial pressure increases, causing:

- Headache

- Nausea and vomiting

- Confusion and disorientation

- Seizures (if severe)

- Coma and brain herniation (if untreated)

Now look at her labs. The **low serum osmolality (242 mOsm/kg)** confirms this is true hyponatremia (dilutional) rather than pseudohyponatremia or hyperglycemia pulling water into the vascular space.

The **urine sodium of 32 mEq/L** and **urine osmolality of 278 mOsm/kg** are inappropriately high. In someone with low serum osmolality, the kidneys should be excreting very dilute urine (urine osmolality <100 mOsm/kg) to get rid of excess water. Instead, her urine is relatively concentrated, indicating ADH is active and preventing water excretion.

Diagnostic Reasoning Questions

How do you approach hyponatremia systematically?

Hyponatremia (sodium <136 mEq/L) is the most common electrolyte abnormality, affecting 15-30% of hospitalized patients. The approach requires three steps:

Step 1: Confirm true hyponatremia

Check serum osmolality:

- **Low osmolality (<275)**: True hyponatremia (hypotonic)

- **Normal osmolality (275-295)**: Pseudohyponatremia (lab artifact from high lipids or proteins) or isotonic hyponatremia (irrigation fluids)

- **High osmolality (>295)**: Hypertonic hyponatremia (hyperglycemia or mannitol pulling water into vascular space, diluting sodium)

Most cases are hypotonic hyponatremia (like this patient).

Step 2: Assess volume status

Examine the patient:

- **Hypovolemic** (dehydrated): dry mucous membranes, poor skin turgor, low blood pressure, high heart rate

- **Euvolemic** (normal volume): normal exam, no edema, normal vital signs

- **Hypervolemic** (fluid overloaded): edema, ascites, elevated JVP

This patient appears euvolemic—no dehydration signs, no edema.

Step 3: Check urine sodium and osmolality

This helps determine the mechanism:

Volume Status	Urine Na	Urine Osm	Causes
Hypovolemic	<20 mEq/L	High	Vomiting, diarrhea, sweating
Hypovolemic	>40 mEq/L	High	Diuretics, salt-wasting nephropathy, adrenal insufficiency
Euvolemic	>40 mEq/L	>100	SIADH, hypothyroidism, glucocorticoid deficiency, drugs
Hypervolemic	<20 mEq/L	High	Heart failure, cirrhosis, nephrotic syndrome

This patient: Euvolemic + Urine Na 32 + Urine Osm 278 = Points toward **SIADH-like picture** from exercise and excessive water intake.

What is SIADH?

Syndrome of Inappropriate Antidiuretic Hormone (SIADH) occurs when ADH is released despite low serum osmolality. ADH tells kidneys to retain water, so excess water can't be excreted, causing dilutional hyponatremia.

Causes of SIADH include:

- Medications (SSRIs, carbamazepine, NSAIDs, PPIs, many others)

- Pulmonary disease (pneumonia, TB, asthma exacerbation)

- CNS disorders (meningitis, encephalitis, stroke, hemorrhage)

- Malignancy (small cell lung cancer, many others secreting ADH)

- Pain, nausea, stress

- **Exercise** (non-osmotic ADH release)

Diagnostic criteria for SIADH:

- Hypotonic hyponatremia (low sodium, low serum osm)

- Urine osmolality >100 mOsm/kg (inappropriately concentrated)

- Urine sodium >40 mEq/L

- Normal volume status (no edema, not dehydrated)

- Normal kidney, thyroid, and adrenal function

This patient's presentation fits SIADH triggered by exercise, pain, and nausea, combined with excessive water intake. It's technically "exercise-associated hyponatremia" but the mechanism overlaps with SIADH.

What are the risks of hyponatremia?

Acute hyponatremia (developing over <48 hours) is dangerous:

- Rapid brain cell swelling

- Increased intracranial pressure

- Seizures, coma, brain herniation, death

- Mortality up to 50% if sodium <120 mEq/L with symptoms (Verbalis et al., 2013)

Chronic hyponatremia (developing over >48 hours) is less immediately dangerous because brain cells adapt by extruding osmotically active substances to reduce cell swelling. However, rapid correction of chronic hyponatremia causes **osmotic demyelination syndrome** (ODS), which can be worse than the hyponatremia itself.

This patient's hyponatremia is **acute** (developed over hours during her run), so aggressive treatment is appropriate and risk of ODS is low.

Sequential Test Results

Additional Tests:

- Thyroid stimulating hormone (TSH): 1.8 mIU/L (normal) - rules out hypothyroidism

- Cortisol: 18 μg/dL (normal: 5-25 μg/dL) - rules out adrenal insufficiency

- Lipid panel: Normal - rules out pseudohyponatremia

Repeat Sodium (30 minutes later):

- Sodium: 116 mEq/L - **DECLINING** despite being in the ED

Her sodium is dropping, and she's becoming more lethargic. This is a neurologic emergency requiring immediate intervention.

What's Happening Here?

This patient has **severe acute exercise-associated hyponatremia** from excessive free water intake during prolonged exercise with non-osmotic ADH release preventing water excretion.

The full pathophysiology:

1. Excessive water intake: Drinking 3-4 liters of water during a 3-4 hour run exceeds most people's sweat losses. Average sweat rate during running is 0.5-1.5 liters/hour. She drank more than she lost, causing net positive fluid balance.

2. Non-osmotic ADH secretion: Exercise is a potent non-osmotic stimulus for ADH release. Add nausea (another strong ADH stimulus), and her kidneys were retaining water despite low serum osmolality.

3. Dilutional hyponatremia: Water intake exceeds excretion → total body water increases → sodium concentration decreases (diluted).

4. Cerebral edema: Water moves into brain cells following osmotic gradients, causing cells to swell. The skull is a rigid container, so brain swelling increases intracranial pressure, causing symptoms.

5. Rapid progression: Once symptoms begin (headache, nausea), they worsen rapidly as brain swelling progresses. Without treatment, seizures, coma, and death can occur within hours.

Exercise-associated hyponatremia affects 10-15% of marathon runners to some degree (mild cases often go unrecognized). Severe symptomatic cases occur in about 1-2% of marathoners. Risk factors include:

- Drinking excessive amounts during exercise (>1.5 liters/hour)

- Exercise duration >4 hours

- Female gender

- Low body weight

- NSAIDs use (increases ADH effect)

- Overzealous hydration driven by fear of dehydration (Hew-Butler et al., 2015)

Final Diagnosis

Severe acute symptomatic exercise-associated hyponatremia with cerebral edema

Treatment and Management

This is a **medical emergency**. Severe symptomatic hyponatremia requires immediate aggressive treatment to prevent death from cerebral herniation.

Immediate Treatment: Hypertonic Saline

3% hypertonic saline IV bolus:

- Give 100 mL of 3% saline over 10 minutes

- Repeat every 10 minutes until symptoms improve or sodium rises 4-6 mEq/L

- Goal: Raise sodium by 4-6 mEq/L in first 1-2 hours (enough to reduce brain swelling and reverse symptoms)

She receives 100 mL of 3% saline immediately, then another 100 mL bolus 10 minutes later.

Within 20 minutes:

- Her mental status begins clearing

- She becomes more alert and oriented

- Headache decreases

- Sodium: 122 mEq/L (increased by 4 mEq/L)

Why hypertonic saline?

Hypertonic (3%) saline contains 513 mEq/L sodium—much higher than serum sodium. It rapidly increases serum osmolality, pulling water out of brain cells and reducing cerebral edema. This reverses symptoms quickly.

Important principles:

For acute symptomatic hyponatremia:

- Aggressive correction is appropriate (4-6 mEq/L in first hours, up to 8-10 mEq/L in first 24 hours)

- Risk of osmotic demyelination syndrome (ODS) is very low when hyponatremia is acute

- Saving the brain from herniation is the priority

For chronic hyponatremia:

- Slow correction is mandatory (maximum 6-8 mEq/L in 24 hours, 12-18 mEq/L in 48 hours)

- Rapid correction causes ODS (demyelination of brain, leading to permanent neurologic damage)

- Need to balance treating symptoms versus causing iatrogenic harm

How do you know if hyponatremia is acute or chronic?

Ask about timing:

- Symptoms began <48 hours ago = likely acute

- Chronic symptoms, known hyponatremia = likely chronic

- Unknown timing = assume chronic and correct slowly (safer)

This patient's hyponatremia definitely developed over hours during her run, so it's acute. Aggressive correction is appropriate.

Ongoing Management:

Fluid restriction:

- Limit free water intake to <800 mL/day until sodium normalizes
- She's allowed only small sips for thirst

Monitor sodium closely:

- Check sodium every 2-4 hours initially
- Adjust treatment based on rate of rise
- Stop hypertonic saline once symptoms resolve and sodium >125 mEq/L

Address underlying cause:

- Stop all water intake
- Once she's urinating (ADH effect wearing off), her kidneys will excrete excess water naturally
- Education about appropriate hydration during exercise

Follow-up

Hour 2:

- Sodium: 124 mEq/L
- Fully alert and oriented
- Headache resolved
- No further hypertonic saline needed

Hour 6:

- Sodium: 128 mEq/L (rising appropriately)
- Feeling much better
- Started urinating large volumes (diuresis as ADH effect wears off and kidneys dump excess water)

Hour 24:

- Sodium: 136 mEq/L (normalized)
- Completely asymptomatic
- Ready for discharge

Discharge: She's educated extensively:

- **Drink to thirst during exercise, not beyond**

- Drinking excessive water during endurance exercise is dangerous

- Sports drinks with sodium are better than plain water for exercise >90 minutes

- Weight loss during exercise is normal and safe (up to 2-3% body weight from sweat)

- Avoid NSAIDs before/during long runs (potentiate hyponatremia)

3 Months Later: She successfully completes her marathon using appropriate hydration strategy (drinking to thirst, consuming sports drinks). No complications. Sodium remains normal.

Teaching Points

Exercise-associated hyponatremia results from excessive water intake, not inadequate sodium intake. The problem is too much water diluting sodium, not sodium deficiency. The well-intentioned advice to "stay hydrated" and "drink before you're thirsty" has caused this problem. Athletes should **drink to thirst**—the body's thirst mechanism is accurate (Hew-Butler et al., 2015).

Symptomatic hyponatremia is a neurologic emergency. Sodium <120 mEq/L with altered mental status, seizures, or coma requires immediate treatment with hypertonic (3%) saline to prevent brain herniation and death. Don't wait for imaging or confirmatory tests—treat based on clinical presentation and sodium level.

Acute vs. chronic hyponatremia determines treatment aggressiveness. Acute hyponatremia (<48 hours) can and should be corrected relatively quickly (4-6 mEq/L in first hours). Chronic hyponatremia must be corrected slowly (maximum 6-8 mEq/L per 24 hours) to prevent osmotic demyelination syndrome. When in doubt, assume chronic and correct slowly.

The approach to hyponatremia requires systematic assessment. Check serum osmolality (confirm true hyponatremia), assess volume status (hypovolemic/euvolemic/hypervolemic), and check urine sodium and osmolality. This three-step approach narrows the differential from dozens of causes to a few likely possibilities.

SIADH is diagnosed by exclusion and specific criteria. Hypotonic hyponatremia + inappropriately concentrated urine (>100 mOsm/kg) + urine sodium >40 mEq/L + euvolemic status + normal kidney/thyroid/adrenal function = SIADH. Many conditions mimic SIADH, so careful evaluation is needed.

Water restriction is the primary treatment for chronic euvolemic hyponatremia. For SIADH and similar conditions, limiting free water to <800-1000 mL/day allows sodium to rise as kidneys excrete excess water slowly. This is safer than rapid correction with hypertonic saline in non-emergent situations.

Hypertonic saline is dangerous if used incorrectly. In chronic hyponatremia, overly aggressive correction causes osmotic demyelination syndrome—permanent brain damage with locked-in syndrome, quadriplegia, and death. Maximum correction rates are 6-8 mEq/L in 24 hours and 12-18 mEq/L in 48 hours for chronic hyponatremia (Verbalis et al., 2013).

Sports drinks are superior to water for prolonged exercise. Plain water during endurance exercise (>90 minutes) increases hyponatremia risk. Sports drinks containing sodium (20-50 mEq/L) help maintain sodium balance while replacing fluids. However, even sports drinks should be consumed to thirst, not excessively.

Related Cases

This case connects to:

- **Case 14: Adrenal Insufficiency** (another cause of hyponatremia with impaired water excretion)

- **Case 6: Thyroid Function Abnormalities** (hypothyroidism causes hyponatremia via SIADH-like mechanism)

- **Case 1: The Confused Diabetic** (another metabolic emergency requiring urgent electrolyte management)

Case 4: The Man with Brown Urine

Clinical Presentation

A 52-year-old man presents to the emergency department complaining of dark brown urine, decreased urine output, and generalized weakness for the past two days. Three days ago, he underwent an intense "boot camp" style workout class—his first vigorous exercise in years. The workout involved hundreds of squats, lunges, and jumping exercises. He felt extremely sore the next day but attributed it to being out of shape.

Yesterday morning, he noticed his urine was dark brown, "like cola or iced tea." He's only urinated twice today despite drinking normal amounts of fluid. He feels weak, nauseated, and his muscles are extremely painful and swollen, especially his thighs and calves. He can barely walk due to muscle pain and stiffness.

His past medical history includes obesity and prediabetes. He takes metformin. He doesn't smoke but drinks alcohol socially. No family history of kidney disease or muscle disorders.

Physical examination reveals an obese man in moderate distress from muscle pain. Vital signs show temperature 37.8°C (100°F), heart rate 102 beats per minute, blood pressure 152/94 mmHg, respiratory rate 18 breaths per minute. His thighs and calves are markedly swollen, tender, and firm to palpation. He has difficulty standing from a seated position due to muscle weakness and pain. The rest of the examination is unremarkable.

Initial Laboratory Findings

Chemistry Panel:

- Glucose: 128 mg/dL (normal: 70-100 mg/dL) - elevated (consistent with his prediabetes)

- Sodium: 138 mEq/L (normal)

- **Potassium: 6.2 mEq/L** (normal: 3.5-5.0 mEq/L) - **ELEVATED**

- Chloride: 104 mEq/L (normal)

- Bicarbonate: 20 mEq/L (normal: 22-28 mEq/L) - slightly low

- **BUN: 42 mg/dL** (normal: 7-20 mg/dL) - **ELEVATED**

- **Creatinine: 3.8 mg/dL** (normal: 0.7-1.3 mg/dL) - **MARKEDLY ELEVATED**

- **Creatine kinase (CK): 185,000 U/L** (normal: 50-200 U/L) - **EXTREMELY ELEVATED**

- **Calcium: 7.8 mg/dL** (normal: 8.5-10.5 mg/dL) - **LOW**

- **Phosphorus: 6.8 mg/dL** (normal: 2.5-4.5 mg/dL) - **ELEVATED**

- **Uric acid: 12.1 mg/dL** (normal: 3.5-7.2 mg/dL) - **ELEVATED**

Complete Blood Count:

- Hemoglobin: 15.2 g/dL (normal)

- Hematocrit: 46% (normal)

- White blood cell count: 14,200/μL (elevated—stress response)

- Platelet count: 285,000/μL (normal)

Urinalysis:

- **Color: Dark brown**

- **Blood: 3+ (large amount) - but no RBCs seen on microscopy** (paradox!)

- Protein: 2+

- Specific gravity: 1.025

- **Myoglobin: Positive** (special test)

- No white blood cells, no bacteria, no casts

Stop and Think

This case presents a clear and dangerous clinical picture: **rhabdomyolysis with acute kidney injury**.

Let's connect the dots:

Rhabdomyolysis = breakdown of skeletal muscle tissue, releasing intracellular contents into the bloodstream.

The key findings:

1. **Extreme CK elevation (185,000 U/L)** - This is the diagnostic hallmark. CK >1,000 U/L suggests rhabdomyolysis; levels >5,000 U/L indicate severe rhabdomyolysis. At 185,000, this is massive muscle breakdown.

2. **Dark brown urine** - Myoglobin (muscle protein) released from damaged muscles gets filtered by kidneys and appears in urine, turning it dark brown or reddish-brown.

3. **Positive urine blood with no RBCs** - The urine dipstick detects heme (in hemoglobin and myoglobin). It's positive for "blood" even though there are no red blood cells—because myoglobin cross-reacts with the test.

4. **Acute kidney injury** - Creatinine 3.8 mg/dL (baseline probably ~1.0) indicates AKI. Myoglobin is directly toxic to kidney tubules. Additionally, volume depletion and intratubular cast formation worsen kidney injury.

5. **Severe muscle pain and swelling** - Physical examination shows extremely tender, swollen muscles (especially thighs and calves). This is the source of muscle breakdown.

6. **Hyperkalemia (6.2 mEq/L)** - Potassium is released from damaged muscle cells. This is dangerous—severe hyperkalemia causes cardiac arrhythmias.

7. **Hypocalcemia (7.8 mg/dL)** - Calcium deposits in damaged muscle tissue (calcium-phosphate precipitation) and is sequestered, lowering serum calcium.

8. **Hyperphosphatemia (6.8 mg/dL)** - Phosphate is released from muscle cell breakdown.

9. **Hyperuricemia (12.1 mg/dL)** - Uric acid is released from nucleotide breakdown in damaged muscles.

The trigger was **exertional rhabdomyolysis**—his intense workout after being deconditioned caused massive muscle damage. This is increasingly common with high-intensity fitness classes, CrossFit-style workouts, and military training in unconditioned individuals.

Diagnostic Reasoning Questions

What causes rhabdomyolysis?

Rhabdomyolysis has many causes, grouped into categories:

1. Physical/Traumatic:

- **Exertion** (extreme exercise, especially eccentric contractions like squats in unconditioned people)
- Crush injuries
- Prolonged immobilization
- Seizures (from muscle contractions)
- Electrical injuries
- Heat stroke

2. Drugs/Toxins:

- Statins (especially with fibrates, cytochrome P450 inhibitors)
- Alcohol
- Cocaine, amphetamines, ecstasy
- Antipsychotics (neuroleptic malignant syndrome)
- SSRIs (serotonin syndrome)

3. Infections:

- Viral (influenza, HIV, coxsackievirus)
- Bacterial (necrotizing fasciitis, toxic shock syndrome)

4. Metabolic:

- Electrolyte abnormalities (severe hypokalemia, hypophosphatemia)
- Hypothyroidism
- Diabetic ketoacidosis
- Hyperosmolar hyperglycemic state

5. Genetic:

- McArdle disease (myophosphorylase deficiency)
- Carnitine palmitoyltransferase II deficiency
- Malignant hyperthermia susceptibility

This patient's cause is **exertional rhabdomyolysis**—the classic presentation after extreme unaccustomed exercise. The hundreds of squats and lunges caused extensive muscle damage in someone who was deconditioned.

How does rhabdomyolysis cause kidney injury?

Three mechanisms contribute:

1. Direct myoglobin toxicity: Myoglobin is filtered by glomeruli and enters renal tubules. In acidic urine, myoglobin precipitates and forms casts that obstruct tubules. Myoglobin also generates free radicals that directly damage tubular cells.

2. Renal vasoconstriction: Muscle breakdown releases vasoactive substances that constrict renal blood vessels, reducing kidney perfusion.

3. Volume depletion: Fluid shifts into damaged, swollen muscles (third-spacing), reducing intravascular volume. This causes prerenal azotemia, worsening kidney injury.

The combination creates acute tubular necrosis (ATN)—the most common cause of AKI in rhabdomyolysis.

What's the risk of kidney failure?

Risk factors for AKI in rhabdomyolysis:

- CK >15,000-20,000 U/L (higher CK = higher risk)
- Dehydration
- Acidic urine (promotes myoglobin precipitation)
- Pre-existing kidney disease
- Sepsis or hypotension

- Use of nephrotoxic drugs

This patient has CK of 185,000 (extremely high) and is clinically volume depleted (decreased urine output, elevated BUN/Cr ratio). His AKI risk is very high. About 30-50% of patients with severe rhabdomyolysis develop AKI; 10-20% require dialysis (Bosch et al., 2009).

What are the other dangers?

Beyond kidney injury:

- **Hyperkalemia** → cardiac arrhythmias and sudden death

- **Compartment syndrome** → severe muscle swelling increases pressure in fascial compartments, compromising blood flow and causing nerve damage. Requires emergency fasciotomy.

- **Disseminated intravascular coagulation** (rare but can occur with massive rhabdomyolysis)

- **Hypocalcemia** initially (calcium deposits in muscle), then **hypercalcemia** during recovery (calcium mobilizes from muscles)

Sequential Test Results

ECG: Sinus tachycardia. **Peaked T waves** (sign of hyperkalemia). Prolonged QRS duration. No life-threatening arrhythmias currently, but hyperkalemia is dangerously high.

Repeat Labs (6 hours after presentation, before treatment):

- Creatinine: 4.2 mg/dL (worsening)

- Potassium: 6.5 mEq/L (worsening)

- Calcium: 7.5 mg/dL (worsening)

- CK: 198,000 U/L (still rising)

Urine Output: Only 150 mL in past 6 hours (oliguria—defined as <400 mL/day or <0.5 mL/kg/hour). This confirms AKI is worsening.

Compartment Pressure Measurements: Orthopedic surgery is consulted due to extreme muscle swelling and pain. Compartment pressures in his calves measure 28 mmHg (normal <15 mmHg). Pressures >30 mmHg indicate compartment syndrome requiring emergency fasciotomy. He's at risk but hasn't crossed that threshold yet. Close monitoring continues.

What's Happening Here?

This patient has **severe rhabdomyolysis** causing **acute kidney injury** (acute tubular necrosis) and **life-threatening hyperkalemia**.

The complete pathophysiology:

1. Muscle breakdown: Extreme, unaccustomed exercise (hundreds of squats and lunges) caused widespread muscle fiber damage, especially in large muscle groups (quadriceps, gluteus, gastrocnemius). Eccentric contractions (lengthening under load, like lowering in a squat) are particularly damaging to unconditioned muscles.

2. Massive CK and myoglobin release: Damaged muscle cells release intracellular contents:

- Creatine kinase (CK) - enzyme marking muscle damage

- Myoglobin - oxygen-carrying protein in muscles

- Potassium - intracellular ion

- Phosphate - intracellular ion

- Uric acid - from nucleotide breakdown

- Calcium sequesters into damaged muscles (causing hypocalcemia)

3. Myoglobinuric acute kidney injury: Myoglobin filters through glomeruli into tubules. In concentrated, acidic urine, myoglobin precipitates and forms obstructive casts. Myoglobin also generates reactive oxygen species that damage tubular epithelium directly. Renal vasoconstriction and volume depletion worsen injury. The result is acute tubular necrosis (ATN).

4. Oliguria and uremia: Kidney function declines rapidly. Urine output drops (oliguria). Creatinine rises. BUN rises. The kidneys can't excrete potassium, phosphate, or uric acid, so these accumulate.

5. Dangerous electrolyte abnormalities:

- Hyperkalemia from muscle breakdown + impaired renal excretion → risk of fatal cardiac arrhythmias

- Hypocalcemia from calcium deposition in damaged muscles → can cause tetany, arrhythmias

- Hyperphosphatemia from muscle breakdown → binds calcium, worsening hypocalcemia

6. Compartment syndrome risk: Severe muscle swelling increases pressure within the fascia surrounding muscles. If pressure exceeds perfusion pressure, blood flow to muscles and nerves stops, causing irreversible damage. This requires emergency surgical decompression (fasciotomy).

Final Diagnosis

Severe rhabdomyolysis (exertional) complicated by:

- **Acute kidney injury (acute tubular necrosis)**

- **Life-threatening hyperkalemia**

- **Electrolyte disturbances (hypocalcemia, hyperphosphatemia)**

- **Risk of compartment syndrome**

Treatment and Management

This is a medical emergency requiring ICU admission and aggressive intervention.

1. Aggressive IV Fluid Resuscitation (MOST IMPORTANT):

Early aggressive hydration is the cornerstone of treatment and the single intervention proven to reduce AKI in rhabdomyolysis.

Protocol:

- **Normal saline (0.9% NaCl) at 500-1,000 mL/hour initially**

- Goal: Maintain urine output >200-300 mL/hour (to flush myoglobin through kidneys)

- Monitor fluid status carefully (CVP monitoring may be needed)

- Continue high-rate fluids until CK <5,000 U/L and myoglobinuria clears

Rationale:

- Dilutes myoglobin concentration in tubules

- Increases urine flow to flush myoglobin out

- Prevents hypovolemia that worsens kidney injury

- Alkalinizes urine (debated—see below)

He receives normal saline at 500 mL/hour initially.

2. Urinary Alkalinization (CONTROVERSIAL):

Some protocols add sodium bicarbonate to IV fluids to alkalinize urine (target urine pH >6.5). The theory is that myoglobin is less likely to precipitate in alkaline urine.

However, evidence is mixed:

- No randomized controlled trials prove benefit

- Risk of worsening hypocalcemia (alkalosis decreases ionized calcium)

- May cause metabolic alkalosis

- Current consensus: Adequate hydration is more important than alkalinization

This patient does NOT receive bicarbonate. Focus is on aggressive fluid resuscitation.

3. Treat Hyperkalemia URGENTLY:

Potassium 6.5 mEq/L with ECG changes (peaked T waves) is an emergency.

Immediate treatments:

- **Calcium gluconate 10% 10 mL IV** (stabilizes cardiac membrane—doesn't lower potassium but prevents arrhythmias)

- **Insulin 10 units IV + D50W 50 mL** (shifts potassium into cells temporarily)

- **Albuterol nebulizer** (shifts potassium into cells)

- **Sodium bicarbonate** if metabolic acidosis present (shifts potassium into cells)

Longer-term potassium removal:

- **Sodium polystyrene sulfonate (Kayexalate)** orally or rectally (removes potassium via GI tract—takes hours)

139

- **Diuretics** if patient responds to fluids (increases renal potassium excretion)
- **Hemodialysis** if severe hyperkalemia refractory to medical management

He receives calcium gluconate, insulin/dextrose, and albuterol. Potassium decreases to 5.8 mEq/L. Continuous cardiac monitoring.

4. Monitor and Support Kidney Function:

- **Urine output hourly** (maintain >200-300 mL/hour)
- **Daily weights** (monitor fluid balance)
- **Electrolytes every 4-6 hours** initially (potassium, calcium, phosphate, magnesium)
- **Daily CK** (should decline with treatment—if rising, suspect ongoing muscle breakdown)
- **Creatinine daily** (tracks kidney function)

If urine output doesn't improve with fluids:

- **Diuretics** (furosemide) may be tried
- **Renal replacement therapy (dialysis)** if:
  - Refractory hyperkalemia
  - Volume overload
  - Severe uremia
  - Metabolic acidosis
  - Persistent oliguria/anuria

5. Pain Control:

His muscle pain is severe. Appropriate analgesia:

- **Acetaminophen** (avoid NSAIDs—nephrotoxic in AKI)
- **Opioids** if needed (careful dosing in kidney injury)
- Muscle relaxants generally avoided

6. Monitor for Compartment Syndrome:

- **Serial compartment pressure measurements** if swelling worsens
- **Neurovascular checks** (pulses, sensation, motor function)
- **Emergency fasciotomy** if pressures >30 mmHg or if neurovascular compromise develops

His compartment pressures remain <30 mmHg, so surgical intervention isn't needed.

7. Treat Hypocalcemia (CAUTIOUSLY):

DO NOT aggressively treat asymptomatic hypocalcemia in rhabdomyolysis. Here's why:

During the initial phase, calcium deposits in damaged muscles (causing low serum calcium). Later, during the recovery phase, this calcium mobilizes back into blood, potentially causing dangerous hypercalcemia. If you give IV calcium during the initial phase, you risk severe hypercalcemia during recovery.

Only treat hypocalcemia if:

- Symptomatic (tetany, seizures)
- Severe (ionized calcium <4.0 mg/dL)
- Life-threatening arrhythmias

His calcium is 7.5 mg/dL (mild), and he's asymptomatic, so **no calcium replacement is given**.

Follow-up

Day 1-2:

- Receives aggressive IV fluids at 500 mL/hour
- Urine output increases to 250 mL/hour (good response)
- CK peaks at 203,000, then begins declining
- Creatinine stabilizes at 4.3 mg/dL
- Potassium controlled at 5.2-5.4 mEq/L with ongoing treatment

Day 3-5:

- CK declining: Day 3: 145,000 → Day 4: 82,000 → Day 5: 38,000
- Creatinine improving: Day 3: 3.9 → Day 4: 3.2 → Day 5: 2.6 mg/dL
- Urine output remains good (200-300 mL/hour)
- Muscle pain and swelling gradually improving
- IV fluid rate reduced to 250 mL/hour as kidney function improves

Day 7:

- CK: 8,200 U/L (approaching normal)
- Creatinine: 1.8 mg/dL (still elevated but recovering)
- Urine clear (no more myoglobinuria)
- Electrolytes normalized
- Able to walk with assistance
- Transferred out of ICU

Day 10:

- CK: 890 U/L (near normal)

- Creatinine: 1.3 mg/dL (approaching baseline)
- Discharged home with instructions

1 Month:

- CK: 180 U/L (normal)
- Creatinine: 1.0 mg/dL (complete recovery of kidney function)
- Full muscle strength and range of motion restored
- Counseled on safe exercise progression

Prognosis and Prevention

Prognosis: With early recognition and aggressive treatment, most patients with exertional rhabdomyolysis recover completely. This patient's kidney function returned to normal within one month. Complete recovery of muscle function typically takes 4-8 weeks.

However, severe cases can cause:

- Permanent kidney damage requiring dialysis (5-10% of severe cases)
- Compartment syndrome with permanent nerve/muscle damage if fasciotomy delayed
- Death from hyperkalemia or complications (mortality 1-5% in exertional rhabdomyolysis, higher in other causes)

Prevention:

- **Gradual exercise progression** (don't jump from sedentary to extreme workouts)
- **Adequate hydration** before, during, and after exercise
- **Avoid exercise in extreme heat**
- **Recognize early symptoms** (severe muscle pain, weakness, dark urine) and seek care immediately
- **Screen for risk factors** (statin use, recent illness, genetic muscle disorders)
- **Educate fitness trainers** about rhabdomyolysis risk in unconditioned participants

Exertional rhabdomyolysis is increasingly recognized with high-intensity interval training, CrossFit, boot camp classes, and military training. The fitness industry needs awareness that pushing deconditioned individuals too hard too fast can cause serious medical emergencies (Bosch et al., 2009).

Teaching Points

Rhabdomyolysis is diagnosed by the triad of muscle pain, weakness, and dark urine, with CK >1,000 U/L. CK elevation is the diagnostic hallmark. CK >5,000 U/L indicates severe rhabdomyolysis with significant AKI risk. Levels can reach >100,000 U/L in severe cases. CK peaks 1-3 days after muscle injury, then declines if no ongoing injury occurs.

Dark brown or reddish-brown urine suggests myoglobinuria. Myoglobin colors urine like "Coca-Cola" or "iced tea." The urine dipstick shows positive for "blood" but microscopy shows no red blood cells—this paradox occurs because myoglobin cross-reacts with the hemoglobin detection on the dipstick. This is a key diagnostic clue.

Aggressive IV hydration is the most important treatment and the only intervention proven to prevent AKI. Start fluids early (ideally within 6 hours of presentation). Use normal saline at 500-1,000 mL/hour initially. Target urine output of 200-300 mL/hour. Continue high-rate fluids until CK <5,000 U/L and myoglobinuria clears. Early aggressive hydration can reduce AKI incidence from 30-50% to 10-20% (Bosch et al., 2009).

Hyperkalemia is the most immediate life threat. Potassium released from damaged muscles accumulates because kidneys can't excrete it (due to AKI). Severe hyperkalemia causes cardiac arrhythmias and sudden death. Check potassium urgently, get ECG, and treat emergently if elevated. Calcium gluconate stabilizes the cardiac membrane (buys time), while insulin/dextrose and albuterol shift potassium into cells.

Do not aggressively treat asymptomatic hypocalcemia in rhabdomyolysis. Calcium deposits in damaged muscles initially, causing low serum calcium. During recovery, this calcium remobilizes, potentially causing dangerous hypercalcemia. Only treat symptomatic or severe hypocalcemia. Over-treatment risks rebound hypercalcemia.

Compartment syndrome requires emergency fasciotomy. Severe muscle swelling increases pressure within fascial compartments. If pressure exceeds perfusion pressure (typically >30 mmHg), blood flow stops, causing irreversible muscle and nerve damage within hours. Emergency surgical decompression (fasciotomy) is required. Monitor for "6 Ps": Pain, Pressure, Pallor, Paresthesias, Pulselessness, Paralysis.

Exertional rhabdomyolysis is increasingly common with high-intensity fitness trends. Extreme workouts in unconditioned individuals cause widespread muscle damage. Eccentric exercises (lowering weight, downhill running, excessive squats) are particularly risky. The fitness industry needs awareness that pushing too hard too fast can cause medical emergencies. Gradual progression and appropriate hydration are essential.

CK trends guide treatment duration. Follow CK daily. It should decline progressively if no ongoing muscle breakdown. If CK rises or plateaus, suspect continued muscle damage or compartment syndrome. Continue aggressive hydration until CK <5,000 U/L and myoglobinuria resolves.

Related Cases

This case connects to:

- **Case 7: Hypokalemia and Cardiac Arrhythmia** (opposite electrolyte problem—hyperkalemia vs. hypokalemia causing cardiac issues)

- **Case 1: The Confused Diabetic** (another medical emergency with electrolyte disturbances)

- **Case 2: The Man with Kidney Stones and Fatigue** (discusses calcium disorders, opposite problem here)

Case 5: The Jaundiced Man with Itching

Clinical Presentation

A 45-year-old man presents to his physician complaining of progressive yellowing of his skin and eyes over the past three weeks, accompanied by intense itching that's worse at night and disrupting his sleep. He's also noticed his urine has become very dark (like tea) and his stools have turned pale, almost white.

He reports mild right upper quadrant abdominal discomfort but denies severe pain. He's lost about 10 pounds over the past month without trying. He denies fever, nausea, or vomiting. No history of hepatitis, blood transfusions, or IV drug use. He drinks 1-2 glasses of wine with dinner but no excessive alcohol. No recent travel or new medications.

Physical examination reveals obvious jaundice of the skin and sclera. He has excoriations (scratch marks) on his arms and trunk from itching. His liver edge is palpable 2 cm below the right costal margin. No splenomegaly. No ascites. No signs of chronic liver disease (spider angiomas, palmar erythema, gynecomastia). Vital signs are normal.

Initial Laboratory Findings

Liver Function Tests (LFTs):

- **Total bilirubin: 12.8 mg/dL** (normal: 0.3-1.2 mg/dL) - **MARKEDLY ELEVATED**

- **Direct (conjugated) bilirubin: 10.2 mg/dL** (normal: 0.0-0.3 mg/dL) - **MARKEDLY ELEVATED**

- Indirect (unconjugated) bilirubin: 2.6 mg/dL

- **Alkaline phosphatase: 685 U/L** (normal: 44-147 U/L) - **MARKEDLY ELEVATED**

- **GGT (gamma-glutamyl transferase): 420 U/L** (normal: 9-48 U/L) - **MARKEDLY ELEVATED**

- **AST: 142 U/L** (normal: 10-40 U/L) - elevated

- **ALT: 135 U/L** (normal: 7-56 U/L) - elevated

- Albumin: 3.8 g/dL (normal: 3.5-5.0 g/dL) - normal

- INR: 1.1 (normal: 0.8-1.2) - normal

Stop and Think

This case shows **obstructive jaundice** (cholestatic pattern). The liver enzyme pattern tells the story:

Cholestatic pattern:

- **Markedly elevated alkaline phosphatase and GGT** (disproportionate to transaminases)

- **Elevated direct (conjugated) bilirubin**

- Moderately elevated AST/ALT

144

Versus hepatocellular pattern:

- Markedly elevated AST/ALT (often >500-1,000 U/L)

- Modest alkaline phosphatase elevation

- Mixed bilirubin elevation

The cholestatic pattern indicates bile flow obstruction. Bile can't drain properly, so bilirubin backs up into blood (causing jaundice), alkaline phosphatase and GGT leak from bile duct epithelium (markedly elevated), and bile doesn't reach intestines (causing pale stools and dark urine).

The **direct (conjugated) bilirubin predominance** (10.2 out of 12.8 total) confirms this is cholestatic/obstructive jaundice, not hemolytic or pre-hepatic jaundice.

Pale stools and dark urine are classic for obstructive jaundice:

- Bile pigments give stool its brown color—without bile reaching intestines, stools turn pale/clay-colored

- Conjugated bilirubin is water-soluble and spills into urine, turning it dark brown

Pruritus (itching) is common in cholestasis from accumulation of bile salts in skin.

The differential for obstructive jaundice includes:

1. **Biliary obstruction**: gallstones (choledocholithiasis), strictures

2. **Pancreatic head mass**: compressing common bile duct (pancreatic cancer, chronic pancreatitis)

3. **Cholangiocarcinoma**: bile duct cancer

4. **Primary sclerosing cholangitis**: autoimmune bile duct disease

5. **Drug-induced cholestasis**: certain medications

6. **Intrahepatic cholestasis**: pregnancy, sepsis, total parenteral nutrition

His presentation (middle-aged, weight loss, painless jaundice) raises concern for **malignancy**—either pancreatic cancer or cholangiocarcinoma.

Sequential Test Results

Additional Laboratory Tests:

- **CA 19-9 (tumor marker): 485 U/mL** (normal: <37 U/mL) - **MARKEDLY ELEVATED**

- CEA: 4.2 ng/mL (normal: <5 ng/mL) - normal

- Hepatitis panel: Negative

- ANA, AMA (antimitochondrial antibody): Negative

Imaging:

Abdominal Ultrasound:

- **Dilated intrahepatic and extrahepatic bile ducts**
- **Mass in pancreatic head measuring 3.2 cm**
- Gallbladder distended but no stones visible

CT Scan Abdomen/Pelvis with Contrast:

- **Pancreatic head mass (3.5 cm) with irregular borders**
- **Dilation of common bile duct and pancreatic duct ("double duct sign")**
- No distant metastases visible
- No ascites

ERCP (Endoscopic Retrograde Cholangiopancreatography):

- Confirms stricture of distal common bile duct from external compression
- Bile duct stent placed to relieve obstruction
- Brushings obtained for cytology

Cytology: Malignant cells consistent with adenocarcinoma

Final Diagnosis

Pancreatic adenocarcinoma (pancreatic head) causing obstructive jaundice

This represents the classic **Courvoisier sign**—painless jaundice with palpable, non-tender gallbladder suggests pancreatic head malignancy obstructing the common bile duct.

Treatment and Follow-up

Pancreatic cancer has poor prognosis. Staging determines treatment:

Staging:

- Localized to pancreas, no vascular involvement, no metastases
- Potentially resectable
- Stage IIB

Treatment:

- **Whipple procedure (pancreaticoduodenectomy):** Surgical resection of pancreatic head, duodenum, part of bile duct, gallbladder
- **Adjuvant chemotherapy:** FOLFIRINOX or gemcitabine-based regimen post-surgery
- Close oncology follow-up

Prognosis: 5-year survival for resectable pancreatic cancer is 20-30% (much better than unresectable disease at <5%)

Teaching Points

Liver enzyme patterns distinguish hepatocellular from cholestatic injury. Hepatocellular pattern: AST/ALT >>alkaline phosphatase (ratio >5:1). Cholestatic pattern: Alkaline phosphatase/GGT >>AST/ALT. Mixed patterns occur but dominant pattern guides differential diagnosis.

Direct (conjugated) vs. indirect (unconjugated) bilirubin helps localize the problem. Indirect hyperbilirubinemia suggests hemolysis or Gilbert syndrome (pre-hepatic). Direct hyperbilirubinemia suggests hepatocellular disease or biliary obstruction (hepatic or post-hepatic).

Painless jaundice with weight loss suggests malignancy. Pancreatic cancer, cholangiocarcinoma, or ampullary carcinoma. Painful jaundice suggests gallstones or cholangitis.

Always image the biliary tree when cholestatic pattern is present. Ultrasound is first-line (cheap, non-invasive). CT or MRCP for detailed anatomy. ERCP for therapeutic intervention (stenting).

Related Cases

- **Case 10: Cushing's Syndrome vs. Disease** (discusses tumor markers)
- **Case 15: Tumor Markers in Cancer Diagnosis** (expanded discussion of CA 19-9 and other markers)

Case 6: The Cold, Tired Woman

Clinical Presentation

A 42-year-old woman presents to her primary care physician complaining of overwhelming fatigue that has progressively worsened over the past six months. She says she's "exhausted all the time" despite sleeping 10-12 hours per night. She can barely get through her workday as a teacher and often naps immediately after getting home.

She's also noticed significant weight gain—about 25 pounds over six months despite no change in diet or exercise. Her hair has become dry and brittle, falling out more than usual. Her skin is extremely dry despite using moisturizer. She feels cold constantly, wearing sweaters even in warm weather when others are comfortable. Her periods have become heavier and more irregular.

She reports difficulty concentrating and memory problems—"brain fog" that makes teaching challenging. Her mood has been low, and she wonders if she's depressed. She's also noticed constipation, muscle aches, and puffiness around her eyes in the morning.

Her past medical history is unremarkable. She takes no medications. No family history of thyroid disease, though her mother has type 1 diabetes (autoimmune). She doesn't smoke or drink alcohol.

Physical examination reveals a slightly overweight woman who appears tired and moves slowly. Vital signs show temperature 36.1°C (97°F—low), heart rate 54 beats per minute (bradycardia), blood pressure 148/92 mmHg (hypertension). Her skin is cool, dry, and pale. Her hair is coarse and thin. Her face appears somewhat puffy, especially around the eyes (periorbital edema). Her thyroid gland is not palpable. She has slow relaxation phase of deep tendon reflexes (delayed relaxation is classic for hypothyroidism). No tremor. The rest of the examination is unremarkable.

Initial Laboratory Findings

Thyroid Function Tests:

- **TSH (thyroid stimulating hormone): 48.5 mIU/L** (normal: 0.4-4.0 mIU/L) - **MARKEDLY ELEVATED**

- **Free T4 (thyroxine): 0.4 ng/dL** (normal: 0.8-1.8 ng/dL) - **VERY LOW**

- Free T3 (triiodothyronine): 1.2 pg/mL (normal: 2.3-4.2 pg/mL) - LOW

Other Laboratory Tests:

- Hemoglobin: 10.8 g/dL (normal: 12.0-16.0 g/dL) - LOW (mild anemia)

- MCV: 96 fL (normal: 80-100 fL) - high normal

- **Total cholesterol: 285 mg/dL** (normal: <200 mg/dL) - **ELEVATED**

- **LDL cholesterol: 195 mg/dL** (normal: <100 mg/dL) - **ELEVATED**

- Triglycerides: 210 mg/dL (normal: <150 mg/dL) - elevated

- **Creatine kinase (CK): 485 U/L** (normal: 50-200 U/L) - **ELEVATED**

- Sodium: 134 mEq/L (normal: 136-145 mEq/L) - slightly low

- Glucose: 92 mg/dL (normal)

Stop and Think

This case screams **hypothyroidism**. The combination of elevated TSH with low free T4 confirms **primary hypothyroidism**.

Let's understand the thyroid axis:

Normal thyroid regulation:

1. Hypothalamus releases TRH (thyrotropin-releasing hormone)

2. TRH stimulates pituitary to release TSH (thyroid-stimulating hormone)

3. TSH stimulates thyroid gland to produce T4 (thyroxine) and T3 (triiodothyronine)

4. T4 and T3 provide negative feedback to pituitary and hypothalamus

Primary hypothyroidism:

- The thyroid gland fails to produce adequate thyroid hormone

- Low T4/T3 → Loss of negative feedback → Pituitary releases massive amounts of TSH trying to stimulate the failing thyroid

- Result: **Very high TSH + Low T4/T3**

Secondary hypothyroidism (rare):

- Pituitary fails to produce TSH

- Result: Low TSH + Low T4/T3

Subclinical hypothyroidism:

- TSH elevated (usually 4.5-10 mIU/L) but T4 still normal

- Early thyroid failure, often progresses to overt hypothyroidism

This patient has **overt primary hypothyroidism** with TSH of 48.5 (massively elevated) and free T4 of 0.4 (very low).

Her symptoms all fit hypothyroidism perfectly:

- **Fatigue and lethargy** → slowed metabolism

- **Weight gain** → decreased metabolic rate, fluid retention

- **Cold intolerance** → decreased heat production from metabolism

- **Dry skin and hair loss** → decreased cellular turnover

- **Constipation** → decreased GI motility

- **Heavy menstrual bleeding** → hormonal effects

- **Cognitive impairment** ("brain fog") → thyroid hormone essential for brain function

- **Depression** → thyroid hormone affects neurotransmitters

- **Bradycardia** → decreased cardiac output and heart rate

- **Hypertension** → increased peripheral vascular resistance

- **Delayed deep tendon reflexes** → slowed nerve conduction

The laboratory abnormalities also fit:

- **Mild anemia** → thyroid hormone stimulates erythropoiesis

- **Elevated cholesterol** → thyroid hormone regulates lipid metabolism; hypothyroidism causes hyperlipidemia

- **Elevated CK** → hypothyroidism causes muscle breakdown (hypothyroid myopathy)

- **Mild hyponatremia** → impaired free water excretion

Diagnostic Reasoning Questions

What causes primary hypothyroidism?

1. Hashimoto's thyroiditis (most common—70-80% of cases):

- Autoimmune destruction of thyroid gland

- Antibodies against thyroid peroxidase (TPO) and thyroglobulin

- Often familial clustering with other autoimmune diseases

- More common in women (5-10:1 female-to-male ratio)

2. Iatrogenic (treatment-induced):

- Radioactive iodine treatment for hyperthyroidism
- Thyroidectomy (surgical removal)
- External beam radiation to neck

3. Medications:

- Lithium (interferes with thyroid hormone synthesis)
- Amiodarone (high iodine content)
- Interferon-alpha
- Tyrosine kinase inhibitors

4. Iodine deficiency:

- Rare in developed countries (salt iodization)
- Still common in developing countries

5. Congenital hypothyroidism:

- Thyroid agenesis or dysgenesis
- Detected on newborn screening

6. Infiltrative diseases (rare):

- Amyloidosis, sarcoidosis, hemochromatosis

This patient's presentation (gradual onset, autoimmune family history) suggests **Hashimoto's thyroiditis**.

How do you confirm Hashimoto's thyroiditis?

Check thyroid antibodies:

- **Anti-TPO (anti-thyroid peroxidase) antibodies** → positive in 90-95% of Hashimoto's
- **Anti-thyroglobulin antibodies** → positive in 60-80% of Hashimoto's

Why does hypothyroidism cause hyperlipidemia?

Thyroid hormone regulates multiple steps in lipid metabolism:

- Increases LDL receptor expression (removing LDL from blood)
- Increases cholesterol excretion via bile
- Increases lipoprotein lipase activity (breaking down triglycerides)

Without adequate thyroid hormone, these processes slow, causing accumulation of cholesterol and triglycerides. Treating hypothyroidism often dramatically improves lipid levels without statin therapy (Duntas, 2002).

What is myxedema coma?

Myxedema coma is severe, life-threatening hypothyroidism presenting with:

- Altered mental status/coma

- Hypothermia (<95°F)

- Bradycardia

- Hypotension

- Hypoventilation

- Hypoglycemia

- Hyponatremia

Triggered by infection, cold exposure, trauma, surgery, or medications. Mortality 20-50% even with treatment. Requires ICU admission and IV thyroid hormone replacement.

This patient is symptomatic but not in myxedema coma. She can be treated outpatient.

Sequential Test Results

Thyroid Antibodies:

- **Anti-TPO antibodies: 520 IU/mL** (normal: <35 IU/mL) - **MARKEDLY ELEVATED**

- Anti-thyroglobulin antibodies: 185 IU/mL (normal: <20 IU/mL) - ELEVATED

Thyroid Ultrasound: Heterogeneous echotexture with decreased vascularity, consistent with chronic thyroiditis (Hashimoto's). No discrete nodules. Gland size is normal to slightly enlarged.

The positive anti-TPO antibodies confirm **Hashimoto's thyroiditis** as the cause of her hypothyroidism.

What's Happening Here?

This patient has **primary hypothyroidism due to Hashimoto's thyroiditis** (chronic autoimmune thyroiditis).

The pathophysiology:

1. Autoimmune destruction: The immune system produces antibodies against thyroid antigens (thyroid peroxidase and thyroglobulin). These antibodies, along with T-cell mediated destruction, gradually damage the thyroid gland over months to years.

2. Progressive thyroid failure: As more thyroid tissue is destroyed, the gland can't produce adequate thyroid hormone. Initially, the gland may compensate (subclinical hypothyroidism—high TSH, normal T4). Eventually, compensation fails (overt hypothyroidism—high TSH, low T4).

3. Pituitary response: The pituitary senses low thyroid hormone and releases massive amounts of TSH trying to stimulate the failing thyroid. TSH remains elevated despite being ineffective because the thyroid tissue is damaged.

4. Metabolic consequences: Thyroid hormone (T3 and T4) regulates metabolism in virtually every cell. Deficiency causes:

- **Decreased basal metabolic rate** → weight gain, cold intolerance, fatigue
- **Decreased cardiac output** → bradycardia, decreased contractility, diastolic hypertension
- **Decreased GI motility** → constipation
- **Decreased protein synthesis** → hair loss, dry skin
- **Accumulation of glycosaminoglycans** → puffy appearance (myxedema)
- **Impaired lipid metabolism** → hyperlipidemia
- **Decreased erythropoiesis** → mild anemia
- **CNS effects** → depression, cognitive impairment, delayed reflexes

5. Secondary effects:

- Muscle breakdown (elevated CK)
- Impaired free water excretion (mild hyponatremia)
- Increased menstrual bleeding (anovulatory cycles)

Hashimoto's thyroiditis is the most common cause of hypothyroidism in iodine-sufficient areas, affecting 1-2% of the population. It's 5-10 times more common in women than men, typically presenting in middle age (30s-50s) (Garber et al., 2012).

Final Diagnosis

Primary hypothyroidism due to Hashimoto's thyroiditis (chronic autoimmune thyroiditis)

Treatment and Management

Levothyroxine (Synthetic T4) Replacement:

This is the standard treatment for hypothyroidism.

Starting dose:

- Young, healthy patients: 1.6 µg/kg body weight daily (typically 100-125 µg daily)
- Older patients or those with cardiac disease: Start low (25-50 µg daily) and increase slowly to avoid cardiac complications

For this 42-year-old healthy woman weighing 80 kg: Starting dose: 1.6 × 80 = 128 µg → Start **levothyroxine 125 µg daily**

Administration:

- Take on empty stomach (30-60 minutes before breakfast)
- Avoid taking with calcium, iron, or antacids (interfere with absorption)
- Take consistently at same time daily

Monitoring:

- Recheck TSH in **6-8 weeks** (it takes 4-6 weeks for steady state after dose change)
- Goal TSH: 0.5-2.5 mIU/L (some patients feel best at lower end of normal range)
- Adjust dose in 12.5-25 μg increments based on TSH
- Once stable, check TSH annually

Important principles:

TSH is the primary monitoring parameter. Free T4 is less useful once treatment is established. TSH reflects tissue thyroid hormone levels better than T4 measurements.

Don't recheck labs too soon. TSH takes 6-8 weeks to equilibrate after dose changes. Checking earlier leads to incorrect dose adjustments.

Symptoms may lag behind TSH normalization. It can take 3-6 months for full symptomatic improvement even after TSH normalizes. Be patient.

Pregnancy considerations: Thyroid hormone requirements increase 30-50% during pregnancy. Women on levothyroxine who become pregnant should increase dose immediately (add 2 extra pills per week) and check TSH urgently. Untreated hypothyroidism during pregnancy risks fetal neurodevelopmental problems (Garber et al., 2012).

Drug interactions: Many medications affect levothyroxine:

- Increase requirements: estrogen, rifampin, phenytoin, carbamazepine
- Decrease absorption: proton pump inhibitors, iron, calcium, sucralfate
- Adjust dose as needed based on TSH

Combination T4/T3 therapy is NOT routinely recommended. Most T3 is produced peripherally from T4 conversion. Adding T3 (Cytomel) to levothyroxine doesn't improve outcomes in most patients and increases risk of side effects (cardiac, bone loss). Reserved for rare cases where patients remain symptomatic despite normalized TSH on T4 alone.

Follow-up

6 Weeks:

- TSH: 2.8 mIU/L (normalized!)
- Free T4: 1.2 ng/dL (normalized)
- She reports feeling "somewhat better" but still fatigued
- Continue same dose

3 Months:

- She feels dramatically better—energy improved, weight down 8 pounds, hair loss stopped
- No longer cold intolerant
- Concentration and memory improved
- Mood much better
- Repeat labs show TSH 1.8 mIU/L, free T4 1.4 ng/dL (excellent control)

6 Months:

- Weight down 18 pounds (lost most of the fluid weight gain)
- Cholesterol: Total 178 mg/dL, LDL 98 mg/dL (normalized without statins!)
- Menstrual periods regular
- CK: 125 U/L (normalized)
- She feels like "herself again"

Ongoing:

- Annual TSH monitoring
- Continues levothyroxine 125 µg daily lifelong
- No adverse effects
- Quality of life excellent

Prognosis

Hypothyroidism is easily treated and patients usually do very well. With appropriate levothyroxine replacement:

- Symptoms resolve completely in 90-95% of patients
- Metabolic abnormalities (hyperlipidemia, anemia) normalize
- Cardiovascular risk decreases
- Quality of life returns to baseline

Hashimoto's thyroiditis is progressive. Thyroid function won't recover. Patients need lifelong thyroid hormone replacement. Antibody levels may decrease over time but don't predict disease progression.

Associated conditions: Hashimoto's thyroiditis increases risk of:

- Other autoimmune diseases (type 1 diabetes, celiac disease, Addison's disease, vitiligo, pernicious anemia)
- Thyroid lymphoma (rare but increased risk—presents as rapidly growing thyroid mass)

Untreated severe hypothyroidism can cause:

- Myxedema coma (mortality 20-50%)

- Heart failure

- Infertility

- Pregnancy complications

- Accelerated atherosclerosis

With treatment, life expectancy is normal.

Teaching Points

TSH is the best screening test for thyroid disease. Elevated TSH indicates hypothyroidism; suppressed TSH indicates hyperthyroidism. Free T4 is added for diagnosis and classification but TSH alone screens effectively. Check TSH in patients with unexplained fatigue, weight changes, depression, hyperlipidemia, or nonspecific symptoms (Garber et al., 2012).

Primary hypothyroidism shows high TSH with low T4. The thyroid gland fails, T4 drops, negative feedback is lost, and TSH rises dramatically. This pattern (TSH ↑↑, T4 ↓) confirms primary hypothyroidism. Secondary hypothyroidism (pituitary failure) shows low TSH with low T4—rare but important to recognize.

Hashimoto's thyroiditis is confirmed by anti-TPO antibodies. Positive anti-TPO antibodies in 90-95% of Hashimoto's cases. Anti-thyroglobulin antibodies are less sensitive. However, antibody testing isn't always necessary—if TSH/T4 pattern confirms hypothyroidism and you're treating anyway, antibody testing doesn't change management. Test when diagnosis uncertain or when documenting autoimmune etiology is important.

Hypothyroidism causes hyperlipidemia. Check TSH in patients with unexplained elevated cholesterol. Treating hypothyroidism often normalizes lipids without statins. Many patients on statins for "high cholesterol" actually have undiagnosed hypothyroidism. TSH should be part of lipid disorder workup (Duntas, 2002).

Levothyroxine is the treatment of choice. Synthetic T4 (levothyroxine) has long half-life (7 days), consistent absorption, and allows once-daily dosing. T3 preparations (Cytomel) have short half-life, cause peaks/troughs, and increase cardiac side effects. Desiccated thyroid (Armour Thyroid) has variable T4/T3 content and inconsistent absorption. Levothyroxine is superior for most patients.

TSH normalization takes 6-8 weeks after dose changes. Don't recheck sooner—TSH equilibrates slowly. Checking at 2-3 weeks leads to inappropriate dose adjustments. Be patient. Similarly, symptoms may take 3-6 months to fully resolve even after TSH normalizes.

Subclinical hypothyroidism (elevated TSH, normal T4) is common and treatment is debated. If TSH is 4.5-10 mIU/L with normal T4 and minimal symptoms, treatment benefit is unclear. Consider treating if: symptoms present, positive TPO antibodies, trying to conceive, TSH >10 mIU/L, or high cardiovascular risk. Otherwise, monitor TSH every 6-12 months—many progress to overt hypothyroidism requiring treatment.

Pregnancy dramatically increases thyroid hormone needs. Women with hypothyroidism who become pregnant need immediate dose increase (typically 30-50% more). Untreated maternal hypothyroidism causes fetal neurodevelopmental problems and pregnancy complications. Check TSH immediately upon pregnancy confirmation and adjust dose to keep TSH <2.5 mIU/L in first trimester, <3.0 mIU/L later (Garber et al., 2012).

Related Cases

This case connects to:

- **Case 3: The Marathon Runner Who Can't Stop Drinking Water** (SIADH—hypothyroidism can cause SIADH-like hyponatremia)

- **Case 12: The Overweight Man with Multiple Problems** (metabolic syndrome—hypothyroidism contributes to metabolic abnormalities)

- **Case 14: The Man Who Collapsed at the Gym** (adrenal insufficiency—can coexist with autoimmune thyroid disease in polyglandular autoimmune syndrome)

Case 7: The Weak Patient with Palpitations

Clinical Presentation

A 67-year-old woman presents to the emergency department complaining of severe muscle weakness, palpitations, and lightheadedness for the past two days. She says her legs feel "like jelly" and she can barely stand from a seated position. She's also experiencing irregular heartbeats that she can feel "fluttering in her chest."

She reports increasing fatigue over the past week, along with nausea and decreased appetite. She's had no vomiting or diarrhea. She's been urinating more frequently than usual.

Her past medical history includes hypertension and osteoarthritis. Her medications include **hydrochlorothiazide (HCTZ) 50 mg daily** for blood pressure (she's been on this for years) and **ibuprofen 800 mg three times daily** for arthritis pain (increased dose about two weeks ago due to worsening joint pain). She doesn't smoke or drink alcohol.

Physical examination reveals an elderly woman who appears weak and uncomfortable. Vital signs show temperature 37.0°C (normal), heart rate 54 beats per minute (bradycardia) with irregular rhythm, blood pressure 162/94 mmHg (hypertension persists despite treatment), respiratory rate 14 breaths per minute. Cardiac examination reveals irregularly irregular rhythm—no P waves on cardiac monitor, consistent with **atrial fibrillation**. She has marked proximal muscle weakness—difficulty rising from a chair without using her arms. Deep tendon reflexes are diminished. The rest of the examination is unremarkable.

Initial Laboratory Findings

Chemistry Panel:

- Glucose: 108 mg/dL (normal)

- Sodium: 138 mEq/L (normal)

- **Potassium: 2.1 mEq/L** (normal: 3.5-5.0 mEq/L) - **CRITICALLY LOW**

- Chloride: 96 mEq/L (normal: 98-107 mEq/L) - slightly low

- **Bicarbonate: 32 mEq/L** (normal: 22-28 mEq/L) - **ELEVATED** (metabolic alkalosis)

- BUN: 28 mg/dL (normal: 7-20 mg/dL) - elevated

- Creatinine: 1.4 mg/dL (normal: 0.6-1.2 mg/dL) - elevated (mild kidney injury)

- **Magnesium: 1.2 mg/dL** (normal: 1.7-2.2 mg/dL) - **LOW**

- Calcium: 9.1 mg/dL (normal)

- Phosphorus: 3.2 mg/dL (normal)

Electrocardiogram (ECG):

- **Atrial fibrillation** with ventricular rate 54 bpm

- **Prominent U waves** (extra waves after T waves—classic for hypokalemia)

- **Flattened T waves**

- **Prolonged QT interval** (measured QTc 520 ms, normal <450 ms in women)

- **ST segment depression**

These ECG changes are all characteristic of severe hypokalemia and place her at high risk for life-threatening ventricular arrhythmias (torsades de pointes, ventricular fibrillation).

Stop and Think

This patient has **severe, symptomatic hypokalemia** (potassium 2.1 mEq/L) with **dangerous cardiac manifestations**. This is a medical emergency.

Potassium is the main intracellular cation. Normal serum potassium is 3.5-5.0 mEq/L, but total body potassium is about 3,500 mEq (98% intracellular). Serum potassium reflects only a tiny fraction of total body stores.

Hypokalemia severity classification:

- **Mild:** 3.0-3.4 mEq/L

- **Moderate:** 2.5-2.9 mEq/L

- **Severe:** <2.5 mEq/L

At 2.1 mEq/L, she has **severe hypokalemia**. But look—she also has **low magnesium (1.2 mg/dL)**. This combination is extremely common and clinically important.

Her symptoms all relate to hypokalemia:

- **Muscle weakness** → potassium essential for muscle cell membrane potential; low K+ causes hyperpolarization and weakness

- **Palpitations and atrial fibrillation** → hypokalemia causes cardiac arrhythmias

- **Polyuria** → hypokalemia impairs kidney concentrating ability

157

The ECG changes are life-threatening. Severe hypokalemia causes:

- Flattened T waves

- Prominent U waves

- ST depression

- Prolonged QT interval

- Risk of ventricular tachycardia, torsades de pointes, ventricular fibrillation

What caused her hypokalemia?

Look at her medications:

1. **Hydrochlorothiazide (thiazide diuretic)** → causes renal potassium wasting

2. **Ibuprofen (NSAID)** → She recently increased the dose

The thiazide diuretic is the primary culprit. Thiazides inhibit sodium-chloride reabsorption in the distal tubule, causing increased sodium delivery to the collecting duct, where sodium reabsorption drives potassium secretion. The result is renal potassium wasting.

The **elevated bicarbonate (32 mEq/L)** indicates **metabolic alkalosis**, which is classic with thiazide diuretics. The mechanism: thiazides cause volume depletion → secondary hyperaldosteronism → increased hydrogen ion secretion and bicarbonate reabsorption → metabolic alkalosis.

The **low magnesium** is also diuretic-induced. Thiazides cause renal magnesium wasting. This is critically important because **hypomagnesemia prevents potassium repletion**. The kidney can't retain potassium effectively when magnesium is low. You must correct magnesium before potassium supplementation will work (Huang & Kuo, 2007).

Diagnostic Reasoning Questions

What are the causes of hypokalemia?

Hypokalemia results from three mechanisms:

1. Decreased intake (rare as sole cause):

- Starvation, anorexia nervosa

- Tea-and-toast diet in elderly

2. Transcellular shift (potassium moves into cells):

- Insulin excess

- Beta-agonists (albuterol)

- Alkalosis

- Refeeding syndrome

- Hypokalemic periodic paralysis (rare genetic disorder)

158

3. Increased losses:

Renal losses (most common):

- **Diuretics** (thiazides, loop diuretics)
- Hyperaldosteronism
- Hypomagnesemia
- Renal tubular acidosis
- Medications (amphotericin B, aminoglycosides)
- Osmotic diuresis (hyperglycemia)

GI losses:

- Vomiting (causes metabolic alkalosis)
- Diarrhea (causes metabolic acidosis)
- Laxative abuse
- Villous adenoma
- VIPoma (rare tumor secreting vasoactive intestinal peptide)

How do you determine the cause?

Check urine potassium:

If hypokalemia is from extrarenal causes (GI losses, decreased intake, transcellular shift), the kidneys should conserve potassium. Urine potassium should be <20 mEq/L.

If hypokalemia is from renal losses (diuretics, hyperaldosteronism), the kidneys are wasting potassium. Urine potassium will be >40 mEq/L despite low serum potassium (inappropriately high).

Acid-base status helps:

Acid-Base	Common Causes
Metabolic alkalosis + hypokalemia	Vomiting, diuretics, hyperaldosteronism
Metabolic acidosis + hypokalemia	Diarrhea, RTA, DKA (after insulin)
Normal pH + hypokalemia	Transcellular shift, GI/renal losses without acid-base disturbance

This patient: **Metabolic alkalosis + hypokalemia** → Points to diuretics (confirmed by medication history).

Why is magnesium important?

Magnesium is essential for potassium homeostasis. About 60% of patients with hypokalemia also have hypomagnesemia. The mechanisms:

1. **Renal potassium wasting:** Low magnesium impairs the kidney's ability to retain potassium (affects ROMK channels in collecting duct)

2. **Similar causes:** Diuretics, diarrhea, and alcoholism cause both potassium and magnesium loss

3. **Refractory hypokalemia:** If you give potassium without correcting magnesium, potassium just gets excreted in urine. The hypokalemia won't correct (Huang & Kuo, 2007).

The rule: Always check magnesium in hypokalemia. If low, replace magnesium first or simultaneously with potassium.

What are the dangers of severe hypokalemia?

1. Cardiac arrhythmias (most dangerous):

- Premature ventricular contractions (PVCs)
- Ventricular tachycardia
- Torsades de pointes (polymorphic VT with prolonged QT)
- Ventricular fibrillation → sudden cardiac death
- Atrial fibrillation (like this patient)
- Potentiation of digoxin toxicity (if patient takes digoxin)

2. Muscle weakness:

- Progressive weakness
- Rhabdomyolysis (severe cases)
- Respiratory muscle weakness → respiratory failure (if K+ <2.0 mEq/L)

3. Kidney effects:

- Polyuria (nephrogenic diabetes insipidus)
- Increased ammonia production → hepatic encephalopathy in cirrhosis

4. GI effects:

- Ileus (decreased GI motility)

5. Metabolic:

- Impaired insulin secretion → hyperglycemia
- Decreased protein synthesis

Sequential Test Results

Additional Laboratory Tests:

- **24-hour urine potassium: 68 mEq/day - ELEVATED** (inappropriate renal potassium wasting)

- Spot urine potassium: 52 mEq/L - inappropriately high

- Aldosterone: 18 ng/dL (normal: 4-31 ng/dL) - normal

- Renin: 4.2 ng/mL/hr (normal: 0.5-3.5 ng/mL/hr) - slightly elevated (appropriate response to volume depletion from diuretics)

- Cortisol: 12 µg/dL (normal)

The elevated urine potassium despite severe hypokalemia confirms **renal potassium wasting**. Combined with metabolic alkalosis and thiazide diuretic use, this confirms **diuretic-induced hypokalemia**.

The normal-to-slightly-elevated renin with normal aldosterone indicates secondary hyperaldosteronism from volume depletion (appropriate response), not primary hyperaldosteronism (which would show very high aldosterone with suppressed renin).

Repeat ECG after initial potassium replacement: Still shows atrial fibrillation but rate improved to 68 bpm. U waves persist but are less prominent. QTc improved to 480 ms (still prolonged but better).

What's Happening Here?

This patient has **severe hypokalemia** and **hypomagnesemia** caused by chronic **thiazide diuretic therapy**, presenting with **life-threatening cardiac arrhythmias** and **profound muscle weakness**.

The complete pathophysiology:

1. Thiazide-induced renal potassium wasting: Hydrochlorothiazide blocks the sodium-chloride cotransporter in the distal convoluted tubule. This increases sodium delivery to the collecting duct, where principal cells reabsorb sodium via ENaC channels. Sodium reabsorption creates a negative luminal potential that drives potassium secretion through ROMK channels. The result: **potassium wasting in urine**.

2. Volume depletion and secondary hyperaldosteronism: Thiazides cause volume depletion (by causing sodium and water loss). The body responds by activating the renin-angiotensin-aldosterone system. Aldosterone further increases potassium secretion in the collecting duct, worsening hypokalemia.

3. Metabolic alkalosis: Thiazides cause volume depletion → increased proximal tubule bicarbonate reabsorption. Aldosterone stimulates hydrogen ion secretion in the collecting duct → more bicarbonate generation. The result: **metabolic alkalosis** (elevated bicarbonate).

Alkalosis worsens hypokalemia by causing potassium to shift into cells in exchange for hydrogen ions moving out.

4. Magnesium depletion: Thiazides also cause renal magnesium wasting via decreased reabsorption in the thick ascending limb and distal tubule. Low magnesium:

- Impairs renal potassium conservation (affects ROMK channel function)

- Makes hypokalemia refractory to treatment

- Independently causes cardiac arrhythmias

161

5. Cardiac manifestations: Potassium is essential for cardiac action potentials. Hypokalemia:

- Hyperpolarizes cardiac cell membranes (makes resting potential more negative)
- Slows repolarization (prolongs action potential duration → prolonged QT interval)
- Increases automaticity and ectopy → arrhythmias
- Precipitates atrial fibrillation, ventricular arrhythmias, sudden death

The ECG changes (flat T waves, prominent U waves, prolonged QT, ST depression) directly result from altered cardiac repolarization.

6. Neuromuscular manifestations: Hypokalemia causes muscle cell hyperpolarization, making them less excitable. This causes:

- Generalized weakness (especially proximal muscles—difficulty rising from chair)
- Decreased reflexes
- Potentially rhabdomyolysis if severe
- Respiratory muscle weakness if potassium <2.0 mEq/L

7. Renal manifestations: Hypokalemia impairs kidney concentrating ability (nephrogenic diabetes insipidus mechanism), causing polyuria.

8. Risk factors for severe hypokalemia on thiazides:

- High thiazide dose (she's on 50 mg HCTZ—relatively high)
- Poor dietary potassium intake
- Concurrent medications (NSAIDs can worsen by causing volume depletion)
- Not taking potassium supplements
- Not using potassium-sparing diuretic adjunct

Final Diagnosis

Severe hypokalemia (2.1 mEq/L) and hypomagnesemia (1.2 mg/dL) induced by thiazide diuretic therapy, complicated by:

- **Life-threatening cardiac arrhythmias (atrial fibrillation, prolonged QT)**
- **Severe proximal muscle weakness**
- **Metabolic alkalosis**
- **Mild prerenal acute kidney injury**

Treatment and Management

This is a **medical emergency** requiring ICU-level monitoring due to cardiac arrhythmia risk.

Immediate Priorities:

1. Continuous Cardiac Monitoring: Severe hypokalemia can cause sudden cardiac death from ventricular arrhythmias. She needs continuous telemetry monitoring until potassium >3.0 mEq/L.

2. STOP the Thiazide Diuretic: Discontinue hydrochlorothiazide immediately. Continue volume depletion and potassium wasting prevents successful repletion.

3. Aggressive Potassium Replacement:

For severe symptomatic hypokalemia with cardiac arrhythmias:

IV potassium chloride:

- **Central line:** Can give 10-20 mEq/hour (faster replacement via central line to avoid peripheral vein irritation)

- **Peripheral IV:** Maximum 10 mEq/hour (higher concentrations cause phlebitis and pain)

- She receives **20 mEq potassium chloride in 100 mL NS over 1 hour via central line**, repeated hourly

Oral potassium (when able to take PO):

- Potassium chloride 40-80 mEq orally (divided doses)

- Can be combined with IV replacement

Monitoring:

- Check potassium every 2-4 hours during aggressive replacement

- Goal: Increase potassium by 0.3-0.5 mEq/L per hour initially

- Once potassium >3.0 mEq/L, can slow replacement rate

Total body potassium deficit estimation: Very rough estimate: For every 1 mEq/L drop in serum K+ below 3.5, total body deficit is ~200-400 mEq. Her potassium is 2.1, so deficit is ~(3.5-2.1) × 300 = ~420 mEq total body deficit.

However, you can't correct this all at once (dangerous to overcorrect). Replace gradually over 24-48 hours.

4. Magnesium Replacement (CRITICAL):

Must replace magnesium or potassium replacement will fail.

IV magnesium sulfate:

- **2 grams (16 mEq) IV over 15-30 minutes** for symptomatic hypomagnesemia with arrhythmias

- Then **6 grams (48 mEq) IV over 24 hours** as continuous infusion

- OR 2 grams IV every 4-6 hours

She receives 2 grams magnesium sulfate IV push, then 6 grams over 24 hours.

5. Monitor for Complications:

- **Cardiac rhythm continuously** (ventricular arrhythmias, torsades de pointes)
- **Respiratory function** (severe hypokalemia can cause respiratory muscle weakness)
- **Kidney function** (potassium replacement can worsen kidney function if given too fast)
- **Overcorrection** (hyperkalemia from excessive replacement—rare but possible)

6. Address Underlying Hypertension with Alternative Agent:

Once potassium stabilizes, she needs a different antihypertensive. Options:

- **ACE inhibitor or ARB** (actually helps retain potassium—opposite effect of thiazides)
- **Calcium channel blocker** (amlodipine)
- **Beta-blocker** (also helps control atrial fibrillation)
- If diuretic is still needed, use with **potassium-sparing diuretic** (amiloride, triamterene) or aldosterone antagonist (spironolactone)

7. NSAIDs: Consider reducing or discontinuing ibuprofen if possible. NSAIDs can worsen hypertension, cause kidney injury, and contribute to electrolyte abnormalities. Consider alternative pain management (acetaminophen, topical NSAIDs, physical therapy).

Follow-up

Hour 4:

- Potassium: 2.6 mEq/L (improved but still very low)
- Magnesium: 1.8 mg/dL (improved)
- Continues aggressive replacement
- Atrial fibrillation persists but heart rate better controlled
- Muscle strength slightly improved

Hour 12:

- Potassium: 3.2 mEq/L (approaching safe range)
- Magnesium: 2.0 mg/dL (normalized)
- ECG: U waves less prominent, QTc 465 ms (improved)
- Muscle strength improving
- Rate of potassium replacement slowed

Day 2:

- Potassium: 3.8 mEq/L (normalized!)
- Magnesium: 2.1 mg/dL (normal)

- Atrial fibrillation spontaneously converted to normal sinus rhythm overnight (common once potassium normalizes)

- ECG: Normal QT interval, T waves normal, U waves resolved

- Muscle strength nearly back to baseline

- Transitioned to oral potassium supplementation

Day 3:

- Potassium stable at 4.1 mEq/L

- Discharged home on:

  o **Lisinopril 10 mg daily** (ACE inhibitor for hypertension—helps retain potassium)

  o **Potassium chloride 40 mEq daily** for 2 weeks (to fully replete body stores)

  o **Magnesium oxide 400 mg daily**

  o HCTZ permanently discontinued

  o Ibuprofen reduced to lowest effective dose, use acetaminophen when possible

2 Weeks:

- Potassium: 4.3 mEq/L (excellent)

- Magnesium: 2.2 mg/dL (excellent)

- Blood pressure: 128/78 mmHg (controlled on lisinopril)

- No arrhythmias, no muscle weakness

- Potassium supplement discontinued

- Continue lisinopril and magnesium

3 Months:

- Potassium remains normal (4.0-4.5 mEq/L) without supplementation

- Blood pressure well-controlled

- No recurrent arrhythmias

- Full strength and function

- Annual monitoring of electrolytes recommended

Teaching Points

Severe hypokalemia (<2.5 mEq/L) is a medical emergency requiring ICU-level monitoring. Cardiac arrhythmias can be fatal. Continuous telemetry, aggressive replacement, and frequent monitoring (every 2-4 hours initially) are essential. Don't send these patients home from the ED with oral potassium—they need admission.

ECG changes in hypokalemia indicate severity and guide urgency. Mild hypokalemia may show subtle T wave flattening. Severe hypokalemia shows prominent U waves, ST depression, prolonged QT, and arrhythmias. The presence of U waves, prolonged QT, or arrhythmias mandates urgent treatment regardless of the exact potassium level.

Always check magnesium in hypokalemia and replace if low. About 40-60% of hypokalemic patients have concurrent hypomagnesemia. Hypokalemia will NOT correct without magnesium replacement because the kidneys can't retain potassium when magnesium is low. Replace magnesium first or simultaneously with potassium (Huang & Kuo, 2007).

Thiazide diuretics are a leading cause of hypokalemia. Especially with high doses, inadequate dietary potassium, and lack of supplementation. Monitor potassium 1-2 weeks after starting thiazides and every 6-12 months thereafter. Consider potassium-sparing diuretics (amiloride, triamterene, spironolactone) as adjuncts to prevent hypokalemia.

The approach to hypokalemia requires determining the cause. Check urine potassium and assess acid-base status. Renal losses (high urine K+ despite low serum K+) include diuretics and hyperaldosteronism. Extrarenal losses (low urine K+) include vomiting and diarrhea. Metabolic alkalosis + hypokalemia suggests vomiting or diuretics. Metabolic acidosis + hypokalemia suggests diarrhea or RTA.

IV potassium replacement has limits and risks. Maximum peripheral IV rate is 10 mEq/hour (higher causes pain and phlebitis). Central line allows up to 20 mEq/hour for life-threatening hypokalemia with cardiac involvement. Never give IV potassium as bolus—always dilute and infuse slowly. Rapid IV potassium can cause cardiac arrest.

Don't overcorrect potassium. Goal is 3.5-4.5 mEq/L, not >5.0 mEq/L. Overcorrection risks hyperkalemia, which is equally dangerous (cardiac arrest). Replace gradually, monitor frequently, and stop when potassium normalizes. Continue oral supplementation for days-weeks to fully replete total body stores.

ACE inhibitors and ARBs are ideal antihypertensives in patients prone to hypokalemia. They block aldosterone effects, promoting potassium retention. This counteracts the potassium-wasting effects of diuretics. Many patients on thiazides who develop hypokalemia can be switched to ACE inhibitors or ARBs with good blood pressure control and normalization of potassium.

Related Cases

This case connects to:

- **Case 4: The Man with Brown Urine** (rhabdomyolysis—discusses hyperkalemia, opposite problem)

- **Case 1: The Confused Diabetic** (DKA—discusses electrolyte shifts with treatment)

- **Case 3: The Marathon Runner Who Can't Stop Drinking Water** (another electrolyte emergency)

Case 8: The Breathless Diabetic

Clinical Presentation

A 58-year-old man with type 2 diabetes presents to the emergency department with severe shortness of breath that has progressively worsened over the past 6 hours. He's breathing rapidly and deeply, feeling like he "can't get enough air." He also reports nausea, vomiting, and severe generalized weakness.

Three days ago, he developed what he thought was a bad flu—fever, body aches, decreased appetite. He continued taking his metformin even though he wasn't eating much. Yesterday, he noticed his urine output decreased dramatically despite drinking fluids. Today, the breathing difficulty began and rapidly worsened.

His past medical history includes type 2 diabetes (on metformin 1000 mg twice daily for 5 years, generally well-controlled), hypertension, and chronic kidney disease stage 3 (baseline creatinine ~1.8 mg/dL). He takes lisinopril and atorvastatin. He doesn't smoke or drink alcohol.

Physical examination reveals a very ill-appearing man in severe respiratory distress. Vital signs show temperature 38.4°C (101°F), heart rate 115 beats per minute, blood pressure 92/58 mmHg (hypotensive), respiratory rate 32 breaths per minute (tachypnea), oxygen saturation 94% on room air. He's breathing rapidly and deeply (Kussmaul respirations—similar to DKA but this is different). He appears dehydrated with dry mucous membranes and poor skin turgor. His mental status is slightly altered—oriented but lethargic. Lung examination reveals bibasilar crackles. Cardiovascular examination is notable for tachycardia. Abdomen is soft with mild diffuse tenderness. The rest of the examination is unremarkable.

Initial Laboratory Findings

Arterial Blood Gas (ABG):

- **pH: 7.18** (normal: 7.35-7.45) - **SEVERELY LOW** (severe acidosis)
- **pCO2: 18 mmHg** (normal: 35-45 mmHg) - **VERY LOW** (respiratory compensation)
- pO2: 96 mmHg (normal: 80-100 mmHg) - normal
- **HCO3 (bicarbonate): 6 mEq/L** (normal: 22-28 mEq/L) - **VERY LOW**

Chemistry Panel:

- Glucose: 165 mg/dL (normal: 70-100 mg/dL) - elevated but not severely
- Sodium: 136 mEq/L (normal)
- **Potassium: 6.1 mEq/L** (normal: 3.5-5.0 mEq/L) - **ELEVATED**
- Chloride: 102 mEq/L (normal)
- Bicarbonate: 6 mEq/L (matches ABG)
- **BUN: 78 mg/dL** (normal: 7-20 mg/dL) - **MARKEDLY ELEVATED**
- **Creatinine: 5.2 mg/dL** (normal: 0.7-1.3 mg/dL; baseline ~1.8) - **MARKEDLY ELEVATED**
- **Anion gap: 28 mEq/L** (normal: 8-12 mEq/L) - **MARKEDLY ELEVATED**
- **Lactate: 18.4 mmol/L** (normal: 0.5-2.0 mmol/L) - **EXTREMELY ELEVATED**

167

Other Tests:

- **Serum osmolality: 305 mOsm/kg** (normal: 275-295 mOsm/kg) - elevated

- White blood cell count: 18,500/μL (elevated—infection)

- Hemoglobin: 16.2 g/dL (elevated—hemoconcentration from dehydration)

- Platelets: 285,000/μL (normal)

Urine:

- Ketones: **Negative** (important—rules out DKA)

- No glucose, protein, blood, or infection

Stop and Think

This case presents **severe metabolic acidosis** with an **elevated anion gap** and **markedly elevated lactate**. The combination of severe acidosis (pH 7.18), high anion gap (28), and lactate of 18.4 mmol/L confirms **severe lactic acidosis**.

Let's work through the acid-base systematically:

Step 1: pH—Is there acidemia or alkalemia? pH 7.18 = **Severe acidemia** (pH <7.35)

Step 2: Primary disturbance—Respiratory or metabolic?

- Low pH + Low HCO3 (6 mEq/L) = **Metabolic acidosis**

- Low pCO2 (18 mmHg) = Respiratory compensation (hyperventilation to blow off CO2)

Step 3: Anion gap—Is this anion gap or non-anion gap metabolic acidosis? Anion gap = Na - (Cl + HCO3) = 136 - (102 + 6) = **28 mEq/L** (very high, normal 8-12)

This is **high anion gap metabolic acidosis** (HAGMA).

Step 4: Identify the cause using MUDPILES mnemonic:

- M: **Methanol**

- U: **Uremia** (kidney failure—his creatinine is 5.2)

- D: **Diabetic ketoacidosis** (ruled out—no ketones, glucose only 165)

- P: Paraldehyde

- I: Isoniazid, Iron

- L: **Lactic acidosis** (lactate 18.4—this is the cause!)

- E: **Ethylene glycol**

- S: **Salicylates** (aspirin)

The **extremely elevated lactate (18.4 mmol/L)** identifies this as **lactic acidosis**. Normal lactate is 0.5-2.0 mmol/L. Lactate >4 mmol/L is severe; >15 mmol/L is life-threatening.

Step 5: What caused the lactic acidosis?

Lactic acidosis is classified as Type A or Type B:

Type A (tissue hypoxia—most common):

- Shock (septic, cardiogenic, hemorrhagic)
- Severe hypoxemia
- Carbon monoxide poisoning
- Severe anemia

Type B (no tissue hypoxia—metabolic):

- **Metformin** (especially with kidney failure)
- Liver failure
- Malignancy
- Medications (NRTIs, linezolid, propofol)
- Toxins (ethanol, methanol, cyanide)
- Inherited metabolic disorders

This patient has:

- **Metformin use** (1000 mg twice daily)
- **Acute on chronic kidney injury** (creatinine 5.2, baseline 1.8)
- **Recent illness** (viral syndrome)
- **Possible sepsis** (fever, hypotension, elevated WBC)

The combination points to **metformin-associated lactic acidosis (MALA)** precipitated by acute kidney injury and possible sepsis.

Here's what happened: Metformin is renally cleared. With his baseline chronic kidney disease (stage 3), metformin was already accumulating slightly. When he developed an acute illness (likely infection based on fever and elevated WBC), he became dehydrated and developed acute kidney injury (creatinine jumped from 1.8 to 5.2). The failing kidneys couldn't excrete metformin, causing it to accumulate to toxic levels. High metformin levels inhibit cellular respiration and cause massive lactic acid production. The sepsis/infection contributed additional lactate production from tissue hypoxia. The result: severe lactic acidosis with lactate of 18.4 mmol/L (DeFronzo et al., 2016).

Diagnostic Reasoning Questions

How do you approach acid-base disorders systematically?

Use the step-wise approach:

1. Check pH: <7.35 = acidemia, >7.45 = alkalemia

2. Determine primary disturbance:

- Metabolic acidosis: Low pH + Low HCO3

- Metabolic alkalosis: High pH + High HCO3

- Respiratory acidosis: Low pH + High pCO2

- Respiratory alkalosis: High pH + Low pCO2

3. Check for compensation:

- Metabolic acidosis → Respiratory compensation (low pCO2 from hyperventilation)

- Metabolic alkalosis → Respiratory compensation (high pCO2 from hypoventilation)

- Respiratory acidosis → Metabolic compensation (high HCO3—kidneys retain bicarbonate)

- Respiratory alkalosis → Metabolic compensation (low HCO3—kidneys excrete bicarbonate)

Expected compensation formulas:

- Metabolic acidosis: Expected $pCO_2 = 1.5 \times HCO_3 + 8 \ (\pm 2)$

  - For this patient: $1.5 \times 6 + 8 = 17$ mmHg (his pCO2 is 18—appropriate compensation)

- If actual pCO2 differs significantly from expected, there's a mixed disorder

4. If metabolic acidosis, calculate anion gap: Anion gap = Na - (Cl + HCO3)

- Normal: 8-12 mEq/L

- High (>12): MUDPILES causes

- Normal (8-12): GI bicarbonate loss (diarrhea), RTA, or early kidney failure

5. If high anion gap, identify the unmeasured anion: Check lactate, ketones, BUN (uremia), toxicology screen, osmolar gap (for toxic alcohols)

What is metformin-associated lactic acidosis (MALA)?

Metformin is a first-line diabetes medication that improves insulin sensitivity. It's generally safe but has a rare (1-5 per 100,000 patient-years), potentially fatal complication: **lactic acidosis**.

Mechanism: Metformin inhibits mitochondrial complex I in the respiratory chain. This:

- Decreases aerobic respiration

- Increases anaerobic metabolism

- Causes lactate accumulation

At therapeutic levels in patients with normal kidney function, this effect is minimal. However, when metformin accumulates to toxic levels (from kidney failure preventing excretion), massive lactic acidosis develops.

Risk factors for MALA:

- **Kidney disease** (CKD, AKI)—most important risk factor

- Liver disease

- Heart failure

- Sepsis or severe infection

- Contrast dye exposure (causes AKI)

- Alcohol use

- Age >65

- Dehydration

Clinical presentation:

- Severe metabolic acidosis (pH often <7.10)

- Extremely high lactate (often >15 mmol/L)

- Nausea, vomiting, abdominal pain

- Kussmaul respirations (deep, rapid breathing to compensate)

- Altered mental status

- Hypotension, shock

- Mortality 30-50% despite treatment

Why did he continue metformin when sick?

This is a common and dangerous mistake. Patients (and sometimes clinicians) don't realize that metformin should be held during acute illness, especially with:

- Vomiting/diarrhea (causes dehydration → AKI)

- Reduced oral intake

- Fever/infection (risk of sepsis and AKI)

- Any condition causing AKI

"Sick day rules" for diabetics on metformin: **HOLD metformin during acute illness**. Restart only after recovery and normal kidney function confirmed (DeFronzo et al., 2016).

How do you distinguish MALA from other causes of lactic acidosis?

Type A lactic acidosis (tissue hypoxia from shock, hypoxemia):

- Evidence of tissue hypoperfusion (hypotension, cool extremities, decreased urine output)

- Lactate usually 4-10 mmol/L (can be higher in severe shock)

- Treat underlying shock

MALA (metformin accumulation):

- History of metformin use + kidney disease

- Often extremely high lactate (>15 mmol/L)

- pH often <7.10

- May have concurrent Type A component (sepsis)

- Metformin level can be measured (but not readily available, so diagnosis is clinical)

D-lactic acidosis:

- Short bowel syndrome or intestinal bacterial overgrowth

- D-lactate (not measured by standard lactate assays)

- Neurologic symptoms out of proportion to acidosis

Sequential Test Results

Blood Cultures: Positive for **Escherichia coli** (Gram-negative bacterium)—confirms **sepsis** as contributory factor

Chest X-ray: Right lower lobe pneumonia

Repeat Labs (4 hours after presentation):

- pH: 7.14 (worsening despite treatment)

- Lactate: 19.2 mmol/L (worsening)

- Creatinine: 5.8 mg/dL (worsening)

- Potassium: 6.5 mEq/L (worsening—dangerous hyperkalemia)

- Bicarbonate: 5 mEq/L (worsening)

Despite aggressive fluid resuscitation and antibiotics, his acidosis and lactate are worsening. His kidney function is deteriorating, preventing metformin excretion and lactate clearance.

What's Happening Here?

This patient has **metformin-associated lactic acidosis (MALA)** precipitated by:

1. **Acute on chronic kidney injury** (creatinine 5.2, baseline 1.8)

2. **Sepsis** (E. coli bacteremia from pneumonia)

3. **Continued metformin use during acute illness**

The complete pathophysiology:

1. Pre-existing CKD: Baseline creatinine 1.8 mg/dL indicates stage 3 chronic kidney disease (GFR ~40-45 mL/min). At this level, metformin clearance is already reduced, causing mild accumulation.

2. Acute illness triggers cascade:

- Develops pneumonia (E. coli bacteremia)

- Becomes dehydrated from fever, decreased intake

- Develops acute kidney injury superimposed on CKD (creatinine rises to 5.2)

- Continues taking metformin despite being sick

3. Metformin accumulation:

- Kidneys can't excrete metformin

- Blood metformin levels rise dramatically

- Toxic levels inhibit mitochondrial complex I

4. Massive lactate production:

- Cells can't perform aerobic respiration (metformin blocks it)

- Shift to anaerobic metabolism

- Produces massive amounts of lactic acid

- Liver can't clear lactate (also metabolizes metformin—overwhelmed)

- Lactate accumulates to 18.4 mmol/L

5. Sepsis contribution:

- Septic shock causes tissue hypoperfusion

- Hypoperfusion → anaerobic metabolism → more lactate production

- Type A (sepsis) + Type B (metformin) lactic acidosis combined

6. Vicious cycle:

- Severe acidosis impairs cardiac function and vasomotor tone

- Worsening shock → more lactate

- Worsening kidney function → less metformin and lactate clearance

- Acidosis continues worsening despite treatment

7. Life-threatening complications:

- Severe acidosis (pH 7.14) causes cardiovascular collapse

- Hyperkalemia (6.5 mEq/L) from acidosis and kidney failure risks cardiac arrest

- Multi-organ failure develops

Final Diagnosis

Metformin-associated lactic acidosis (MALA) precipitated by:

- **Acute on chronic kidney injury** (AKI on CKD stage 3)

- **Sepsis** (E. coli bacteremia from pneumonia)
- **Continued metformin use during acute illness**

Contributing factors:

- **Severe lactic acidosis** (lactate 18.4-19.2 mmol/L)
- **Life-threatening hyperkalemia** (6.5 mEq/L)
- **Septic shock**

Treatment and Management

This is a **life-threatening emergency** requiring ICU care and likely dialysis.

Immediate Priorities:

1. Discontinue Metformin: Stop immediately (obviously—should have been stopped 3 days ago when illness started).

2. Aggressive Fluid Resuscitation:

- **Normal saline 1-2 liters rapidly** (despite kidney failure risk, he needs volume for shock)
- Goal: Improve tissue perfusion, increase renal clearance if possible
- Monitor for fluid overload (he has AKI, so kidneys won't excrete fluid well)

3. Broad-Spectrum Antibiotics for Sepsis:

- **Ceftriaxone 2g IV + azithromycin** (for community-acquired pneumonia with bacteremia)
- Blood cultures guide antibiotic adjustment
- Source control (treat pneumonia)

4. Treat Hyperkalemia URGENTLY: Potassium 6.5 mEq/L is immediately life-threatening:

- **Calcium gluconate 10% 10 mL IV** (cardiac membrane stabilization)
- **Insulin 10 units IV + D50W 50 mL** (shift K+ into cells)
- **Albuterol nebulizer**
- Consider **sodium bicarbonate** (also helps acidosis, though controversial—see below)

5. Sodium Bicarbonate (CONTROVERSIAL):

For severe metabolic acidosis (pH <7.1), sodium bicarbonate is sometimes given to temporize:

- **150 mEq (3 ampules) in 850 mL D5W, infuse over 1-2 hours**
- Goal: Raise pH to ~7.20 (NOT to normal—just enough to improve cardiac function)

Controversy:

- No proven mortality benefit in acidosis

- Risk of paradoxical intracellular acidosis, sodium overload, hypernatremia

- May worsen lactic acidosis by increasing lactate production

- Generally NOT recommended for lactic acidosis

However, in severe MALA with pH <7.10 and cardiovascular instability, some centers use bicarbonate as a bridge to definitive therapy (hemodialysis).

6. HEMODIALYSIS (DEFINITIVE TREATMENT):

Emergent hemodialysis is the treatment of choice for MALA because it:

- **Removes metformin** (dialyzable)

- **Removes lactate** (dialyzable)

- **Corrects acidosis** (bicarbonate-based dialysate)

- **Removes potassium** (treats hyperkalemia)

- **Treats fluid overload** (if present)

Indications for emergent dialysis in MALA:

- pH <7.10

- Lactate >20 mmol/L

- Refractory shock despite vasopressors

- AKI with oliguria/anuria

- Severe hyperkalemia refractory to medical management

- Failure to improve with supportive care

This patient meets criteria (pH 7.14, lactate 19.2, AKI, hyperkalemia).

Hemodialysis is started within 2 hours of ED presentation.

7. Vasopressors for Shock:

- **Norepinephrine** infusion for hypotension despite fluids

- Goal MAP (mean arterial pressure) >65 mmHg

8. Supportive Care:

- ICU monitoring

- Mechanical ventilation if respiratory failure develops

- Correct electrolytes

- Treat coexisting conditions

Follow-up

Hour 6 (during hemodialysis):

- pH: 7.22 (improving)
- Lactate: 14.8 mmol/L (declining)
- Potassium: 5.1 mEq/L (improving)
- Blood pressure stabilizing on vasopressors

Day 1 (after 8 hours hemodialysis):

- pH: 7.32 (much improved)
- Lactate: 6.2 mmol/L (dramatically improved)
- Bicarbonate: 16 mEq/L (recovering)
- Creatinine: 4.1 mg/dL (improving as AKI resolves)
- Potassium: 4.5 mEq/L (normalized)
- Mental status clearing
- Off vasopressors

Day 3:

- pH: 7.38 (normalized)
- Lactate: 2.1 mmol/L (normalized)
- Creatinine: 2.8 mg/dL (still elevated but improving)
- Blood cultures clearing on antibiotics
- Extubated (was intubated day 1 for airway protection)
- Transferred out of ICU

Day 7:

- Creatinine: 2.0 mg/dL (approaching baseline)
- Pneumonia resolving on antibiotics
- Tolerating regular diet
- Ambulating with assistance
- Ready for discharge

Discharge (Day 10):

- Creatinine: 1.9 mg/dL (near baseline of 1.8)
- All other labs normalized
- Completed antibiotic course for pneumonia

- **Metformin permanently discontinued**
- Started on insulin for diabetes management
- Extensive education provided on:
    - **NEVER restart metformin** (given history of MALA and CKD)
    - Sick day management for diabetes
    - When to hold medications during illness
    - Signs of infection requiring urgent care

3 Months:

- Full recovery
- Creatinine stable at 1.8 mg/dL (back to baseline)
- Diabetes controlled on insulin regimen
- No recurrence of lactic acidosis
- Understanding of medication safety and sick day rules

Prognosis

MALA has high mortality (30-50%) even with appropriate treatment. Survivors often have prolonged ICU stays and may develop permanent kidney damage requiring dialysis.

Factors predicting poor outcome:

- pH <7.0
- Lactate >20-25 mmol/L
- Age >65
- Severe sepsis/shock
- Delayed recognition and treatment
- Inability to perform dialysis

This patient survived because:

- Relatively early recognition (within hours of severe symptoms)
- Aggressive treatment including emergent dialysis
- Appropriate antibiotics for sepsis
- ICU-level supportive care
- Younger age (58) and no severe cardiac disease

Prevention is key:

- Screen for contraindications before prescribing metformin (CKD stage 4-5, liver disease, heart failure)

- Regular monitoring of kidney function (annually, or every 3-6 months in CKD)

- Patient education about sick day rules (HOLD metformin during acute illness)

- Discontinue metformin before procedures involving contrast dye (hold 48 hours before and after)

- Consider alternative diabetes medications in high-risk patients

Teaching Points

Lactic acidosis causes severe metabolic acidosis with markedly elevated anion gap and elevated lactate. Normal lactate is 0.5-2.0 mmol/L. Lactate >4 mmol/L is elevated; >15 mmol/L is life-threatening. The extremely high lactate (>15-20 mmol/L) with severe acidosis (pH <7.10) is characteristic of MALA, distinguishing it from other causes of high anion gap metabolic acidosis.

Approach acid-base disorders systematically using the step-wise method. (1) Check pH (acidemia vs. alkalemia), (2) Determine if primary disturbance is respiratory or metabolic, (3) Check for appropriate compensation, (4) If metabolic acidosis, calculate anion gap, (5) If high anion gap, identify the unmeasured anion using MUDPILES mnemonic plus lactate measurement. This systematic approach prevents diagnostic errors.

MUDPILES mnemonic identifies causes of high anion gap metabolic acidosis. Methanol, Uremia, Diabetic ketoacidosis, Paraldehyde, Isoniazid/Iron, Lactic acidosis, Ethylene glycol, Salicylates. In practice, the most common causes are lactic acidosis, ketoacidosis (diabetic or alcoholic), kidney failure, and toxic ingestions. Always measure lactate and check for ketones when evaluating high anion gap acidosis.

Metformin is contraindicated in moderate-to-severe kidney disease. Current guidelines recommend avoiding metformin when eGFR <30 mL/min (stage 4-5 CKD) and using with caution when eGFR 30-45 mL/min (stage 3b CKD). This patient with CKD stage 3a (eGFR ~40-45) was at borderline risk at baseline, but AKI pushed him into dangerous territory. Regular monitoring of kidney function is essential for patients on metformin (DeFronzo et al., 2016).

Metformin should be held during acute illness. "Sick day rules" for diabetics on metformin: Hold the medication during any acute illness causing dehydration, reduced oral intake, vomiting/diarrhea, or risk of kidney injury. Don't restart until patient recovers and kidney function is confirmed normal. Many cases of MALA are precipitated by continuing metformin during acute illness.

Hemodialysis is the definitive treatment for severe MALA. Metformin and lactate are both dialyzable. Emergent hemodialysis removes accumulated metformin, clears lactate, corrects acidosis, and treats complications (hyperkalemia, fluid overload). Indications for emergent dialysis include pH <7.10, lactate >20 mmol/L, refractory shock, or failure to improve with supportive care. Don't delay dialysis in severe MALA—mortality increases with delayed treatment.

Sodium bicarbonate therapy in lactic acidosis is controversial and not routinely recommended. While bicarbonate raises pH temporarily, it doesn't address the underlying problem (lactate production and impaired clearance). It may worsen outcomes by causing paradoxical intracellular acidosis, sodium/volume overload, and increased lactate production. Most guidelines recommend against routine bicarbonate use. It's sometimes used as a temporizing measure in severe acidosis (pH <7.0-7.1) with cardiovascular instability while arranging definitive treatment (dialysis).

Kussmaul respirations (rapid, deep breathing) indicate metabolic acidosis with respiratory compensation. The body tries to correct metabolic acidosis by hyperventilating to blow off CO2 (creating respiratory alkalosis to offset metabolic acidosis). Kussmaul breathing occurs in DKA, lactic acidosis, uremia, and other causes of severe metabolic acidosis. It's a sign of severe acid-base disturbance requiring urgent evaluation.

Type A lactic acidosis (tissue hypoxia) is more common than Type B (metabolic). Type A results from inadequate oxygen delivery (shock, severe hypoxemia, severe anemia, carbon monoxide poisoning). Type B occurs without tissue hypoxia (metformin, liver failure, malignancy, thiamine deficiency, toxins). This patient had both Type A (sepsis) and Type B (metformin) contributing to his extraordinarily high lactate. Treating the underlying cause is essential—antibiotics and source control for sepsis, dialysis to remove metformin.

Related Cases

This case connects to:

- **Case 1: The Confused Diabetic** (DKA—another diabetes complication with severe metabolic acidosis and high anion gap)

- **Case 4: The Man with Brown Urine** (rhabdomyolysis—discusses acid-base disturbances and kidney injury)

- **Case 14: The Man Who Collapsed at the Gym** (adrenal insufficiency—can cause metabolic acidosis)

Case 9: The Man with Purple Urine

Clinical Presentation

A 32-year-old man presents to the emergency department with severe, cramping abdominal pain that began suddenly 6 hours ago and has progressively worsened. He describes the pain as "the worst pain of my life," rated 10/10, diffuse across his entire abdomen but with no specific location. The pain comes in waves but never completely resolves.

He's also experiencing nausea and has vomited three times. He reports feeling extremely anxious and agitated. Over the past day, he's noticed his urine has turned dark reddish-brown, almost purple, which alarmed him. He denies any trauma, recent illnesses, or new medications.

Interestingly, he mentions having similar episodes of abdominal pain about twice per year for the past 5 years, though never this severe. These episodes usually last 2-3 days and resolve on their own. His doctor previously did extensive workup (CT scans, endoscopy) but never found a cause. He was told it might be "irritable bowel syndrome."

His past medical history is otherwise unremarkable. He takes no regular medications. He occasionally uses ibuprofen. He smoked marijuana last night (first time in months), wondering if that could be related. No family history of similar symptoms, though his father had some kind of "nerve problem" that caused weakness.

Physical examination reveals an anxious, distressed young man writhing in pain. Vital signs show temperature 37.4°C (normal), heart rate 108 beats per minute (tachycardia), blood pressure 152/96 mmHg (hypertension from pain), respiratory rate 20 breaths per minute. Abdominal examination is remarkable for diffuse tenderness without guarding, rebound, or rigidity (suggesting pain is not from peritonitis). Bowel sounds are present but decreased. Neurologic examination reveals mild proximal muscle weakness in his arms and legs. No rashes. The rest of the examination is unremarkable.

Initial Laboratory Findings

Chemistry Panel:

- Glucose: 102 mg/dL (normal)

- **Sodium: 128 mEq/L** (normal: 136-145 mEq/L) - **LOW**

- Potassium: 3.8 mEq/L (normal)

- Chloride: 98 mEq/L (normal)

- Bicarbonate: 24 mEq/L (normal)

- BUN: 18 mg/dL (normal)

- Creatinine: 1.0 mg/dL (normal)

Complete Blood Count:

- Hemoglobin: 14.2 g/dL (normal)

- White blood cell count: 12,500/μL (slightly elevated—stress response)

- Platelet count: 305,000/μL (normal)

Liver Function Tests:

- AST: 42 U/L (normal: 10-40 U/L) - slightly elevated

- ALT: 38 U/L (normal)

- Alkaline phosphatase: 95 U/L (normal)

- Total bilirubin: 1.4 mg/dL (normal: 0.3-1.2 mg/dL) - slightly elevated

- Direct bilirubin: 0.3 mg/dL (normal)

Urinalysis:

- **Color: Dark reddish-brown to purple**

- **Porphobilinogen (PBG): Strongly positive** (special test)

- **Aminolevulinic acid (ALA): Elevated** (special test)

- Protein: Trace

- No blood, no RBCs, no infection

- **Urine darkens further on standing in light** (classic finding)

Imaging:

- CT abdomen/pelvis: No evidence of bowel obstruction, perforation, appendicitis, or other acute pathology. Normal-appearing organs.

Stop and Think

This case presents a diagnostic puzzle that many clinicians miss: severe abdominal pain with negative imaging, psychiatric symptoms, dark/purple urine, mild hyponatremia, and recurrent similar episodes over years. The urine findings are the key—**positive porphobilinogen (PBG)** confirms the diagnosis of **acute intermittent porphyria (AIP).**

Porphyrias are rare inherited disorders of heme biosynthesis. Heme is essential for hemoglobin, cytochrome P450 enzymes, and other proteins. The heme synthesis pathway involves eight enzymatic steps. Deficiency in any enzyme causes accumulation of precursor molecules (porphyrins or porphyrin precursors), which are toxic.

Acute intermittent porphyria (AIP) results from **porphobilinogen deaminase (PBGD) deficiency** (also called hydroxymethylbilane synthase deficiency). This is the third enzyme in the heme synthesis pathway.

Pathophysiology:

1. PBGD enzyme is deficient (50% activity in heterozygotes)

2. During acute attacks, demand for heme increases (from medications, hormones, fasting, stress, infection)

3. Early pathway enzymes (ALA synthase) are upregulated

4. Porphobilinogen (PBG) and aminolevulinic acid (ALA) accumulate

5. These precursors are neurotoxic

6. Causes acute neurovisceral symptoms

Classic triad of AIP:

1. **Abdominal pain** (85-95% of attacks)

2. **Neuropsychiatric symptoms** (anxiety, confusion, hallucinations, seizures)

3. **Peripheral neuropathy** (weakness, paresthesias)

Additional features:

- **Dark/red urine** from porphobilinogen (darkens on standing or light exposure due to polymerization)

- **Hyponatremia** (SIADH is common during attacks)

- **Tachycardia and hypertension** (autonomic dysfunction)

- **Constipation** (from autonomic neuropathy affecting GI motility)

- Recurrent attacks triggered by:

  o Medications (especially cytochrome P450 inducers)

  o Hormonal changes (menstrual cycle, pregnancy, oral contraceptives)

  o Fasting/low-carb diets

  o Alcohol

  o Stress, infection

  o Smoking (including marijuana)

This patient's marijuana use last night may have triggered this attack. Cannabis can precipitate porphyria attacks, though the mechanism isn't fully understood (Bonkovsky et al., 2014).

Diagnostic Reasoning Questions

What are the porphyrias and how are they classified?

Porphyrias are grouped by primary symptom manifestation:

Acute porphyrias (neurovisceral symptoms):

1. **Acute intermittent porphyria (AIP)** - most common acute porphyria

2. Hereditary coproporphyria (HCP)

3. Variegate porphyria (VP)

4. ALA dehydratase deficiency porphyria (very rare)

Cutaneous porphyrias (skin photosensitivity):

1. Porphyria cutanea tarda (PCT) - most common porphyria overall

2. Erythropoietic protoporphyria (EPP)

3. Congenital erythropoietic porphyria (very rare)

Some porphyrias (VP, HCP) cause both acute attacks and skin symptoms.

AIP causes **only neurovisceral symptoms, NO skin involvement**. This distinguishes it from VP and HCP.

How do you diagnose acute porphyria?

During an acute attack:

Urine tests (most important):

- **Spot urine PBG (porphobilinogen):** Markedly elevated (often 50-100× normal)

- **Spot urine ALA (aminolevulinic acid):** Elevated

- **Urine porphyrins:** May be elevated

- Fresh urine may appear normal but turns dark red/brown/purple on standing in light

Positive urine PBG during symptoms is diagnostic of an acute porphyria attack. This is the key screening test.

Between attacks:

- Urine PBG may be normal or only mildly elevated

- **Genetic testing** confirms diagnosis and identifies specific mutation

- **Erythrocyte PBGD enzyme activity:** Reduced to ~50% (but normal in 10-20% of AIP patients due to mutations affecting only hepatic enzyme)

Blood tests during attack:

- Plasma or serum porphyrins: Elevated

- Hyponatremia (SIADH)

- Mild liver enzyme elevations

Why is diagnosis often delayed?

AIP is rare (prevalence ~1 in 20,000) and easily missed because:

- Abdominal pain mimics common surgical emergencies

- Imaging is normal (pain is neurologic, not from structural pathology)

- Psychiatric symptoms lead to psychiatric diagnoses

- Many patients undergo unnecessary surgeries before diagnosis

- Average delay from symptom onset to diagnosis is 15 years!

The key is **thinking of porphyria** when you see unexplained abdominal pain with negative imaging plus neuropsychiatric symptoms, especially with dark urine or recurrent episodes (Bonkovsky et al., 2014).

What triggers acute porphyria attacks?

Medications (most common): Many drugs are porphyrinogenic (induce ALA synthase, increasing heme demand):

- Barbiturates, phenytoin, carbamazepine (strong triggers)

- Sulfonamide antibiotics

- Alcohol

- Some hormones (progesterone, synthetic estrogens)
- Many others (consult porphyria drug database before prescribing)

Hormonal factors:

- Menstrual cycle (attacks often premenstrual)
- Pregnancy
- Oral contraceptives

Nutritional:

- Fasting, low-calorie diets, low-carbohydrate diets
- Increases heme demand as body needs cytochrome P450 for gluconeogenesis

Other:

- Infections
- Stress (physical or emotional)
- Tobacco and cannabis use
- Dehydration

Safe medications in porphyria:

- Acetaminophen, aspirin, NSAIDs (generally safe)
- Penicillins, cephalosporins
- Opioids (needed for pain management)
- Propofol (safe anesthetic)
- Many others

Always check drug safety in porphyria before prescribing: www.porphyriafoundation.org or www.drugs-porphyria.org

Sequential Test Results

Confirmatory Testing:

24-hour Urine Collection:

- **Porphobilinogen (PBG): 385 mg/24h** (normal: <2 mg/24h) - **EXTREMELY ELEVATED**
- **Aminolevulinic acid (ALA): 95 mg/24h** (normal: <7 mg/24h) - **MARKEDLY ELEVATED**
- Total porphyrins: Elevated

Plasma Porphyrins:

- Elevated (consistent with acute porphyria)

Genetic Testing:

- **HMBS (PBGD) gene mutation identified** - confirms hereditary acute intermittent porphyria

- Heterozygous mutation (one normal, one abnormal copy)

Family Testing: His father is tested and found to carry the same HMBS mutation (explaining his "nerve problem"—likely had mild porphyria attacks).

What's Happening Here?

This patient is experiencing an **acute attack of acute intermittent porphyria (AIP),** likely triggered by marijuana use.

The complete pathophysiology:

1. Genetic predisposition: He inherited a mutation in the HMBS gene (encoding porphobilinogen deaminase enzyme) from his father. This enzyme deficiency is present lifelong, but symptoms are intermittent.

2. Trigger (marijuana use): Cannabis use increases heme demand (mechanism not fully clear). With only 50% enzyme activity, the pathway can't keep up. ALA synthase (first enzyme in pathway) gets upregulated to produce more heme.

3. Precursor accumulation: The bottleneck at PBGD enzyme causes porphobilinogen (PBG) and aminolevulinic acid (ALA) to accumulate to toxic levels.

4. Neurotoxic effects: PBG and ALA are directly neurotoxic. They cause:

- **Autonomic neuropathy** → abdominal pain (visceral nerve dysfunction), tachycardia, hypertension, constipation

- **Peripheral motor neuropathy** → muscle weakness (can progress to quadriplegia if severe)

- **Central nervous system effects** → anxiety, confusion, hallucinations, seizures

- **SIADH** → hyponatremia

The **abdominal pain** is visceral neuropathic pain from autonomic nervous system dysfunction, NOT from intra-abdominal pathology. This is why imaging is normal.

5. Dark urine: Porphobilinogen is colorless when freshly excreted but spontaneously polymerizes to form porphyrins (red/brown pigments) on standing, especially with light exposure. This causes the characteristic dark reddish-brown to purple urine.

6. Attack duration: Without treatment, attacks last days to weeks. With treatment (hemin infusion), attacks resolve within days. Untreated severe attacks can cause permanent neurologic damage or death from respiratory paralysis.

7. Between attacks: Patients are often completely asymptomatic between attacks. PBG and ALA levels normalize or remain only mildly elevated.

Final Diagnosis

Acute intermittent porphyria (AIP) with acute neurovisceral attack triggered by cannabis use

Treatment and Management

Acute Attack Management:

1. Discontinue Triggers:

- Stop all potentially porphyrinogenic drugs
- In this case, ensure no further marijuana use

2. High-Dose Glucose (Carbohydrate Loading):

- **Dextrose 10% IV at 300-500 grams/day** (e.g., D10W at 125-200 mL/hour)
- Suppresses ALA synthase (reduces heme precursor production)
- Effective for mild attacks
- Start immediately while arranging hemin

3. Hemin Infusion (Definitive Treatment):

Hemin (Panhematin) 3-4 mg/kg IV daily for 4 days

- Hemin is heme in solution
- Provides exogenous heme, suppressing ALA synthase via negative feedback
- Reduces PBG and ALA production
- Usually causes rapid symptom improvement (within 24-48 hours)
- Must be given through central line or large peripheral vein (causes phlebitis)
- Mix with human albumin to prevent degradation
- Given over 30-60 minutes
- Side effects: Phlebitis, coagulopathy (transient), rare renal toxicity

Indications for hemin:

- Severe or prolonged symptoms
- Progressive neurologic signs (weakness, respiratory compromise)
- Failure to respond to glucose loading within 24-48 hours
- Recurrent attacks

He receives hemin 3 mg/kg IV daily starting on hospital day 1.

4. Aggressive Pain Management: Pain is severe and opioids are needed:

- **Morphine or hydromorphone IV** (safe in porphyria)
- Adequate doses to control pain

186

- Opioids are NOT porphyrinogenic

5. Antiemetics:

- **Ondansetron or promethazine** (safe in porphyria)
- Control nausea/vomiting

6. Treat Hyponatremia (SIADH):

- Usually mild and doesn't require specific treatment
- If severe (<125 mEq/L), fluid restriction
- SIADH resolves as attack resolves

7. Monitor Neurologic Function:

- Serial muscle strength testing
- Respiratory function (vital capacity, negative inspiratory force)
- If weakness progresses, may need mechanical ventilation
- Some patients develop Guillain-Barré-like ascending paralysis

8. Avoid Unsafe Medications:

- No barbiturates, phenytoin, sulfa drugs
- Check porphyria drug database before any new medication
- Use safe anesthetics if surgery needed (propofol is safe)

Prevention of Future Attacks:

1. Patient Education:

- Detailed list of unsafe medications (provide wallet card)
- Avoid fasting, maintain adequate carbohydrate intake
- Avoid alcohol and recreational drugs (including marijuana)
- Manage stress
- Medical alert bracelet

2. For Women with Menstrual-Related Attacks:

- GnRH analogs to suppress menstruation
- Prophylactic hemin infusions

3. For Frequent Attacks:

- Prophylactic weekly hemin infusions
- Liver transplantation (curative but reserved for severe refractory cases)

187

- Gene therapy (experimental)

4. Genetic Counseling:

- Autosomal dominant inheritance
- 50% chance of passing mutation to each child
- Family members should be tested

Follow-up

Day 2 (after first hemin infusion and glucose loading):

- Abdominal pain significantly improved (now 4/10)
- Nausea resolved
- Anxiety much better
- Urine still dark but clearing
- Sodium: 132 mEq/L (improving)

Day 4 (after completing 4 days of hemin):

- Abdominal pain resolved
- Neurologic examination normal
- Urine color normalizing
- PBG level declining
- Ready for discharge

Discharge:

- Extensive education on porphyria triggers and management
- Medical alert bracelet
- Written list of safe/unsafe medications
- Emergency action plan for future attacks (go to ED immediately, bring porphyria card)
- Genetic counseling appointment
- Hematology/porphyria specialist follow-up

Long-term:

- No further marijuana use
- Avoids alcohol and fasting
- Has had two more attacks over next 5 years (triggered by viral infections)
- Each attack treated successfully with hemin

- Now on prophylactic quarterly hemin infusions due to frequent attacks
- Good quality of life between attacks

Teaching Points

Acute intermittent porphyria presents with the triad of abdominal pain, neuropsychiatric symptoms, and peripheral neuropathy. Severe abdominal pain with negative imaging plus psychiatric symptoms should trigger consideration of porphyria. Dark/reddish urine that turns purple on standing is pathognomonic. Hyponatremia from SIADH is common. Think of porphyria in unexplained abdominal pain, especially with recurrent episodes (Bonkovsky et al., 2014).

Urine porphobilinogen (PBG) during an acute attack is the key diagnostic test. Markedly elevated PBG (often 50-100× normal) during symptoms confirms acute porphyria. Fresh urine may appear normal but turns dark on standing in light. Spot urine PBG is a simple screening test. If positive, confirm with 24-hour urine PBG/ALA and genetic testing. Between attacks, PBG may normalize, so test during symptoms.

Many medications trigger porphyria attacks. Barbiturates, anticonvulsants (phenytoin, carbamazepine), sulfa antibiotics, alcohol, and many other drugs induce ALA synthase and precipitate attacks. Before prescribing any medication to a porphyria patient, check drug safety at www.porphyriafoundation.org. Safe options include most penicillins, cephalosporins, acetaminophen, NSAIDs, and opioids.

Hemin infusion is the definitive treatment for acute attacks. Hemin (exogenous heme) suppresses ALA synthase via negative feedback, reducing toxic precursor production. Give hemin 3-4 mg/kg IV daily for 4 days for severe attacks or those not responding to glucose. Most patients improve dramatically within 24-48 hours. Glucose loading (D10W IV) helps mild attacks by also suppressing ALA synthase.

Fasting and low-carbohydrate diets trigger attacks. Caloric restriction and low carbohydrate intake increase heme demand (gluconeogenesis requires cytochrome P450 enzymes). Patients should maintain adequate calorie and carbohydrate intake. High-carbohydrate diet (350+ grams/day) may help prevent attacks. This is one condition where low-carb diets are dangerous.

AIP causes neurologic symptoms without skin involvement. This distinguishes AIP from variegate porphyria and hereditary coproporphyria (which cause both acute attacks and photosensitivity). Porphyria cutanea tarda causes only skin symptoms, no acute attacks. If a patient has photosensitivity, it's not AIP—consider other porphyrias.

Diagnosis is often delayed 10-20 years with patients undergoing unnecessary surgeries. Average time from first symptoms to diagnosis is 15 years. Many patients have exploratory laparotomies for suspected appendicitis or other surgical emergencies before porphyria is considered. Raising awareness among physicians can prevent diagnostic delays and unnecessary interventions.

Acute porphyria is inherited autosomal dominant with incomplete penetrance. About 50% of mutation carriers never have symptoms (latent porphyria). Women are more likely to have attacks than men (hormonal influences). First-degree relatives should undergo genetic testing to identify carriers, who can then avoid triggers even if currently asymptomatic.

Related Cases

This case connects to:

- **Case 3: The Marathon Runner Who Can't Stop Drinking Water** (hyponatremia from SIADH, different cause)

- **Case 14: The Man Who Collapsed at the Gym** (another rare endocrine/metabolic emergency)

- **Case 8: The Breathless Diabetic** (discusses approach to severe metabolic derangements)

Case 10: The Marathon Runner's Collapse

Chief Complaint: "I can't stop cramping"

Sarah, a 28-year-old recreational marathon runner, is brought to the medical tent after collapsing at mile 22. She's conscious but experiencing severe muscle cramps in both legs and appears confused. The temperature is 85°F with high humidity.

Initial Assessment:

- Appears volume depleted

- Muscle fasciculations visible

- Altered mental status

Laboratory Results:

Sodium: 118 mmol/L (136-145)

Potassium: 3.2 mmol/L (3.5-5.0)

Chloride: 82 mmol/L (98-106)

CO2: 22 mmol/L (22-29)

Glucose: 72 mg/dL (70-100)

BUN: 28 mg/dL (7-20)

Creatinine: 1.4 mg/dL (0.6-1.2)

Serum Osmolality: 245 mOsm/kg (280-295)

Urine Sodium: <20 mmol/L

Urine Osmolality: 450 mOsm/kg

The Exercise-Associated Hyponatremia Pattern:

This case illustrates exercise-associated hyponatremia (EAH), a potentially fatal condition affecting endurance athletes. The pathophysiology involves excessive free water intake combined with non-osmotic ADH secretion triggered by exercise stress.

190

Key Diagnostic Features:

1. **Hypotonic hyponatremia** (low sodium with low serum osmolality)

2. **Inappropriately concentrated urine** (urine osmolality >100 despite hypotonicity)

3. **Clinical context** (prolonged endurance exercise)

4. **Volume status assessment critical** (can be hypovolemic, euvolemic, or hypervolemic)

The Tricky Differential:

Many assume marathon runners are always dehydrated, but EAH often results from overhydration. Sarah drank water at every station, following outdated advice to "drink as much as possible." Her kidneys, under the influence of exercise-induced ADH, couldn't excrete the excess water.

Volume Assessment Clues:

- **Hypovolemic EAH**: Elevated BUN/Cr ratio, orthostatic changes

- **Euvolemic EAH**: Normal BUN/Cr, no edema

- **Hypervolemic EAH**: Edema, weight gain from baseline

Sarah shows mild volume depletion (elevated BUN/Cr ratio) despite excessive water intake – she lost sodium through sweat but replaced only water.

Treatment Approach:

The treatment depends critically on symptom severity:

Mild symptoms (fatigue, nausea):

- Fluid restriction

- Oral sodium supplementation

- Monitor closely

Moderate symptoms (confusion, headache):

- 3% hypertonic saline 100 mL bolus

- Can repeat x2 if needed

- Target 4-6 mmol/L increase in first hour

Severe symptoms (seizures, coma):

- 3% hypertonic saline 100 mL over 10 minutes

- Repeat up to twice at 10-minute intervals

- Goal: Increase sodium by 4-6 mmol/L urgently

Critical Safety Points:

Correction speed matters, but context is key:

- Acute hyponatremia (<48 hours) can be corrected quickly

- Chronic hyponatremia requires careful correction (<10-12 mmol/L per 24 hours)

- EAH is always acute – aggressive initial correction is safe and necessary

Sarah received 100 mL of 3% saline with improvement in confusion. Her sodium rose to 123 mmol/L after one hour. She was transitioned to normal saline and oral sodium tablets, with full recovery over 24 hours.

Prevention Pearls:

- Drink to thirst, not on schedule

- Include sodium replacement during prolonged exercise

- Weight gain during race indicates overhydration

- Sports drinks aren't sufficient – sodium content too low

Case 11: The Teenager Who Can't Wake Up

Chief Complaint: "She won't respond to us"

Emma, a 17-year-old high school senior, is brought by ambulance after her parents couldn't wake her for school. They found an empty bottle of extra-strength acetaminophen in her room. She had seemed stressed about college applications but hadn't expressed suicidal thoughts.

Presentation Timeline:

- Last seen normal: 10 PM previous night

- Found unconscious: 7 AM (9 hours later)

- Arrives at ED: 8 AM (10 hours post-presumed ingestion)

Initial Laboratory Results:

Acetaminophen level: 180 μg/mL (therapeutic: 10-30)

Time since ingestion: ~10 hours (estimated)

AST: 92 U/L (10-40)

ALT: 88 U/L (10-40)

Total Bilirubin: 1.2 mg/dL (0.2-1.0)

PT/INR: 13.8 sec / 1.2 (11-13 sec / 0.8-1.1)

Basic Metabolic Panel:

Glucose: 68 mg/dL (70-100)

BUN: 18 mg/dL (7-20)

Creatinine: 0.9 mg/dL (0.6-1.2)

pH: 7.32 (7.35-7.45)

Lactate: 2.8 mmol/L (0.5-2.0)

The Rumack-Matthew Nomogram Challenge:

The Rumack-Matthew nomogram guides treatment decisions but requires known ingestion time. With uncertain timing, we must think differently.

If ingestion was 10 hours ago:

- Level of 180 µg/mL is well above treatment line (~140 at 10 hours)

- Indicates significant toxicity

- N-acetylcysteine (NAC) must start immediately

But what if ingestion was earlier?

- 16 hours ago: Still above treatment line

- 20 hours ago: Catastrophically high

- The further back, the worse the prognosis

Evolving Hepatotoxicity Stages:

Stage I (0-24 hours):

- Nausea, vomiting, malaise

- Labs often normal initially

- This is the critical treatment window

Stage II (24-48 hours):

- Clinical improvement (the "honeymoon period")

- Rising transaminases

- PT/INR begins prolonging

Stage III (48-96 hours):

- Fulminant hepatic failure

- AST/ALT can exceed 10,000

- Coagulopathy, encephalopathy, renal failure
- Death or transplant without treatment

Stage IV (4 days-2 weeks):

- Recovery if patient survives
- Complete resolution usual if treated early

Emma is in late Stage I/early Stage II – liver enzymes rising, mild coagulopathy starting.

Laboratory Monitoring Protocol:

Initial and every 12-24 hours:

- Acetaminophen level (until undetectable)
- AST, ALT, bilirubin
- PT/INR
- Creatinine
- Glucose
- Phosphate (marker of severe toxicity)
- Lactate
- Blood gas if acidotic

Treatment Beyond NAC:

While NAC is life-saving, comprehensive management includes:

NAC protocol:

- Loading dose: 150 mg/kg over 1 hour
- Second dose: 50 mg/kg over 4 hours
- Third dose: 100 mg/kg over 16 hours
- Continue if liver injury evident

Supportive care:

- Glucose for hypoglycemia
- Vitamin K for coagulopathy
- Consider activated charcoal if <4 hours
- Transplant evaluation if fulminant failure develops

Prognostic Indicators – The King's College Criteria:

Poor prognosis if:

- pH <7.3 after fluid resuscitation
- OR all three of:
  - PT >100 seconds (INR >6.5)
  - Creatinine >3.4 mg/dL
  - Grade III/IV encephalopathy

Emma's early treatment with NAC led to complete recovery. Her transaminases peaked at AST 2,100, ALT 2,400 on day 3, with full normalization by day 10. The psychiatric team addressed her underlying depression.

Critical Pearls:

- "Therapeutic" acetaminophen levels can be toxic with chronic use
- Fasting, alcohol use, and malnutrition deplete glutathione, increasing toxicity
- Massive ingestion (>30 grams) may require extended NAC treatment
- Check acetaminophen level in all intentional overdoses – often unreported

---

Case 12: The Executive's Hidden Disease

Chief Complaint: "I need my physical form signed"

Robert, a 52-year-old bank executive, comes for his annual physical required for life insurance. He mentions feeling more tired lately but attributes it to long work hours. He admits to "a few drinks" most evenings to unwind.

Physical Examination:

- Spider angiomas on chest
- Palmar erythema
- No asterixis
- Slight hepatomegaly

Comprehensive Metabolic Panel:

Glucose: 108 mg/dL (70-100)

BUN: 8 mg/dL (7-20)

Creatinine: 0.7 mg/dL (0.7-1.3)

Sodium: 138 mmol/L (136-145)

Potassium: 3.6 mmol/L (3.5-5.0)

Chloride: 102 mmol/L (98-106)

CO2: 24 mmol/L (22-29)

Liver Function Tests:

AST: 124 U/L (10-40)

ALT: 52 U/L (10-40)

ALP: 142 U/L (40-120)

Total Bilirubin: 2.1 mg/dL (0.2-1.0)

Direct Bilirubin: 0.8 mg/dL (0.0-0.3)

Albumin: 3.2 g/dL (3.5-5.0)

Total Protein: 7.8 g/dL (6.3-8.2)

Additional Tests:

GGT: 186 U/L (5-55)

PT/INR: 14.8 sec / 1.4

MCV: 104 fL (80-100)

The AST:ALT Ratio Story:

The 2:1 AST:ALT ratio (124:52 = 2.4) screams alcohol-related liver disease. This pattern occurs because:

1. **Alcohol directly damages mitochondria** (where AST concentrates)

2. **Alcohol depletes pyridoxal phosphate** (cofactor for ALT > AST)

3. **AST has longer half-life** when released from damaged hepatocytes

Classic Patterns:

- **AST:ALT >2:1**: Alcoholic liver disease (70-80% specific)

- **AST:ALT <1**: Viral hepatitis, NAFLD

- **Both massively elevated**: Acute hepatic necrosis

Supporting Laboratory Evidence:

The complete picture reveals chronic alcohol abuse:

Direct markers:

- **Elevated GGT** (186): Induced by alcohol, sensitive but not specific

196

- **Macrocytosis** (MCV 104): Direct toxic effect on RBC maturation
- **AST:ALT ratio >2**: Classic for alcoholic hepatitis

Indirect markers suggesting advanced disease:

- **Hypoalbuminemia** (3.2): Decreased synthetic function
- **Elevated INR** (1.4): Impaired coagulation factor synthesis
- **Hyperbilirubinemia** (2.1): Mixed pattern suggesting hepatocellular dysfunction
- **Low BUN** (8): Decreased hepatic urea synthesis

Staging the Disease – Child-Pugh Score:

Parameter	1 Point	2 Points	3 Points	Robert's Score
Bilirubin	<2	2-3	>3	2 points
Albumin	>3.5	2.8-3.5	<2.8	2 points
INR	<1.7	1.7-2.3	>2.3	1 point
Ascites	None	Mild	Moderate	1 point
Encephalopathy	None	Grade I-II	Grade III-IV	1 point

Total: 7 points = Child-Pugh B (moderate disease)

MELD Score Calculation:

$$MELD = 3.78 \times \ln(bilirubin) + 11.2 \times \ln(INR) + 9.57 \times \ln(creatinine) + 6.43$$

$$Robert's\ MELD = 3.78 \times \ln(2.1) + 11.2 \times \ln(1.4) + 9.57 \times \ln(0.7) + 6.43 = 10$$

This indicates 6% three-month mortality – significant but not requiring immediate transplant evaluation.

Additional Testing Reveals:

Hepatitis Panel: Negative

Iron Studies:

  Ferritin: 428 ng/mL (20-250)

  Transferrin Saturation: 38% (20-50%)

Alpha-fetoprotein: 8 ng/mL (<10)

Ceruloplasmin: Normal

Alpha-1 antitrypsin: Normal

Calculated Values:

AST/Platelet Ratio Index (APRI): 1.8 (>1 suggests significant fibrosis)

FIB-4 Score: 3.2 (>3.25 suggests advanced fibrosis)

The Complete Diagnosis:

Robert has alcoholic liver disease with evidence of:

1. Active alcoholic hepatitis (AST:ALT ratio, elevated GGT)

2. Cirrhosis (low albumin, elevated INR, elevated APRI/FIB-4)

3. Portal hypertension (spider angiomas, low platelets implied by APRI)

4. No evidence of hepatocellular carcinoma (normal AFP)

Management Based on Laboratory Values:

Immediate interventions:

- Alcohol cessation counseling

- Thiamine, folate supplementation

- Monitor for alcohol withdrawal

Ongoing monitoring every 3-6 months:

- Liver function tests

- CBC (watch for thrombocytopenia)

- Alpha-fetoprotein (HCC screening)

- Ultrasound every 6 months

Robert's case illustrates how routine laboratory tests can unmask serious disease in "healthy" executives seeking routine clearance.

Case 13: The Construction Worker's Mysterious Weakness

Chief Complaint: "I keep dropping my tools"

Carlos, a 45-year-old construction worker, presents with three weeks of progressive weakness. He's been dropping tools, struggling to climb ladders, and his wife notes his voice sounds different. He takes lisinopril for hypertension and recently started spironolactone for resistant hypertension.

Vital Signs:

- BP: 165/95 (on medications)

- Heart rate: 52 bpm, regular

- Respiratory rate: 14

Initial Laboratory Results:

Sodium: 140 mmol/L (136-145)

Potassium: 6.9 mmol/L (3.5-5.0) - CRITICAL

Chloride: 108 mmol/L (98-106)

CO_2: 18 mmol/L (22-29)

BUN: 45 mg/dL (7-20)

Creatinine: 2.3 mg/dL (0.7-1.3)

Glucose: 98 mg/dL (70-100)

Baseline creatinine (6 months ago): 1.2 mg/dL

Immediate EKG Findings:

- Peaked T waves
- Prolonged PR interval
- Widened QRS (118 ms)
- Bradycardia

The Hyperkalemia Emergency:

Potassium of 6.9 mmol/L with EKG changes represents a cardiac emergency. The progression of EKG changes with rising potassium:

1. **5.5-6.5**: Peaked T waves
2. **6.5-7.5**: PR prolongation, P wave flattening
3. **7.0-8.0**: QRS widening
4. **>8.0**: Sine wave pattern → cardiac arrest

Carlos shows changes suggesting K+ actually >7.0 despite lab value of 6.9.

The Perfect Storm – Multiple Hits:

Carlos developed hyperkalemia through multiple mechanisms:

1. **Decreased renal excretion**:
   - Acute on chronic kidney disease (Cr 1.2 → 2.3)
   - Lisinopril (blocks aldosterone via ACE inhibition)
   - Spironolactone (direct aldosterone antagonist)

2. **Possible cellular shift**:

  o Metabolic acidosis (low CO_2)

Pseudohyperkalemia Checklist:

Before treating, quickly verify this is real:

- No hemolysis noted on sample

- No severe leukocytosis (>100,000)

- No severe thrombocytosis (>1,000,000)

- EKG changes confirm true hyperkalemia

Emergency Treatment Sequence:

Priority 1 - Cardiac Protection (0-5 minutes):

Calcium gluconate 10% 10 mL IV over 2-3 minutes

- Stabilizes cardiac membranes

- Works in 1-3 minutes

- Lasts 30-60 minutes

- Can repeat if EKG doesn't improve

- Does NOT lower potassium

Priority 2 - Shift Potassium Intracellularly (5-30 minutes):

1. Regular insulin 10 units IV + Dextrose 50% 25g IV

  - Onset: 10-20 minutes

  - Lowers K+ by 0.5-1.5 mmol/L

  - Monitor glucose hourly x4

2. Albuterol 10-20 mg nebulized

  - Onset: 30 minutes

  - Lowers K+ by 0.5-1.0 mmol/L

  - Additive with insulin

3. Sodium bicarbonate 50 mEq IV (if acidotic)

  - Only effective if pH <7.35

  - Controversial benefit

Priority 3 - Remove Potassium from Body (30+ minutes):

1. Furosemide 40-80 mg IV (if making urine)

2. Sodium polystyrene sulfonate 15-30g PO/PR

   - Slow onset (2-6 hours)

   - Risk of intestinal necrosis

3. Hemodialysis if:

   - K+ >7.0 with refractory EKG changes

   - Anuric

   - Failed medical management

Laboratory Monitoring During Treatment:

- Potassium every 2 hours until <5.5

- Glucose hourly x4 after insulin

- Basic metabolic panel every 4 hours

- Continuous cardiac monitoring

Carlos's Response:

After calcium and insulin/glucose:

- EKG normalized in 15 minutes

- K+ decreased to 5.8 after 2 hours

- Medications adjusted: stopped spironolactone, reduced lisinopril

- Nephrology consulted for CKD management

Preventing Recurrence:

1. **Medication review**: Avoid K-sparing diuretics with ACE/ARB

2. **Dietary counseling**: Low potassium diet

3. **Laboratory monitoring**: Check K+ within 1 week of medication changes

4. **Patient education**: Recognize weakness as warning sign

Case 14: The Bruising Librarian

Chief Complaint: "I bruise when someone looks at me"

Patricia, a 68-year-old librarian, comes in covered with bruises. She's noticed increasing bruising over three months, bleeding gums when brushing teeth, and prolonged bleeding from paper cuts. She takes warfarin for atrial fibrillation but swears she hasn't changed her dose.

Physical Examination:

- Multiple ecchymoses at various stages

- Petechiae on lower extremities

- No hepatosplenomegaly

- No lymphadenopathy

Coagulation Cascade Testing:

PT: 42 seconds (11-13) - CRITICAL

INR: 4.8 (goal 2-3 for AFib)

aPTT: 38 seconds (25-35)

Platelet count: 189,000/μL (150,000-400,000)

Mixing Study (1:1 with normal plasma):

PT immediately: 14 seconds (corrects)

PT after 2-hour incubation: 13 seconds (remains corrected)

Factor Levels:

Factor II: 18% (70-120%)

Factor VII: 12% (70-120%)

Factor IX: 82% (70-120%)

Factor X: 22% (70-120%)

Decoding the Coagulation Results:

The pattern tells a specific story:

1. **Prolonged PT, normal/mildly elevated aPTT** = Extrinsic pathway problem

2. **Mixing study corrects** = Factor deficiency (not inhibitor)

3. **Factors II, VII, X low; IX normal** = Vitamin K deficiency or warfarin effect

This is classic warfarin pattern, but why the sudden change?

The Dietary History Detective Work:

"What's different in the last three months?"

Patricia reveals she started a "health kick" after her friend's heart attack:

- Eliminated leafy greens ("too much vitamin K interferes with warfarin")
- Started CoQ10 supplement
- Began drinking green tea (stopped 2 weeks ago)
- Started antibiotics for UTI 1 week ago

The Warfarin Perfect Storm:

Multiple factors conspired to increase her INR:

1. **Antibiotic effect** (most likely culprit):
   - Killed gut bacteria that produce vitamin K
   - Possible drug interaction

2. **Dietary vitamin K depletion**:
   - Avoided vitamin K foods
   - Paradoxically increased warfarin sensitivity

3. **Supplement interactions**:
   - Green tea (stopped) was actually protecting her

Understanding Vitamin K-Dependent Factors:

The "1972" rule for vitamin K-dependent factors:

- Factors II, VII, IX, X (2, 7, 9, 10 = "1972")
- Protein C and S

Warfarin blocks vitamin K epoxide reductase, preventing activation of these factors.

Factor Half-Lives Explain the Timeline:

Factor   Half-Life Clinical Effect

Factor VII 6 hours   First to drop, PT prolongs first

Factor IX 24 hours   aPTT affected later

Factor X   48 hours   Common pathway affected

Factor II 72 hours   Last to normalize

This explains why:

- PT is more sensitive to warfarin (Factor VII drops first)

203

- Effects persist days after stopping warfarin
- Vitamin K takes time to work

Management Based on INR and Bleeding:

INR 4-5, no bleeding:

- Hold warfarin 1-2 doses
- Reduce weekly dose by 10-20%

INR 5-9, no significant bleeding:

- Hold warfarin
- Consider vitamin K 1-2.5 mg PO

INR >9 or any serious bleeding:

- Hold warfarin
- Vitamin K 5-10 mg IV slowly
- Consider fresh frozen plasma or PCC if life-threatening

Patricia's Management:

Given INR 4.8 with minor bleeding:

1. Held warfarin x2 days
2. Vitamin K 2 mg PO
3. Completed antibiotic course
4. Counseled on consistent vitamin K intake

Follow-up Laboratory Monitoring:

- Day 3: INR 2.8
- Week 1: INR 2.4 (resumed warfarin at lower dose)
- Week 2: INR 2.2 (therapeutic)

Critical Warfarin Pearls:

1. **Consistent vitamin K intake > Low vitamin K intake**
2. **Check INR within 3-5 days of any medication change**
3. **Antibiotics are common culprits for INR changes**
4. **"Natural" doesn't mean "safe" with warfarin**
5.

Case 15: The Anxious Teacher's Racing Heart

Chief Complaint: "My heart won't stop pounding"

Jennifer, a 34-year-old elementary teacher, presents with six months of palpitations, 20-pound weight loss despite increased appetite, tremors, and anxiety. She's been told she has "anxiety from job stress" and prescribed lorazepam, which hasn't helped.

Vital Signs:

- Heart rate: 118 bpm, irregularly irregular
- BP: 148/72 mmHg
- Temperature: 37.8°C (100°F)
- BMI: 19 (was 23 six months ago)

Physical Examination:

- Exophthalmos
- Lid lag
- Fine tremor
- Smooth, diffuse goiter
- Warm, moist skin
- Hyperactive reflexes

Thyroid Function Cascade:

TSH: <0.01 mIU/L (0.4-4.0) - CRITICAL LOW

Free T4: 4.8 ng/dL (0.8-1.8)

Free T3: 8.2 pg/mL (2.3-4.2)

The TSH-First Algorithm:

TSH is the most sensitive thyroid test because of the negative feedback loop:

- Small increases in thyroid hormone → Large decreases in TSH
- The pituitary is exquisitely sensitive to thyroid hormone changes

TSH Interpretation Framework:

- **<0.1**: Overt hyperthyroidism or suppression
- **0.1-0.4**: Subclinical hyperthyroidism or normal variant
- **0.4-4.0**: Normal (some say 0.4-2.5 optimal)

- **4.0-10**: Subclinical hypothyroidism
- **>10**: Overt hypothyroidism

Determining the Cause - Additional Testing:

TSH Receptor Antibodies (TRAb): 18 IU/L (<1.75)

Thyroid Peroxidase Antibodies (TPO): 89 IU/mL (<35)

Thyroglobulin Antibodies: 45 IU/mL (<40)

Thyroid Uptake Scan:

- Diffuse increased uptake (45% at 24 hours, normal 10-30%)

- No cold or hot nodules

Diagnosis: Graves' Disease

The antibody pattern confirms autoimmune hyperthyroidism:

- **TRAb positive**: Pathognomonic for Graves'
- **TPO positive**: General thyroid autoimmunity
- **Diffuse uptake**: Entire gland is hyperactive

Differentiating Causes of Hyperthyroidism:

Condition	TSH	FT4/FT3	Uptake Scan	TRAb
Graves' Disease	↓↓	↑↑	Diffuse ↑	Positive
Toxic Multinodular Goiter	↓↓	↑	Patchy ↑	Negative
Toxic Adenoma	↓↓	↑	Single hot nodule	Negative
Thyroiditis	↓↓	↑	↓ or absent	Negative
Factitious	↓↓	↑	↓	Negative

Additional Laboratory Abnormalities in Hyperthyroidism:

Complete Blood Count:

- WBC: 3,800/μL (mild leukopenia)

- Hemoglobin: 11.2 g/dL (mild anemia)

Comprehensive Metabolic Panel:

- Calcium: 10.8 mg/dL (8.5-10.5) - mild elevation

- Alkaline Phosphatase: 142 U/L (40-120) - bone turnover

- ALT: 68 U/L (10-40) - thyroid hepatopathy

- Glucose: 118 mg/dL (70-100) - increased gluconeogenesis

Lipid Panel:

- Total Cholesterol: 112 mg/dL (paradoxically low)

- LDL: 58 mg/dL

- HDL: 42 mg/dL

The Cardiovascular Connection:

Thyroid hormone effects on the heart:

- Increases heart rate and contractility

- Decreases systemic vascular resistance

- Can cause atrial fibrillation (10-25% of hyperthyroid patients)

- Risk of high-output heart failure if untreated

Jennifer's EKG shows atrial fibrillation with rapid ventricular response.

Treatment Monitoring:

Baseline before starting methimazole:

- CBC with differential (watch for agranulocytosis)

- Liver function tests (hepatotoxicity risk)

- Beta-hCG (teratogenic medication)

After starting treatment:

Week 2: CBC

Week 4: TSH, FT4, CBC, LFTs

Week 8: TSH, FT4

Then every 4-12 weeks until euthyroid

The Agranulocytosis Warning:

Methimazole's most feared side effect occurs in 0.3%:

- Usually within first 3 months

- Presents with fever, sore throat

- Absolute neutrophil count <500
- Requires immediate drug discontinuation

Jennifer was instructed: "If you develop fever or sore throat, stop the medication and get a CBC immediately."

Treatment Response Timeline:

- Week 4: FT4 normalizes, TSH still suppressed
- Week 8: Symptoms improving, heart rate controlled
- Month 3: TSH 0.2, FT4 normal (TSH lags behind)
- Month 6: TSH 1.8, FT4 normal (biochemical remission)

Long-term Monitoring Reveals:

After 18 months of treatment, attempting to taper methimazole:

TSH: 0.08 mIU/L

FT4: 1.9 ng/dL (upper normal)

TRAb: 14 IU/L (still positive)

High TRAb predicts relapse. Jennifer opted for radioactive iodine ablation.

Post-Ablation Monitoring:

- TSH and FT4 every 4-6 weeks
- 80% become hypothyroid within 1 year
- Requires lifelong levothyroxine replacement
- Monitor for Graves' ophthalmopathy worsening
-

Summary: What These 15 Cases Teach Us

Through these comprehensive chemistry cases, we've explored the full spectrum of laboratory medicine's diagnostic power:

Critical Values Recognition:

- Potassium 6.9: Immediate cardiac threat requiring staged intervention
- INR 4.8: Bleeding risk requiring vitamin K and warfarin adjustment
- Sodium 118: Symptomatic hyponatremia needing controlled correction
- TSH <0.01: Thyrotoxicosis requiring prompt treatment

Pattern Recognition Mastery:

- AST:ALT ratio >2:1 pointing to alcoholic liver disease

- Vitamin K-dependent factor deficiency indicating warfarin effect

- Hypotonic hyponatremia with concentrated urine suggesting SIADH

- TRAb positivity confirming Graves' disease

Clinical Context Integration:

- Marathon runner's hyponatremia differs from chronic SIADH

- Acetaminophen timing changes treatment urgency

- Multiple medications creating hyperkalemia perfect storm

- Dietary changes affecting warfarin stability

Laboratory Monitoring Strategies:

- Serial acetaminophen levels guiding NAC duration

- Factor half-lives explaining warfarin reversal timeline

- TSH lag phenomenon in hyperthyroidism treatment

- CBC surveillance for methimazole agranulocytosis

These cases emphasize that **laboratory values never exist in isolation**. Each result must be interpreted within the complete clinical picture - the patient's symptoms, medications, timing, and trajectory. A sodium of 120 might require emergent hypertonic saline in a seizing patient or gentle fluid restriction in an asymptomatic one. An INR of 4.8 might need reversal with vitamin K and plasma, or just holding warfarin depending on bleeding status.

Most importantly, these cases demonstrate that **laboratory medicine is dynamic**. Values change, patterns evolve, and our interpretation must adapt accordingly. The AST that's double the ALT today might reverse tomorrow. The critically low sodium requiring ICU admission might become chronically stable at 125 next month. The suppressed TSH might take months to recover even after thyroid hormones normalize.

Master these patterns, understand these principles, and you'll transform from someone who reports laboratory values to someone who interprets their clinical significance. That's the difference between a technician and a true laboratory medicine professional.

What You've Learned from Chemistry Cases

You've worked through 15 diverse chemistry and metabolic disorder cases covering:

- **Metabolic emergencies**: DKA, hyponatremia, rhabdomyolysis

- **Electrolyte disorders**: hypercalcemia, hypokalemia, hyperkalemia

- **Endocrine diseases**: hypothyroidism, Cushing's syndrome, adrenal insufficiency

- **Liver and biliary disease**: obstructive jaundice patterns

- **Kidney injury**: prerenal, intrinsic (ATN), diagnostic approach

- **Acid-base disturbances**: metabolic acidosis, lactic acidosis

- **Lipid disorders**: severe hypertriglyceridemia, metabolic syndrome

- **Tumor markers**: principles, interpretation, clinical use

The systematic approach to chemistry cases you've developed—identifying primary abnormalities, determining mechanisms, looking for patterns, considering clinical context—will serve you throughout your career in laboratory medicine.

Bringing It All Together

You've now completed three intensive chapters covering 30 complex cases across hematology and clinical chemistry. Each case taught specific diagnostic skills, but more importantly, you've developed broader competencies that transfer across all laboratory disciplines.

Pattern recognition has become instinctive. You now see microcytic anemia and immediately think iron deficiency versus thalassemia. Severe hyperglycemia with metabolic acidosis triggers "DKA" before you even check ketones. Cholestatic liver enzyme patterns point you toward biliary obstruction. These automatic associations—developed through repeated exposure to cases—will accelerate your real-world diagnostic process.

Systematic thinking has replaced guesswork. When faced with hyponatremia, you don't panic or randomly order tests. You check osmolality, assess volume status, measure urine sodium and osmolality, and systematically narrow the differential. When you see elevated calcium, you immediately measure PTH to distinguish hyperparathyroidism from other causes. This structured approach prevents diagnostic errors and unnecessary testing.

Clinical context has become second nature. You've learned that laboratory values never exist in isolation. A glucose of 485 mg/dL means something very different in a known diabetic who stopped insulin versus a previously healthy person. A hemoglobin of 10 g/dL is concerning in a man but might be baseline for someone with hereditary spherocytosis. Age, medications, symptoms, family history, and clinical presentation all influence interpretation.

You understand mechanisms, not just facts. You know *why* DKA causes hyperkalemia (acidosis shifts potassium out of cells) and *why* that reverses with treatment (insulin drives potassium back into cells). You understand *why* rhabdomyolysis causes hypocalcemia initially (calcium deposits in damaged muscle) and *why* aggressive calcium replacement is dangerous (risk of rebound hypercalcemia). This mechanistic understanding helps you anticipate complications and explain findings that don't fit textbook patterns.

You've developed clinical judgment about urgency. Not every abnormal lab requires emergency intervention. Mild chronic anemia in thalassemia trait needs education, not transfusion. Mild hypercalcemia from hyperparathyroidism can be worked up outpatient. But severe symptomatic hyponatremia, hyperkalemia with ECG changes, and DKA with pH <7.0 are true emergencies requiring immediate action. You've learned to distinguish "abnormal but stable" from "abnormal and life-threatening."

You appreciate the limits of laboratory testing. No test is perfect. False positives and false negatives occur. Pseudohyponatremia from lab artifact mimics true hyponatremia. Pseudothrombocytopenia from platelet clumping falsely suggests thrombocytopenia. Elevated PSA doesn't always mean prostate cancer. You've learned to correlate laboratory findings with clinical presentation, repeat unexpected results, and use confirmatory testing appropriately.

You've seen how one abnormality cascades into others. Severe hyperglycemia in DKA causes osmotic diuresis, which causes dehydration, which causes prerenal kidney injury, which impairs electrolyte excretion, which causes hyperkalemia and other electrolyte derangements. Understanding these cascades helps you anticipate complications and order appropriate monitoring tests.

You've learned that treatment affects lab results. PTH testing during acute hypercalcemia gives different information than PTH tested weeks later. Protein C and protein S assays are unreliable during acute thrombosis or anticoagulation. Potassium levels fluctuate rapidly during DKA treatment. Timing matters. You've learned when to test, when to retest, and how to interpret results in the context of ongoing treatment.

You understand the difference between screening and diagnostic testing. TSH screens for thyroid disease in asymptomatic people. Once thyroid dysfunction is suspected, you add free T4, free T3, and thyroid antibodies for diagnosis and classification. Hemoglobin A1c screens for diabetes but glucose and oral glucose tolerance tests diagnose it. Tumor markers like PSA are controversial for screening but valuable for monitoring known cancer. Each test has appropriate and inappropriate uses.

You've learned to communicate results effectively. Critical values (potassium 6.8 mEq/L, hemoglobin 5.2 g/dL, sodium 118 mEq/L) require immediate phone calls to clinicians. Incidental findings (mild anemia, borderline glucose) can be reported routinely. Your role includes not just generating accurate numbers but ensuring clinicians understand what those numbers mean and what action is needed.

Common Threads Across Cases

Several principles emerged repeatedly across these cases:

Electrolyte disturbances affect multiple organ systems. Hyponatremia causes neurologic symptoms. Hyperkalemia causes cardiac arrhythmias. Hypocalcemia causes neuromuscular irritability. Electrolytes aren't just chemistry values—they're essential for cellular function throughout the body. Understanding their physiologic roles helps you predict clinical manifestations.

Endocrine disorders often present with vague, nonspecific symptoms. Fatigue, weakness, weight changes, mood disturbances—these could be anything. But when you find abnormal thyroid function, cortisol levels, or parathyroid hormone, suddenly those vague symptoms make sense. Laboratory testing often provides the key to diagnosing endocrine disease that clinical examination alone would miss.

Many conditions present with anemia, but the MCV guides your differential. Microcytic anemia (low MCV): iron deficiency, thalassemia, anemia of chronic disease. Normocytic anemia (normal MCV): acute blood loss, hemolysis, kidney disease, bone marrow disorders. Macrocytic anemia (high MCV): B12/folate deficiency, liver disease, hypothyroidism, myelodysplastic syndrome. This simple categorization narrows your differential immediately.

The kidney affects and is affected by many conditions. Dehydration from DKA causes prerenal AKI. Rhabdomyolysis causes intrinsic AKI (acute tubular necrosis). Hypercalcemia impairs kidney concentrating ability. Kidney failure causes hyperkalemia, metabolic acidosis, anemia, and hyperphosphatemia. The kidney is the great integrator—it responds to systemic disease and its dysfunction affects multiple systems.

Acid-base disorders follow predictable compensatory patterns. Metabolic acidosis (low pH, low HCO_3) triggers respiratory compensation (hyperventilation to lower CO_2). Respiratory acidosis (low pH, high CO_2) triggers metabolic compensation (kidneys retain HCO_3). Understanding these relationships helps you distinguish primary disorders from compensatory responses and identify mixed acid-base disturbances.

Malignancy presents in myriad ways. Pancreatic cancer causes obstructive jaundice. Multiple myeloma causes hypercalcemia and anemia. Leukemia causes cytopenias and circulating blasts. Small cell lung cancer causes SIADH. Cancer affects laboratory values through direct organ invasion, paraneoplastic syndromes, and systemic effects. Always consider malignancy in unexplained laboratory abnormalities, especially with weight loss or constitutional symptoms.

Medications cause numerous laboratory abnormalities. Diuretics cause hypokalemia. NSAIDs cause kidney injury and hyperkalemia. Metformin causes lactic acidosis. Statins cause rhabdomyolysis. Thiazides cause hypercalcemia. A complete medication history is essential when evaluating any laboratory abnormality. Drug-induced problems are common and usually reversible if identified early.

Family history provides crucial diagnostic clues. Thalassemia, hereditary spherocytosis, Factor V Leiden, familial hyperlipidemia, hereditary hemochromatosis—all have genetic components. A family history of early heart attacks, blood clots, anemia, kidney stones, or endocrine disorders should trigger consideration of inherited conditions. Many diagnoses that seem mysterious become obvious with family history.

Moving Forward in Your Laboratory Career

These foundational cases in hematology and chemistry prepare you for advanced practice in laboratory medicine. As you progress, you'll encounter:

Rare diseases that don't fit textbook patterns. The systematic diagnostic approach you've learned here applies to unusual presentations. Start with what you know, consider mechanisms, and work through possibilities systematically.

Complex cases with multiple abnormalities. Real patients often have several conditions simultaneously—diabetes plus kidney disease plus heart failure, each affecting laboratory values. You've learned to untangle complex presentations by addressing primary problems first and understanding how conditions interact.

New tests and technologies. Laboratory medicine evolves constantly. New molecular tests, advanced flow cytometry panels, mass spectrometry methods, and point-of-care devices change practice. The fundamental principles you've learned—understanding what tests measure, how to interpret results, and how to integrate with clinical information—transfer to new technologies.

Quality assurance and laboratory management. Beyond interpreting results, laboratory professionals ensure testing quality, troubleshoot instrument problems, validate new methods, and maintain

212

accreditation. Understanding the clinical significance of tests (which you've developed through these cases) informs quality decisions about acceptable performance, critical result policies, and test utilization.

Consultation and collaboration. Clinicians will ask for your expertise interpreting complex results, selecting appropriate tests, and troubleshooting unexpected findings. The depth of knowledge you've gained through working these cases positions you to provide valuable consultation, improving patient care beyond just generating accurate numbers.

Final Thoughts on Clinical Reasoning

The cases in these chapters weren't just about learning facts—they trained your clinical reasoning. This skill develops through deliberate practice: forming hypotheses, gathering data, revising your thinking based on new information, and learning from mistakes.

Every case you encounter in practice—whether you diagnose it correctly immediately or struggle through confusion to eventual understanding—builds expertise. The difference between novices and experts isn't just knowledge volume. Experts recognize patterns faster, generate better hypotheses, and efficiently test those hypotheses through targeted testing.

You've started that journey. These 45 cases provided deliberate practice in diagnostic reasoning. Keep this approach as you transition to real practice:

Always start with the clinical story. Numbers without context are just numbers. A 28-year-old diabetic who stopped insulin and now has glucose 485 mg/dL tells a very different story than a 75-year-old with new-onset glucose 485 mg/dL (probably hyperosmolar hyperglycemic state, not DKA).

Generate differential diagnoses systematically. Don't jump to the first plausible explanation. List possibilities, consider which findings support or refute each, and test the most likely hypotheses.

Think mechanistically. Understanding pathophysiology helps you predict what you'll find on testing and anticipate complications. When mechanisms don't match your findings, reconsider your diagnosis.

Recognize when you're uncertain. The best clinicians and laboratory professionals acknowledge uncertainty and seek additional information rather than forcing data to fit preconceived diagnoses. "I'm not sure, let's get more information" is often the right answer.

Learn from every case. When you're wrong, figure out why. When you're right, understand what clues led you there. Keep a learning journal or discuss interesting cases with colleagues. This reflective practice accelerates expertise development.

Stay current. Medicine advances rapidly. New diseases emerge (like VEXAS syndrome discovered in 2020). Treatment guidelines change (like the evolution of hyponatremia correction limits). Technologies improve (like next-generation sequencing in hematologic malignancies). Commit to lifelong learning through journals, conferences, and professional organizations.

Maintain humility. Laboratory medicine involves inherent uncertainty. Tests have limits. Rare presentations occur. Patients don't always follow textbook patterns. Approach each case with curiosity rather than overconfidence. The most dangerous laboratory professional is the one who never questions their interpretations.

You're ready for the next stage. Chapter 4 awaits with cases in microbiology and infectious diseases, where you'll apply similar diagnostic reasoning to identify organisms, interpret antibiotic susceptibilities, and manage infectious complications. The skills you've developed working through hematology and chemistry cases—systematic thinking, pattern recognition, mechanistic understanding, clinical integration—transfer directly to microbiology and beyond.

Keep learning. Keep thinking. Keep questioning. This is how expertise develops—one case at a time, one insight at a time, one diagnostic success (or instructive failure) at a time. You've built a strong foundation. Now build on it throughout your career in laboratory medicine.

The patients you'll help diagnose through accurate, thoughtful laboratory testing are depending on your expertise. The work you do matters. A correctly identified diagnosis, a timely critical value call, an insightful test recommendation—these directly impact patient outcomes. Take that responsibility seriously, and approach each case with the systematic thinking and clinical curiosity you've developed here.

Chapter 4: Transfusion Medicine and Immunohematology

The blood bank phone rings at 2 AM. "We need O-negative stat for trauma room one. Patient's bleeding out." The technologist's fingers fly across the keyboard, checking inventory. Three units available. She grabs them, performs the emergency release protocol, and rushes them to the OR. Twenty minutes later, another call: "Patient's having a reaction. Temp spiked to 103, pressure's dropping." Now the real detective work begins.

Blood transfusion saves lives, but it's also one of medicine's most complex interventions. Every unit of blood is essentially an organ transplant, carrying hundreds of antigens that can trigger immune responses ranging from mild fever to catastrophic hemolysis. The blood bank isn't just a refrigerator full of blood bags – it's a sophisticated immunology laboratory where life-and-death decisions happen every hour.

These eight cases will walk you through the intricate world of transfusion medicine, where a single antibody can complicate treatment for decades, where compatible blood isn't always safe blood, and where the difference between crossmatch compatible and truly compatible can mean everything.

Case 1: The Emergency Department's Blood Type Mystery

Chief Complaint: Motor vehicle accident with massive bleeding

Tyler, a 22-year-old college student, arrives unconscious after a head-on collision. He's lost an estimated 2 liters of blood, BP 70/40, heart rate 140. The trauma team needs blood immediately.

Initial Blood Bank Results:

Forward Typing (Patient cells + reagent):

Anti-A: 4+ agglutination

Anti-B: 0 (no agglutination)

Anti-D: 3+ agglutination

Reverse Typing (Patient serum + reagent cells):

A1 cells: 0 (no agglutination) - UNEXPECTED

B cells: 4+ agglutination

The Discrepancy That Could Kill

Forward typing says A-positive. Reverse typing suggests... something else entirely. In trauma, there's no time for investigation – but giving the wrong blood type could be fatal.

The blood bank technologist recognizes a classic pattern: **forward and reverse typing don't match**. This discrepancy must be resolved before type-specific blood can be safely given.

Working Through the ABO Discrepancy

Expected pattern for blood type A:

- Anti-A: Positive (has A antigen)

- Anti-B: Negative (no B antigen)

- A1 cells: Negative (has anti-B antibodies)

- B cells: Positive (has anti-B antibodies)

Tyler shows A antigen on cells but no anti-A in serum – impossible for a typical type A patient.

Additional Testing Reveals:

Patient age confirmation: 22 years old

Direct antiglobulin test (DAT): Negative

Antibody screen: Negative

A2 cell testing: 0 (no agglutination)

Room temperature incubation: Still no anti-A

Previous blood type (found in records): A-positive at age 5

The Subgroup Solution

Tyler has **A-subgroup** blood, likely A3 or Ax. These weak A variants produce less A antigen, and patients often lack the expected anti-A1 antibodies. The forward typing detected his weak A antigen (strong reaction with potent reagents), but his serum lacks the anti-A1 that 80% of A-subgroup patients produce.

Clinical significance:

- **As a recipient**: Can receive A or O blood safely

- **As a donor**: Blood types as A but might be missed in emergencies

- **For this trauma**: A-positive blood is safe

Massive Transfusion Protocol Activated

While the subgroup investigation proceeded, the trauma team couldn't wait:

Initial emergency release:

- 2 units O-negative uncrossmatched (universal donor)

- Type and screen sent simultaneously

After blood type confirmed:

- Switched to A-positive blood
- 6 units RBCs, 6 units FFP, 1 unit platelets (1:1:1 ratio)

The Forward-Looking Protocol

Tyler received 14 units of blood products total. Post-transfusion testing shows:

Mixed field agglutination in forward typing (his A3 cells + transfused normal A cells)

DAT: Negative (no immune reaction)

Hemoglobin: 9.2 g/dL (adequate)

Documentation for future: "A-subgroup (A3/Ax), can receive A or O blood"

Critical Lessons from Tyler's Case:

1. **Discrepancies demand investigation** but emergency needs override
2. **O-negative blood buys time** for complex workups
3. **Subgroups are rare but real** – about 1% of type A patients
4. **Documentation prevents future confusion**
5. **Massive transfusion is more than RBCs** – plasma and platelets matter

---

Case 2: The Third Pregnancy

Presenting Concern: "My doctor says my blood is attacking my baby"

Maria, 28 years old, is 10 weeks pregnant with her third child. She's Rh-negative, her husband is Rh-positive. Her first pregnancy was uncomplicated. Her second ended in stillbirth at 34 weeks. Now her antibody screen is positive.

Initial Antibody Testing:

Blood type: O-negative

Antibody screen: Positive

Direct antiglobulin test: Negative

Antibody Identification Panel:

Anti-D titer: 1:32 (critical titer ≥1:16)

Anti-C: Negative

Anti-E: Negative

Anti-K: Negative

The Timeline That Tells The Story

First pregnancy (2019):

- Uncomplicated delivery
- RhoGAM given at 28 weeks and delivery
- Baby: A-positive

Second pregnancy (2021):

- No prenatal care until 20 weeks
- Presented at 34 weeks with decreased fetal movement
- Stillbirth, severely anemic baby
- Antibody screen done postpartum: Anti-D detected

Current pregnancy:

- Early prenatal care
- Already sensitized with anti-D titer 1:32

Understanding Rh Sensitization

Maria became sensitized during or after her first pregnancy. Despite RhoGAM, about 0.1% of Rh-negative women still develop anti-D. Possible reasons:

1. **RhoGAM failure** (rare but possible)
2. **Large fetomaternal hemorrhage** exceeding RhoGAM coverage
3. **Delayed or missed RhoGAM** administration
4. **Previous unrecognized pregnancy loss**

Once sensitized, RhoGAM won't help – the immune system already recognizes Rh-positive cells as foreign.

Managing This High-Risk Pregnancy

Paternal testing:

Father's blood type: A-positive

Rh genotype: D/D (homozygous)

Conclusion: All offspring will be Rh-positive

Fetal monitoring protocol:

- Antibody titers every 4 weeks until 24 weeks, then every 2 weeks

- If titer ≥1:16 or rises 2 dilutions: Begin fetal surveillance

Week 18 - Middle Cerebral Artery Doppler:

Peak systolic velocity: 1.6 MoM (>1.5 suggests moderate-severe anemia)

Decision: Cordocentesis for direct fetal blood sampling

Cordocentesis Results:

Fetal blood type: O-positive (at risk)

Fetal hemoglobin: 6.2 g/dL (severe anemia)

Fetal bilirubin: 4.8 mg/dL (elevated)

Decision: Intrauterine transfusion required

The Intrauterine Transfusion Process

Blood product preparation:

- O-negative blood (matching mother)
- CMV-negative
- Irradiated (prevent TA-GVHD)
- Leukoreduced
- Fresh (<5 days old)
- Hematocrit 75-85% (concentrated)

Volume calculation:

- Estimated fetal blood volume: 150 mL
- Target: Raise Hgb from 6 to 11 g/dL
- Volume needed: 40 mL packed cells

Serial Transfusions Save a Life

Maria's baby received four intrauterine transfusions:

- Week 18: Hgb 6.2 → 11.0
- Week 21: Hgb 7.8 → 11.5
- Week 24: Hgb 8.1 → 12.0
- Week 27: Hgb 8.5 → 12.2

Delivery at 32 weeks:

- Baby's blood: 90% donor O-negative cells
- Direct antiglobulin test: Strongly positive

- Required phototherapy but no exchange transfusion
- Healthy discharge at 3 weeks

Prevention for Future Pregnancies

For Maria's next pregnancy:

1. Anti-D already present – will affect all Rh-positive babies
2. Earlier monitoring starting at 10 weeks
3. Consideration of IVF with PGD for Rh-negative embryos
4. Psychological support given previous stillbirth

Case 3: The Delayed Reaction

Day 1 Post-Op: "I feel great, when can I go home?" **Day 8 Post-Op:** "I can barely breathe, and my urine looks like Coca-Cola"

Robert, 67, had uncomplicated knee replacement surgery. He received 2 units of packed red cells for post-op anemia (Hgb 7.2). Discharged day 3 feeling well. Now he's back with severe fatigue, jaundice, and dark urine.

Current Laboratory Values:

Hemoglobin: 6.8 g/dL (was 10.2 at discharge)

Total bilirubin: 4.2 mg/dL (0.2-1.0)

Indirect bilirubin: 3.8 mg/dL

LDH: 892 U/L (140-280)

Haptoglobin: <10 mg/dL (30-200)

Direct antiglobulin test: Positive (IgG)

Urinalysis:

Blood: 3+

RBCs: 0-2/hpf

Diagnosis: Hemoglobinuria (not hematuria)

The Blood Bank Investigation

Pre-transfusion (8 days ago):

Blood type: O-positive

Antibody screen: Negative

Crossmatch: Compatible with 2 units

Current testing:

Blood type: Still O-positive (ruling out ABO error)

Antibody screen: POSITIVE (new finding)

Direct antiglobulin test: Positive

Eluate testing: Pan-reactive with all cells

Antibody Identification Panel Results:

Testing patient's serum against panel cells:

Cell 1 (D+C+E-c+e+, K-, Fy(a)+, Jk(a)+): 3+

Cell 2 (D+C-E+c+e-, K+, Fy(a)-, Jk(a)+): 3+

Cell 3 (D-C-E-c+e+, K-, Fy(a)+, Jk(a)-): Negative

Cell 4 (D+C+E-c-e+, K-, Fy(a)-, Jk(a)+): 3+

...continues through 11 cells

The Smoking Gun: Anti-Jk(a)

Pattern analysis reveals antibody reacting with all Jk(a)+ cells. The patient is Jk(a)-Jk(b)+.

Classic Kidd antibody characteristics:

- **Appears and disappears** (titer drops below detectable)
- **Delayed hemolytic reactions** (3-14 days post-transfusion)
- **Severe when re-exposed** (anamnestic response)
- **Often missed in antibody screens** if titer low

Reconstructing What Happened

1. **Remote sensitization**: Robert likely received blood years ago (found a 1998 surgery record)
2. **Antibody disappeared**: Dropped below detectable levels
3. **Re-exposure**: The 2 units were Jk(a)+

221

4. **Anamnestic response**: Antibody surged back, destroying transfused cells

5. **Delayed hemolysis**: Peak destruction at day 7-10

Management of Delayed Hemolytic Reaction

Supportive care:

- IV fluids to protect kidneys from hemoglobin

- Monitor for dropping hemoglobin

- Avoid transfusion unless critical

When transfusion necessary:

- Must be Jk(a)-negative blood

- Only 23% of population is Jk(a)-

- Crossmatch with current sample

- May need rare blood from reference lab

Robert's hemoglobin stabilized at 6.8 g/dL. With supportive care, he recovered without additional transfusion. His medical record now permanently flagged: **"Anti-Jk(a) antibody - requires Jk(a)-negative blood"**

The Kidd Killer Pattern

Why Kidd antibodies are so dangerous:

1. **Complement activating** - cause intravascular hemolysis

2. **Dosage effect** - react stronger with homozygous cells

3. **Evanescent** - disappear then reappear

4. **Common antigen** - 77% of donors are Jk(a)+

Case 4: Trauma Bay Chaos

Initial Report: "Multiple GSWs, ETA 3 minutes, requesting trauma activation"

David, 34, arrives with four gunshot wounds to the torso. He's losing blood faster than it can be replaced. BP unmeasurable, heart rate 160, Glasgow Coma Scale 7.

Massive Transfusion Protocol (MTP) Activation

The blood bank prepares for chaos. MTP means delivering blood products in specific ratios rapidly and repeatedly until bleeding stops or the patient dies.

Round 1 (First 10 minutes):

6 units O-positive RBCs (uncrossmatched)

6 units FFP (AB or A, low-titer anti-B)

1 pooled platelet unit

The 1:1:1 Ratio Revolution

Traditional approach: Give RBCs first, add plasma and platelets if coagulopathy develops Modern MTP: Balanced resuscitation from the start

Evidence from PROPPR trial (Holcomb et al., 2015):

- 1:1:1 ratio reduces death from exsanguination at 24 hours

- Prevents dilutional coagulopathy

- Reduces total blood product use

Laboratory Values at 30 Minutes:

Hemoglobin: 5.2 g/dL

Platelets: 42,000/µL

INR: 2.1

Fibrinogen: 88 mg/dL (150-400)

pH: 7.18

Lactate: 8.2 mmol/L

Temperature: 35.2°C

The Lethal Triad Emerges

David shows the trauma triad of death:

1. **Acidosis** (pH 7.18)

2. **Hypothermia** (35.2°C)

3. **Coagulopathy** (INR 2.1, low fibrinogen)

Each worsens the others. Cold impairs clotting. Acidosis impairs clotting. Poor clotting increases blood loss, worsening acidosis and hypothermia.

Round 2 Modifications:

4 units RBCs (now type-specific A-positive)

4 units FFP

1 pooled platelet unit

2 units cryoprecipitate (for fibrinogen)

1 gram tranexamic acid (antifibrinolytic)

Monitoring During MTP

Every 30 minutes:

- CBC
- PT/INR, aPTT
- Fibrinogen
- Blood gas
- Lactate
- Temperature

Thromboelastography (TEG) guides therapy:

R time: 12 min (prolonged - needs FFP)

K time: 4 min (prolonged - needs cryoprecipitate)

Alpha angle: 45° (low - needs fibrinogen)

MA: 42 mm (low - needs platelets)

LY30: 8% (mild hyperfibrinolysis)

Emergency Release Blood Complications

After 8 units of O-positive emergency blood, David (type A) now has mixed field:

- Forward typing shows both A and O cells
- Must continue O-positive or A-positive
- Cannot switch to A-negative (has anti-B from O plasma)

Two Hours Later - Achieving Control

Total products transfused:

- 18 units RBCs
- 16 units FFP
- 3 pooled platelets
- 4 units cryoprecipitate
- 2 grams tranexamic acid
- 3 amps calcium chloride

Final labs:

Hemoglobin: 8.8 g/dL

Platelets: 95,000/μL

INR: 1.4

Fibrinogen: 182 mg/dL

pH: 7.34

Temperature: 36.8°C

Bleeding controlled. David survived.

Post-Resuscitation Complications to Monitor

Next 24-48 hours watch for:

- TRALI (transfusion-related acute lung injury)

- TACO (transfusion-associated circulatory overload)

- Hyperkalemia from stored RBCs

- Citrate toxicity causing hypocalcemia

- Alloimmunization to multiple antigens

Case 5: The Untypeable Patient

Blood Bank Alert: "Cannot determine patient blood type - multiple antibodies detected"

Linda, 58, needs surgery for colon cancer. Pre-op blood bank testing has been running for 6 hours with no resolution.

Initial Testing Chaos:

Forward typing:

Anti-A: 2+ with mixed field

Anti-B: Negative

Anti-D: 1+ weak

Reverse typing:

A1 cells: 2+

B cells: 4+

O cells: 1+ (should be negative!)

Antibody screen: Positive in all 3 cells

Autocontrol: Positive

Direct antiglobulin test: Positive (IgG and C3)

The Warm Autoantibody Problem

Linda has warm autoimmune hemolytic anemia (WAIHA) with autoantibodies coating her cells and circulating in her plasma. These antibodies react with all cells, making blood typing and crossmatching nearly impossible.

Advanced Testing Techniques:

Elution to remove antibodies from cells:

1. Wash patient cells x6 with saline

2. Treat with chloroquine to dissociate IgG

3. Re-test forward typing:

   o Anti-A: Negative

   o Anti-B: Negative

   o Anti-D: 4+ (true positive)

   o Conclusion: O-positive

Adsorption to remove plasma antibodies:

1. Incubate patient serum with pooled O cells

2. Antibodies bind to adsorbing cells

3. Test supernatant against panel

4. Reveals underlying alloantibodies

After 3 Differential Adsorptions:

Underlying alloantibodies identified:

- Anti-E (titer 1:4)

- Anti-K (titer 1:2)

- Warm autoantibody (still present but weaker)

The Transfusion Dilemma

Linda needs E-negative, K-negative blood, but her autoantibody means:

- No units will be crossmatch compatible

- Must give "least incompatible" blood

- Risk of hemolysis with any transfusion

Phenotype-matched approach:

- Extended phenotype patient's cells

- Find units matching Rh and Kell phenotype

- Reduces risk of additional alloantibodies

Patient's Extended Phenotype:

Rh: D+C+E-c+e+ (R1R1)

Kell: K-k+

Duffy: Fy(a+b-)

Kidd: Jk(a+b+)

MNS: M+N+S-s+

Transfusion Strategy:

1. Find O-positive, E-negative, K-negative units

2. Match Rh phenotype if possible (C+c+e+)

3. Perform biological crossmatch:

   o Infuse 10-15 mL over 5 minutes

   o Monitor vitals

   o If stable, continue transfusion

Surgery Day Preparations:

Blood bank prepared:

- 4 units O-positive, E-neg, K-neg, C+e+ blood

- All units "least incompatible"

- Consent obtained for incompatible transfusion

- Extra plasma for potential hemolysis

Surgery proceeded with 2 units transfused. Post-op:

- Hemoglobin rose appropriately (7.2 to 9.1)

- LDH and bilirubin stable (no excess hemolysis)

- DAT remained positive (expected)

Case 6: The Monthly Transfusion Patient

Chief Complaint: "My regular transfusion isn't working anymore"

Michael, 24, has beta-thalassemia major, receiving monthly transfusions since age 2. He usually feels energetic post-transfusion, but the last three sessions left him exhausted. His hemoglobin barely rises despite receiving blood.

Pre-Transfusion Testing Today:

Hemoglobin: 6.2 g/dL (target >9)

Antibody screen: Positive (new - was negative 4 months ago)

Direct antiglobulin test: Negative

Antibody identification reveals:

- Anti-E (titer 1:64)

- Anti-Fy(a) (titer 1:8)

- Anti-S (titer 1:4)

The Multi-Antibody Challenge

After ~200 lifetime transfusions, Michael has developed multiple alloantibodies. Each antibody eliminates compatible donors:

- E-negative: 70% of donors
- Fy(a)-negative: 34% of donors
- S-negative: 45% of donors
- Must be negative for ALL three: ~11% of donors

Historical Review Reveals Pattern:

Age 8: Developed anti-K

Age 14: Developed anti-C

Age 19: Developed anti-Jk(b)

Age 24: Now anti-E, anti-Fy(a), anti-S

Each transfusion exposed him to foreign antigens, gradually limiting his donor pool.

Phenotype-Matched Protocol Implementation

New strategy: Instead of basic ABO/Rh matching, provide extended phenotype-matched blood:

- Match for C, c, E, e, K, Fy(a), Fy(b), Jk(a), Jk(b), S, s

- Reduces new antibody formation by 75%
- Requires rare donor program participation

Finding Compatible Blood:

The blood bank's search:

1. Local inventory: 0 compatible units
2. Regional supplier: 2 units found (shipped overnight)
3. National rare donor registry: 8 additional units located
4. International registry: Backup option if needed

Compatible unit phenotype required:

O-positive (patient's type)

C-, E-, e+, K-, Fy(a)-, Jk(b)-, S-

Phenotype frequency: 1 in 912 donors

Managing the Chronic Transfusion Patient

Modified transfusion protocol:

- Transfuse 3 units every 5 weeks (instead of 2 every 4)
- Maintain higher pre-transfusion Hgb (7-8 instead of 6-7)
- Reduces antibody stimulation from donor exposure

Immunosuppression consideration:

- Rituximab to prevent new antibodies
- Risk-benefit for lifelong transfusion need
- Reserved for patients with antibodies to high-frequency antigens

Six Months Later:

With phenotype-matched blood:

- No new antibodies developed
- Hemoglobin maintained at target
- Transfusion reactions eliminated
- Quality of life improved

Michael now carries a rare blood card listing his antibodies and required phenotype for emergencies.

Case 7: The Breathless Recovery

Post-Op Hour 2: "Something's wrong. She can't breathe."

Sarah, 45, just received her second unit of FFP after liver resection. Suddenly she's gasping, oxygen saturation plummeting from 98% to 82%. Pink frothy sputum appears. Chest X-ray shows bilateral infiltrates that weren't there an hour ago.

Initial Assessment:

Vital signs:

- BP: 128/76 (not hypotensive)

- Heart rate: 110

- Temperature: 37.2°C (no fever)

- O2 saturation: 82% on room air → 88% on 100% O2

Blood gas:

- pH: 7.35

- PaO2: 58 mmHg (on 100% O2)

- P/F ratio: 58 (severe ARDS)

BNP: 45 pg/mL (rules out cardiac cause)

Echo: Normal cardiac function

The TRALI Investigation

Transfusion-Related Acute Lung Injury suspected. TRALI is acute lung injury within 6 hours of transfusion without other risk factors.

Diagnostic criteria met:

1. Acute onset (during transfusion)

2. Hypoxemia (P/F ratio <300)

3. Bilateral infiltrates on imaging

4. No evidence of cardiac overload

5. No other ALI risk factors

6. Temporal relationship to transfusion

Blood Bank's Detective Work

Donor investigation for the implicated FFP unit:

Donor: 32-year-old female

Pregnancy history: G3P3 (3 pregnancies)

Last pregnancy: 2 years ago

Previous report: None

HLA antibody testing on donor:

HLA Class I antibodies: Positive

HLA Class II antibodies: Positive

Specificity: Anti-HLA-A2, Anti-HLA-B8

Patient's HLA type: A2, B8 (perfect storm)

The Mechanism Explained

Donor's anti-HLA antibodies (from pregnancies) reacted with Sarah's white cells:

1. Antibodies bound patient neutrophils

2. Neutrophils activated and sequestered in lungs

3. Released inflammatory mediators

4. Capillary leak syndrome developed

5. Acute lung injury resulted

Management Without Making It Worse

What NOT to do:

- Don't give diuretics (this isn't fluid overload)

- Don't give more blood products unless critical

- Don't give steroids (no proven benefit)

Supportive care:

- Mechanical ventilation with lung-protective strategy

- PEEP optimization

- Conservative fluid management

- Monitor for improvement

The Other Transfusion Reactions to Rule Out

Reaction	Timing	Fever	BP	Lungs	Key Test
TRALI	<6 hours	No	Normal	Bilateral infiltrates	HLA antibodies
TACO	During/immediately	No	High	Bilateral infiltrates	Elevated BNP
Allergic	During	No	Low	Wheezing	Tryptase
Febrile	During/after	Yes	Normal	Clear	White cell antibodies
Septic	Hours-days	Yes	Low	Variable	Blood culture
Hemolytic	Immediate	Yes	Low	Clear	DAT, hemolysis markers

Outcome and Prevention

Sarah's course:

- Day 1: Required intubation
- Day 3: Infiltrates improving
- Day 5: Extubated
- Day 7: Discharged home

Prevention strategies implemented:

1. Donor deferred from plasma donation
2. Male-only plasma policy consideration
3. Never-pregnant female plasma preferred
4. Patient notification for future transfusion awareness

The TRALI Paradox

TRALI is:

- Leading cause of transfusion death
- Completely unpredictable
- Not prevented by crossmatching
- Donor-specific (same donor could cause TRALI in one patient, not another)
- Decreasing with male-predominant plasma

Case 8: The Yellow Baby

Delivery Room: "Baby's jaundiced already. That's not normal, right?"

Baby Chen, 8 hours old, already yellow. Mom is O-negative, baby is A-positive. The pediatrician's concern grows when initial bilirubin comes back at 8.2 mg/dL at 8 hours of life.

Hemolytic Disease Workup:

Baby's blood:

- Type: A-positive

- Direct antiglobulin test: 3+ positive

- Hemoglobin: 10.2 g/dL (low for newborn)

- Reticulocytes: 12% (elevated)

- Indirect bilirubin: 7.8 mg/dL

Mother's blood:

- Type: O-negative

- Antibody screen: Negative for unexpected antibodies

- Anti-A titer: 512 (high titer)

- Anti-B titer: 256 (high titer)

ABO Incompatibility vs Rh Disease

This is ABO hemolytic disease, not Rh:

- Mom O, baby A = ABO incompatible

- Mom's natural anti-A (IgG portion) crossed placenta

- Attacking baby's A-positive cells

- Usually milder than Rh disease

- Can occur in first pregnancy

Why ABO is usually milder:

1. A and B antigens not fully developed at birth

2. Antigens present on other tissues (absorb antibody)

3. Usually IgG2 (doesn't activate complement well)

Bilirubin Trajectory Crisis

Hour-specific bilirubin levels:

8 hours: 8.2 mg/dL (>95th percentile)

12 hours: 10.1 mg/dL

18 hours: 12.8 mg/dL

24 hours: 15.2 mg/dL (approaching exchange level)

Using Bhutani nomogram: High-risk zone, steep trajectory

Phototherapy Initiated But Failing

Despite intensive phototherapy:

30 hours: 17.8 mg/dL

36 hours: 19.2 mg/dL

Exchange transfusion threshold at 36 hours: 20 mg/dL

Emergency Exchange Transfusion Preparation

Blood product selection:

- Type: O-negative (matches mom, won't be hemolyzed)
- Fresh (<5 days old)
- CMV-negative
- Irradiated
- Hematocrit 50-60%
- Crossmatch with mom's serum

Volume calculations:

Baby weight: 3.2 kg

Blood volume: 85 mL/kg × 3.2 = 272 mL

Double-volume exchange: 544 mL

Aliquot size: 20 mL in-out cycles

The Exchange Process

Via umbilical vein catheter:

1. Withdraw 20 mL baby's blood
2. Infuse 20 mL donor blood
3. Repeat 27 times
4. Monitor vitals, glucose, calcium

Labs during exchange:

- Every 100 mL: Electrolytes, calcium

- End: Bilirubin, CBC, glucose

Post-Exchange Results:

Immediate post:

- Bilirubin: 8.4 mg/dL (from 19.2)

- Hemoglobin: 14.5 g/dL

- Platelets: 180,000 (watch for thrombocytopenia)

6 hours post (rebound check):

- Bilirubin: 11.2 mg/dL (expected rebound)

- Continue phototherapy

Why Exchange Transfusion Works

Double-volume exchange removes:

- 85% of baby's antibody-coated cells

- 50% of available bilirubin

- Maternal antibodies from plasma

Replaces with:

- Cells that won't be hemolyzed (O type)

- Fresh plasma without anti-A

- Normal adult hemoglobin

Long-term Follow-up Reveals

Week 1:

- Bilirubin normalized

- Mild anemia developed (Hgb 9.8)

- No transfusion needed

Month 1:

- DAT still positive but weakening

- Hemoglobin recovering (10.5)

- Normal development

Month 3:

- DAT negative

- No residual effects

- Mom counseled about future pregnancy risk

Prevention for Next Pregnancy

For mom's future pregnancies:

1. Check antibody titers early

2. Consider IVIG if titers >512

3. Early delivery consideration (37-38 weeks)

4. Immediate phototherapy at birth

5. Have exchange setup ready

Summary: Mastering Transfusion Medicine

Through these eight cases, you've witnessed the complexity of modern transfusion medicine. This isn't just about matching A to A or B to B anymore. Every transfusion decision involves sophisticated immunology, risk assessment, and sometimes life-or-death calculations made in seconds.

Pattern Recognition Excellence:

You've learned to recognize critical patterns:

- Forward and reverse typing discrepancies signaling subgroups or antibodies

- Rising antibody titers predicting hemolytic disease severity

- The classic presentation of delayed hemolytic reactions

- TRALI's distinctive acute respiratory distress pattern

Antibody Investigation Mastery:

From Linda's warm autoantibody making her "untypeable" to Michael's growing collection of alloantibodies limiting his donor pool, you've seen how antibodies complicate transfusion. Each antibody tells a story – previous transfusions, pregnancies, or autoimmune disease.

Emergency Response Protocols:

David's massive transfusion showed you that modern trauma resuscitation is about balanced component therapy. The 1:1:1 ratio isn't just a number – it's based on battlefield medicine translated to civilian trauma. Tyler's ABO discrepancy during trauma demonstrated that sometimes you give O-negative first and ask questions later.

Specialized Populations:

Different patients need different approaches:

- Chronically transfused patients need phenotype matching

- Pregnant women need careful antibody monitoring

236

- Newborns need specially processed blood
- Autoimmune patients need "least incompatible" units

Safety Systems:

Every case reinforced that transfusion safety requires:

- Meticulous patient identification
- Careful antibody investigation
- Appropriate product selection
- Vigilant reaction monitoring
- Comprehensive documentation

The Human Element:

Behind every unit of blood is a donor. Behind every transfusion is a patient whose life might depend on your expertise. The pregnant mother terrified her antibodies will harm another baby. The trauma patient who'll never know how many strangers' blood saved them. The thalassemia patient whose quality of life depends on finding those rare compatible units.

Modern transfusion medicine stands at the intersection of immunology, hematology, and critical care. These cases show that blood banking isn't just about having blood on the shelf – it's about having the right blood, prepared the right way, given at the right time, with the right monitoring.

Every antibody identified prevents a reaction. Every protocol followed saves a life. Every discrepancy investigated avoids a catastrophe. That's the real work of transfusion medicine – being the guardian between the gift of blood and the patient who needs it.

Chapter 5: Clinical Microbiology and Infectious Diseases

The lab tech squints at the blood agar plate under the light. Those tiny beta-hemolytic colonies weren't there yesterday. She grabs the Gram stain reagents, already suspecting what she'll find. Minutes later, her suspicion confirms: Gram-positive cocci in chains. The patient's blood is growing Streptococcus. She dials the ICU. "Doctor, we have a critical result."

Microbiology labs are where invisible threats become visible. Where a single colony on a plate can explain why someone's dying. Where the difference between Gram-positive and Gram-negative determines which antibiotics might save a life. Unlike chemistry results that pop out of machines in minutes, micro takes patience. Bacteria grow on their own schedule. But when they finally show themselves, the entire clinical picture often snaps into focus.

These fifteen cases will take you through the detective work of clinical microbiology. You'll see how a urine sample tells the story of antibiotic resistance spreading through a nursing home. How a traveler's diarrhea reveals a parasite picked up three countries ago. How molecular diagnostics can identify a pathogen in hours that culture would take weeks to grow. This is where laboratory medicine meets infectious disease, and timing is everything.

Case 1: The Fever Without a Source

Day 3 in ICU: "We've cultured everything. Still no answers."

Marcus, 58, came to the ED with confusion and fever. Three days later, he's intubated, on three pressors, and circling the drain. Every culture is negative, but his white count keeps climbing.

Initial Presentation:

- Temperature: 39.8°C (103.6°F)

- Heart rate: 124 bpm

- Blood pressure: 82/45 (on norepinephrine)

- Respiratory rate: 28

- O2 saturation: 91% on 60% FiO2

Laboratory Results Day 1:

WBC: 18,400/μL (87% neutrophils, 8% bands)

Hemoglobin: 10.2 g/dL

Platelets: 89,000/μL

Lactate: 4.2 mmol/L

Procalcitonin: 12.5 ng/mL (severe bacterial infection likely)

CRP: 287 mg/L

Blood cultures x2 sets: No growth at 24 hours

Urine culture: No growth

Sputum culture: Normal respiratory flora

The SOFA Score Climb

Marcus meets septic shock criteria:

- Suspected infection (fever, elevated WBC)

- Organ dysfunction (SOFA score 11)

- Hypotension requiring vasopressors

- Lactate >2 despite fluid resuscitation

But where's the infection?

Day 3 - Expanded Investigation:

Additional cultures:

- Blood cultures x2 more sets: Still negative

- CSF: Normal cell count, negative culture

- Stool: Negative for pathogens

Molecular diagnostics ordered:

BioFire FilmArray Blood Culture ID Panel: Pending

Multiplex respiratory PCR: Negative

Urinary antigens:

- Streptococcus pneumoniae: Negative

- Legionella: Negative

The History That Changes Everything

Marcus's wife mentions something new: "He helped his brother fix a flooded basement two weeks ago. Waded through sewage water. Cut his leg on something down there."

Physical exam reveals a small, healing laceration on the right shin. No obvious cellulitis, minimal erythema. The wound looks benign. But...

Day 4 - The Break in the Case:

Blood culture (anaerobic bottle only): Growth detected at 76 hours

Gram stain: Gram-negative rods

Subculture: Grows only on chocolate agar in CO_2

Identification: Capnocytophaga canimorsus

Source: Dog saliva (brother's dog licked the wound)

The Fastidious Organism Problem

C. canimorsus characteristics that delayed diagnosis:

- Slow growing (3-7 days)

- Requires CO_2 enrichment

- Fastidious (needs special media)

- Often missed on routine culture

- Can cause fulminant sepsis in asplenic or immunocompromised

Marcus had an unreported splenectomy 20 years ago after trauma.

Antimicrobial Susceptibility Testing Challenges:

Beta-lactamase: Negative

Penicillin: Sensitive (MIC 0.06)

Ampicillin/sulbactam: Sensitive

Ceftriaxone: Sensitive

Fluoroquinolones: Variable

Note: No CLSI breakpoints established

Using PK/PD principles for guidance

Treatment and Outcome:

Switched from broad-spectrum coverage to targeted therapy:

- Penicillin G 4 million units q4h

- Rapid improvement within 24 hours

- Extubated day 6

- Discharged day 10

Lessons from Marcus:

This case demonstrates several critical micro principles:

1. **Negative cultures don't mean no infection** - Some organisms need special conditions

2. **History details matter** - Dog exposure was key

3. **Immunocompromised state affects everything** - Splenectomy made him vulnerable

4. **Extended incubation sometimes necessary** - Not all bacteria grow in 24-48 hours

5. **Fastidious organisms require patience** - And knowledge of their growth requirements

---

Case 2: The Worst Headache Ever

Emergency Department: "She says it feels like her head's exploding"

Jennifer, 19, college sophomore, brought in by roommates. Sudden severe headache, neck stiffness, and now a spreading rash. The triage nurse takes one look at the petechial rash and hits the isolation button.

Rapid Assessment:

- Temperature: 39.2°C

- Nuchal rigidity present

- Kernig's sign positive

- Petechial rash on trunk and extremities

- Glasgow Coma Scale: 13 (confused)

STAT Lumbar Puncture:

CSF Appearance: Cloudy

Opening pressure: 32 cm H2O (elevated)

Cell count:

- WBC: 2,840/μL (95% neutrophils)

- RBC: 10/μL

Chemistry:

- Protein: 248 mg/dL (15-45)

- Glucose: 18 mg/dL (40-70)

- Serum glucose: 98 mg/dL

241

- CSF:serum glucose ratio: 0.18 (should be >0.6)

Gram stain: Gram-negative diplococci seen

The Clock Starts Ticking

Bacterial meningitis suspected. Mortality increases each hour antibiotics are delayed. Started empirically:

- Ceftriaxone 2g IV q12h

- Vancomycin 20 mg/kg IV q8h

- Dexamethasone 10 mg IV q6h

CSF Culture and Beyond:

Growth at 18 hours: Neisseria meningitidis

Serogroup: B (by latex agglutination)

Antimicrobial susceptibility:

- Penicillin: Sensitive (MIC 0.03)

- Ceftriaxone: Sensitive (MIC <0.008)

- Ciprofloxacin: Sensitive (for prophylaxis)

The Public Health Emergency

N. meningitidis triggers immediate action:

- Reportable within 24 hours

- Contact tracing initiated

- Prophylaxis for close contacts

Defining Close Contacts:

Who needs prophylaxis?

- Household members

- Roommates (both suite-mates)

- Anyone with direct respiratory secretion exposure

- Sexual partners in past 7 days

Prophylaxis options:

- Ciprofloxacin 500 mg PO x1 (adults)

- Rifampin 600 mg PO q12h x 4 doses

- Ceftriaxone 250 mg IM x1

Molecular Epidemiology:

Public health lab performs:

Multilocus sequence typing (MLST): ST-32 complex

Clonal complex: Associated with serogroup B outbreaks

PorA type: P1.5-1,2-2

FetA type: F1-5

Matches ongoing college outbreak strain

Jennifer's Course:

Day 2:

- Mental status improving
- Switched to penicillin G monotherapy
- Rash evolving to purpura

Day 4:

- Repeat LP: WBC dropping, cultures negative
- Hearing assessment: Bilateral intact
- Started on physical therapy

Day 10:

- Discharged home
- Cognitive testing scheduled
- University notified for outbreak control

Prevention Discussion:

Jennifer asks: "Could the vaccine have prevented this?"

Meningococcal vaccines available:

- **MenACWY**: Covers serogroups A, C, W, Y (she had this)
- **MenB**: Covers serogroup B (she didn't have this)

Her infection was serogroup B – the vaccine she didn't receive could have prevented it.

Case 3: The UTI That Wouldn't Quit

Clinic Visit #4: "Doctor, I've taken three different antibiotics. Nothing works."

Patricia, 72, has had burning with urination for six weeks. Three courses of antibiotics provided temporary relief, but symptoms always return.

Antibiotic History:

1. Nitrofurantoin x5 days - Symptoms improved then returned
2. Ciprofloxacin x7 days - No improvement
3. Trimethoprim/sulfamethoxazole x10 days - Partial improvement

Current Urine Analysis:

Appearance: Cloudy

pH: 8.0 (alkaline)

Specific gravity: 1.018

Protein: 1+

Blood: Trace

Nitrite: Positive

Leukocyte esterase: Positive

WBC: >50/hpf

RBC: 5-10/hpf

Bacteria: Many

Urine Culture Results:

Organism: >100,000 CFU/mL Escherichia coli

Antimicrobial Susceptibility:

Ampicillin: Resistant

Ampicillin/sulbactam: Resistant

Cefazolin: Resistant

Ceftriaxone: Resistant

Ciprofloxacin: Resistant

Levofloxacin: Resistant

Trimethoprim/sulfa: Resistant

Nitrofurantoin: SENSITIVE

Gentamicin: Sensitive

Meropenem: Sensitive

Fosfomycin: Sensitive

ESBL: Positive

The ESBL Problem

Extended-spectrum beta-lactamase (ESBL) producing *E. coli*:

- Resistant to all penicillins and cephalosporins

- Often resistant to fluoroquinolones

- Increasing in community-acquired UTIs

- Limited oral options

But wait – she took nitrofurantoin and it's sensitive. Why did it fail?

The Complicating Factor:

Renal ultrasound reveals:

- Right hydronephrosis

- 8mm stone in right ureter

- Post-void residual: 150 mL

This isn't just a UTI – it's a complicated UTI with obstruction.

Treatment Approach:

Immediate:

- Fosfomycin 3g PO once

- Urology referral for stone management

After stone removal:

- Ertapenem 1g IV daily x5 days (outpatient IV therapy)

- Then fosfomycin 3g PO every 3 days x3 doses

The Bigger Picture - Resistance Mechanisms:

Patricia's isolate tested for resistance genes:

CTX-M-15: Positive (most common ESBL gene)

TEM: Positive

SHV: Negative

AmpC: Negative

Carbapenemase: Negative (thank goodness)

Risk Factors for ESBL:

Patricia had several:

- Recent antibiotics (selects for resistance)
- Recurrent UTIs
- Recent hospitalization (3 months ago)
- Nursing home residence

Six Months Later:

Patricia returns with another UTI:

Same organism: ESBL E. coli

New resistance: Now fosfomycin resistant too

Still sensitive: Meropenem, amikacin

Molecular typing: Same strain as before

Conclusion: Persistence, not reinfection

Prevention Strategies Implemented:

1. **Suppressive therapy**: Nitrofurantoin 50 mg daily
2. **Non-antibiotic prevention**:
   - Vaginal estrogen cream
   - Cranberry supplement
   - Improved bathroom access at nursing home
3. **Surveillance cultures**: Monthly while on suppression

Case 4: The Cough That Wouldn't Stop

Week 6 of symptoms: "I've tried everything. Still coughing."

Robert, 48, accountant, has been coughing for six weeks. Two rounds of azithromycin, one of levofloxacin. Chest X-ray showed "atypical pneumonia." Nothing's helped.

Current Presentation:

- Productive cough with white sputum

- No fever

- Night sweats occasionally

- Lost 8 pounds

- Never smoked

- No known TB exposure

Initial Workup:

Chest X-ray: Right upper lobe infiltrate with cavitation

CBC: Normal

HIV: Negative

Sputum Gram stain: Many WBCs, no organisms seen

Routine culture: Normal respiratory flora

The Missing Diagnosis

Three sputum samples for AFB (acid-fast bacilli):

Day 1: AFB smear negative

Day 2: AFB smear negative

Day 3: AFB smear 1+ positive (rare bacilli seen)

Molecular Diagnostics Speed Things Up:

Xpert MTB/RIF assay on sputum:

- *Mycobacterium tuberculosis* detected

- Rifampin resistance NOT detected

- Results in 2 hours vs. weeks for culture

Starting Treatment Before Culture Confirmation:

Based on positive molecular test:

- Isoniazid 300 mg daily

- Rifampin 600 mg daily

- Pyrazinamide 1500 mg daily

- Ethambutol 1200 mg daily

Culture Confirmation at 3 Weeks:

MGIT (liquid culture): Positive at 18 days

Löwenstein-Jensen (solid): Growth at 21 days

Identification: M. tuberculosis confirmed

Drug Susceptibility (4 weeks):

- Isoniazid: Sensitive

- Rifampin: Sensitive

- Pyrazinamide: Sensitive

- Ethambutol: Sensitive

- Streptomycin: Sensitive

Contact Investigation Reveals Source:

Public health investigation finds:

- Coworker diagnosed with TB 8 months ago

- Shared small office space

- Poor ventilation

- 12 employees exposed

Testing of contacts:

- 5/12 positive tuberculin skin tests

- 3/5 positive QuantiFERON-Gold

- All chest X-rays negative

- Latent TB treatment started

The Slow-Growing Challenge

Why TB is tricky:

- Generation time: 12-24 hours (vs. 20 minutes for *E. coli*)

- Requires special media (egg or liquid with supplements)

- Biosafety level 3 lab needed

- Drug susceptibility takes weeks

Monthly Monitoring:

Month 2:

- Sputum AFB smear negative
- Culture pending
- Pyrazinamide discontinued (standard protocol)

Month 4:

- Culture negative (conversion documented)
- Continue isoniazid and rifampin

Month 6:

- Treatment completed
- Final chest X-ray: Residual scarring
- Declared cured

Case 5: The Hospital's Unwelcome Guest

Day 14 post-surgery: "Every time we stop antibiotics, his fever returns"

Thomas, 68, had routine cardiac surgery two weeks ago. Now he's back with fever, and his sternal wound looks angry. The edges are separating, and there's purulent drainage.

Wound Culture Initial Results:

Gram stain: Many WBCs, Gram-positive cocci in clusters

Growth at 24 hours:

- Moderate Staphylococcus species

- Catalase: Positive

- Coagulase: Negative

The Critical Question: Pathogen or Contaminant?

Coagulase-negative staph could be:

- Skin contamination (common)
- True pathogen (in prosthetic material)

Thomas has prosthetic valve and sternal wires.

Species Identification Changes Everything:

MALDI-TOF result: Staphylococcus lugdunensis

Not S. epidermidis as initially suspected

This changes management completely

Why *S. lugdunensis* Matters:

Unlike other coagulase-negative staph:

- Aggressive like *S. aureus*
- Forms biofilms readily
- Causes endocarditis
- Requires aggressive treatment

Blood Cultures Turn Positive:

2/2 sets growing S. lugdunensis

Time to positivity: 14 hours

Suggests high-grade bacteremia

Antimicrobial Susceptibility:

Oxacillin: RESISTANT (mecA positive)

Vancomycin: Sensitive (MIC 1.0)

Daptomycin: Sensitive

Linezolid: Sensitive

Rifampin: Sensitive

Gentamicin: Sensitive

Echocardiogram Findings:

Transesophageal echo shows:

- 8mm vegetation on prosthetic valve
- Mild valvular regurgitation
- No abscess

Diagnosis: Prosthetic valve endocarditis with sternal osteomyelitis

Treatment Complexity:

Standard therapy insufficient for prosthetic material:

- Vancomycin 15 mg/kg IV q12h
- PLUS Rifampin 300 mg PO TID

- PLUS Gentamicin 1 mg/kg IV q8h x2 weeks

Surgical debridement of sternum required

The Biofilm Problem:

Prosthetic material infections are tough because:

1. Bacteria form biofilms
2. Antibiotics penetrate poorly
3. Immune cells can't access bacteria
4. Often requires device removal

Six-Week Treatment Course:

Weekly surveillance:

- Blood cultures (remained negative after day 3)
- Vancomycin troughs (goal 15-20)
- Renal function (creatinine rose from 1.0 to 1.6)
- Gentamicin levels

Outcome:

After 6 weeks IV therapy:

- Wound healed
- Valve function preserved (no surgery needed)
- Suppressive therapy: Doxycycline indefinitely
- Monthly labs for monitoring

Case 6: The Traveler's Revenge

Chief Complaint: "I haven't stopped running to the bathroom in five days"

Sandra, 34, returned from Peru eight days ago. The diarrhea started on day 3 of her trip but has worsened since returning home. She's having 8-10 watery stools daily with cramping.

Travel History:

- Two-week trek through rural Peru
- Drank bottled water "mostly"
- Ate street food regularly

- Swam in local rivers
- No malaria prophylaxis

Initial Stool Studies:

Appearance: Watery, no blood

WBC: Few

RBC: None

Ova and parasites x1: No parasites seen

Bacterial culture: Pending

C. difficile toxin: Negative

Rotavirus/Adenovirus: Negative

Day 2 - Stool Culture Results:

Salmonella species isolated

Serotype: Salmonella Typhi

Antimicrobial susceptibility:

Ampicillin: Resistant

Trimethoprim/sulfa: Resistant

Ciprofloxacin: INTERMEDIATE (MIC 0.5)

Ceftriaxone: Sensitive

Azithromycin: Sensitive

Not Just Traveler's Diarrhea - It's Typhoid

S. Typhi differs from other Salmonella:

- Causes systemic disease (enteric fever)
- Human-only reservoir
- Reportable immediately
- Can cause chronic carrier state

Additional Findings:

Blood cultures: 1/2 positive for S. Typhi

Rose spots: Present on trunk (pathognomonic)

Relative bradycardia: HR 72 with fever 39°C

The Fluoroquinolone Resistance Problem

Intermediate ciprofloxacin resistance (0.5 μg/mL):

- Treatment failure likely with standard dosing
- Common in South Asia and South America
- Must use alternative therapy

Treatment choice:

- Azithromycin 1g daily x5 days
- Or Ceftriaxone 2g IV daily x7-14 days

Day 5 - Not Improving, Stool O&P Repeated:

Modified acid-fast stain: Positive

Organism: Cyclospora cayetanensis also present

Co-infection discovered!

Dual Infection Management:

For Cyclospora:

- Trimethoprim/sulfamethoxazole DS BID x7 days
- (Despite Salmonella resistance, different mechanism)

For Typhoid:

- Continue azithromycin
- Monitor for complications

Public Health Investigation:

Contact tracin reveals:

- Travel group of 8 people
- 5/8 developed similar symptoms
- Same street vendor identified
- Local health authorities notified

The Carrier State Concern:

Follow-up required:

- Stool cultures at 1 month
- If positive, chronic carrier workup
- Gallbladder ultrasound (chronic carriage site)
- May need prolonged antibiotics

Three Months Later:

Sandra's follow-up:

- Three negative stool cultures
- Not a chronic carrier
- Full recovery
- Travel medicine referral for future trips

Case 7: The Immunocompromised Host's Mystery Fever

Oncology Ward: "His counts are recovering, but he's getting sicker"

David, 52, is day +18 post stem cell transplant for AML. His neutrophils are finally recovering (ANC 800), but he's developed fever and chest pain.

Current Status:

- Temperature: 38.4°C
- On broad-spectrum antibiotics already
- Meropenem + vancomycin x10 days
- New pleuritic chest pain
- Oxygen requirement increasing

Chest CT Findings:

Multiple nodular infiltrates with "halo sign" - ground-glass opacity surrounding nodules. Classic for angioinvasive fungal infection.

Fungal Workup Initiated:

Serum galactomannan: 2.8 (positive >0.5)

Serum (1,3)-beta-D-glucan: 324 pg/mL (positive >80)

Sputum culture: Septate hyphae with acute angle branching

Blood cultures: No growth

Bronchoscopy with BAL:

BAL fluid:

- Galactomannan: 4.2 (strongly positive)

- KOH prep: Septate hyphae seen

- Culture pending

- PCR: Aspergillus fumigatus detected

Invasive Aspergillosis Confirmed

Risk factors in David:

- Prolonged neutropenia

- High-dose steroids for GVHD

- Broad-spectrum antibiotics

- Stem cell transplant

Antifungal Susceptibility (Finally, at Day 7):

A. fumigatus isolated

Voriconazole: Sensitive (MIC 0.5)

Posaconazole: Sensitive

Isavuconazole: Sensitive

Amphotericin B: Sensitive

Treatment Approach:

First-line therapy:

- Voriconazole loading: 6 mg/kg IV q12h x2 doses

- Then 4 mg/kg IV q12h

- Therapeutic drug monitoring required

Target trough: 2-5 µg/mL

The Azole Resistance Emergence

Some centers seeing 5-10% azole resistance:

- Environmental pressure from agricultural azoles

- TR34/L98H mutation most common

- Requires susceptibility testing

- May need combination therapy

Week 2 - Worsening Despite Therapy:

Repeat galactomannan: 3.4 (increasing)

Voriconazole trough: 1.2 (subtherapeutic)

CYP2C19 genotype: Rapid metabolizer

Explains low levels despite standard dosing

Adjusted Approach:

- Increased voriconazole dose to 5 mg/kg
- Added anidulafungin 200 mg load, then 100 mg daily
- Combination therapy for severe disease

Monitoring Response:

Weekly markers:

- Galactomannan trend (best indicator)
- CT imaging monthly
- Liver enzymes (voriconazole toxicity)
- Visual symptoms (voriconazole side effect)

Three-Month Outcome:

After 12 weeks therapy:

- Galactomannan normalized (<0.5)
- CT: Residual scarring only
- Switched to oral posaconazole
- Continue through immunosuppression

Case 8: The New Resistance Nightmare

ICU Day 21: "We're running out of antibiotics to try"

Margaret, 74, has been in the ICU for three weeks with ventilator-associated pneumonia. She's been on multiple antibiotics, but keeps growing resistant organisms.

Current Culture Results:

Sputum culture:

>100,000 CFU/mL Klebsiella pneumoniae

Susceptibility profile:

ALL BETA-LACTAMS: Resistant

Ciprofloxacin: Resistant

Gentamicin: Resistant

Amikacin: Resistant

Tigecycline: Intermediate

Colistin: SENSITIVE (MIC 1.0)

The Carbapenemase Test:

Modified Hodge test: Positive Carba NP test: Positive Molecular testing: KPC (Klebsiella pneumoniae carbapenemase) detected

This is carbapenem-resistant Enterobacteriaceae (CRE).

Limited Options:

Treatment started:

- Colistin 5 mg/kg loading dose
- Then 2.5 mg/kg q12h (adjusted for renal function)
- PLUS Meropenem 2g q8h (high-dose despite resistance)
- PLUS Tigecycline 100 mg q12h

The Colistin Complexity:

Colistin (polymyxin E) challenges:

- Nephrotoxicity in 30-50%
- Neurotoxicity risk
- Poor lung penetration
- Heteroresistance common
- No established breakpoints initially

Day 5 - New Problem:

Repeat culture: Same organism

New finding: Colistin MIC 8 (now resistant)

Developed resistance during therapy

Searching for Options:

Expanded susceptibility testing:

Ceftazidime/avibactam: SENSITIVE (MIC 4)

Meropenem/vaborbactam: Sensitive (MIC 2)

Plazomicin: Sensitive

Fosfomycin: Variable

Newer Agent Success:

Switched to:

- Ceftazidime/avibactam 2.5g IV q8h
- Discontinued colistin
- Continued high-dose meropenem

Infection Control Emergency:

CRE requires strict isolation:

- Contact precautions
- Single room
- Dedicated equipment
- Environmental cultures
- Staff screening

Three other ICU patients subsequently found colonized.

The Resistance Mechanism Arms Race:

Margaret's isolate:

- KPC-2 carbapenemase (most common in US)
- Porin mutations (decreased permeability)
- Efflux pump overexpression

But ceftazidime/avibactam works because:

- Avibactam inhibits KPC
- Restores ceftazidime activity

Two-Week Outcome:

After switching therapy:

- Clinical improvement by day 4
- Repeat cultures negative

- Successfully extubated
- But remains colonized

Long-term: CRE colonization persists months to years.

Case 9: The Telling Vegetation

Admission Note: "Four weeks of fever, new murmur detected"

James, 42, injection drug user, presents with month-long fever, weight loss, and malaise. Exam reveals new systolic murmur and splinter hemorrhages.

Initial Blood Cultures:

4/4 bottles positive

Time to positivity: 8 hours (all bottles)

Gram stain: Gram-positive cocci in clusters

Preliminary ID: Staphylococcus aureus

Catalase: Positive

Coagulase: Positive

The Critical Next Test:

Oxacillin screen: POSITIVE (MRSA)

mecA gene PCR: Positive

Vancomycin MIC: 2.0 µg/mL (concerning)

Duke Criteria for Endocarditis:

Major criteria (2/2 met):

- Positive blood cultures with typical organism
- Echo showing 1.8 cm vegetation on tricuspid valve

Minor criteria (3/5 met):

- IVDU predisposition
- Fever >38°C
- Vascular phenomena (septic pulmonary emboli)

Definite endocarditis diagnosed.

259

The Vancomycin MIC Problem:

MIC = 2.0 technically "sensitive" but:

- Associated with treatment failure
- Mortality doubles vs. MIC ≤1.0
- Consider alternative therapy

Alternative Testing Reveals More:

Daptomycin: Sensitive (MIC 0.5)

Ceftaroline: Sensitive

Linezolid: Sensitive

Tedizolid: Sensitive

Treatment Decision:

Given vancomycin MIC 2.0 and severe disease:

- Daptomycin 10 mg/kg daily (high dose)
- PLUS Gentamicin 1 mg/kg q8h x2 weeks
- Not vancomycin despite "sensitivity"

Week 1 - Persistent Bacteremia:

Daily blood cultures still positive through day 5

Daptomycin increased to 12 mg/kg

Added rifampin 600 mg daily

The Source Control Issue:

TEE shows:

- Vegetation growing to 2.3 cm
- Severe tricuspid regurgitation
- Multiple septic emboli to lungs

Cardiac surgery consulted but declined ("IVDU, will reinfect")

Clearance Finally:

Day 8: First negative blood cultures

Day 10: Confirmed clearance

Continue 6 weeks from clearance date

Outpatient IV Therapy Challenge:

IVDU history complicates discharge:

- PICC line in active user risky
- Daily supervised therapy required
- Addiction medicine involved
- Methadone program enrollment

Six-Week Course Completed:

Final outcome:

- Blood cultures remained negative
- Vegetation decreased to 1.2 cm
- Tricuspid regurgitation moderate
- Enrolled in addiction treatment

But 20% will have recurrence within a year.

Case 10: The Post-Antibiotic Disaster

Hospital Day 12: "She finished antibiotics yesterday. Today she has severe diarrhea."

Carol, 81, was admitted with pneumonia, treated successfully with levofloxacin. Now has profuse watery diarrhea, cramping, and fever.

Initial Assessment:

Temperature: 38.6°C

WBC: 24,000/μL (was 8,000 yesterday)

Creatinine: 1.8 mg/dL (baseline 1.0)

Albumin: 2.4 g/dL

Stool: Liquid, foul-smelling

Bristol stool chart: Type 7

Frequency: 12 episodes in 24 hours

C. difficile Testing:

GDH antigen: Positive

Toxin A/B EIA: Positive

PCR confirmation: Positive (Ct value 18 - high burden)

The Testing Algorithm Matters:

Why multi-step testing?

- GDH sensitive but not specific

- Toxin EIA specific but not sensitive

- PCR sensitive but detects colonization too

- Algorithm improves accuracy

Carol is GDH+/Toxin+ = True infection

Severity Stratification:

WBC >15,000: Yes (24,000)

Creatinine >1.5x baseline: Yes (1.8 from 1.0)

Albumin <2.5: Yes (2.4)

Classification: SEVERE C. difficile infection

Treatment Based on Severity:

For severe CDI:

- Vancomycin 125 mg PO QID x10 days

- Not metronidazole (inferior for severe disease)

Day 3 - Worsening Despite Treatment:

WBC: 35,000/μL

Lactate: 2.8 mmol/L

Abdominal CT: Colonic wall thickening, ascites

Now fulminant CDI

Escalated Management:

- Vancomycin 500 mg PO QID

- PLUS Metronidazole 500 mg IV q8h
- PLUS Vancomycin enemas 500 mg QID
- Surgical consultation
- Consider fecal transplant

The Hypervirulent Strain Question:

Strain typing performed:

Ribotype 027 (NAP1/BI)

Binary toxin: Positive

Increased toxin A/B production confirmed

This explains severity - epidemic hypervirulent strain.

Day 10 - Finally Improving:

After aggressive therapy:

- WBC trending down (18,000)
- Diarrhea decreasing (4 episodes/day)
- Creatinine improving (1.3)

Completed 14-day course.

The Recurrence Problem:

Week 3 post-treatment:

- Diarrhea returns
- C. diff testing positive again
- First recurrence

Treatment for recurrence:

- Vancomycin taper and pulse:
  - 125 mg QID x10 days
  - 125 mg BID x7 days
  - 125 mg daily x7 days
  - 125 mg every 2-3 days x2-8 weeks

Prevention Measures:

For Carol and the unit:

- Contact isolation

- Soap and water (not alcohol sanitizer)

- Bleach for environmental cleaning

- Antibiotic stewardship reinforced

- Probiotics considered (evidence mixed)

Case 11: The Confusing STI Panel

Urgent Care: "I need everything tested. I made a mistake last month."

Brandon, 26, requests comprehensive STI testing after unprotected encounter 4 weeks ago. Now has dysuria and urethral discharge.

Initial Testing:

Urethral swab Gram stain:

- >10 WBC per high-power field

- Gram-negative intracellular diplococci seen

Urine NAAT (nucleic acid amplification test):

- Neisseria gonorrhoeae: POSITIVE

- Chlamydia trachomatis: POSITIVE

Dual Infection Treatment:

CDC guidelines for coinfection:

- Ceftriaxone 500 mg IM x1 (increased from 250 mg due to resistance)

- PLUS Doxycycline 100 mg PO BID x7 days

Additional Testing Ordered:

HIV 4th generation: Negative

RPR: Reactive (titer 1:32)

Confirmatory TP-PA: Positive

Hepatitis B surface antigen: Negative

Hepatitis C antibody: Negative

The Syphilis Diagnosis:

RPR 1:32 with positive TP-PA confirms syphilis. Physical exam reveals:

- Painless penile chancre (missed initially)
- Non-tender inguinal lymphadenopathy

Stage: Primary syphilis

Treatment Addition:

- Benzathine penicillin G 2.4 million units IM x1

The Antimicrobial Resistance Crisis:

Brandon's isolates sent for susceptibility:

N. gonorrhoeae:

- Ceftriaxone: Sensitive (MIC 0.06)

- Cefixime: Intermediate (MIC 0.125)

- Ciprofloxacin: Resistant

- Tetracycline: Resistant

- Penicillin: Resistant (beta-lactamase positive)

Test of Cure Complexity:

When to retest?

- Gonorrhea/Chlamydia: Only if symptoms persist
- Syphilis: RPR at 6 and 12 months

For syphilis, expect 4-fold RPR decline by 6 months.

Three Months Later - Reinfection:

Brandon returns with discharge again:

GC/CT testing: GC positive, CT negative

Different resistance pattern suggests reinfection

Partner notification critical

The Pre-Exposure Prophylaxis Discussion:

Given recurrent STIs, discussed:

- HIV PrEP (Truvada or Descovy)
- Would prevent HIV but not bacterial STIs

- Requires quarterly monitoring
- Kidney function and STI testing q3 months

Case 12: The Expanding Rash

Day 10 of symptoms: "Started as a bullseye, now I feel terrible"

Rachel, 38, presents with expanding rash that began after camping in Connecticut. Now has fever, headache, and joint pain.

Classic Presentation:

- Erythema migrans: 12 cm targetoid rash
- Recent tick exposure (removed embedded tick)
- Endemic area for Lyme disease
- Constitutional symptoms developing

Laboratory Testing Approach:

For early Lyme with erythema migrans:

- Clinical diagnosis
- Serology often negative early
- Treatment shouldn't await testing

But testing ordered given systemic symptoms:

Lyme antibody screen (EIA): Positive

Western blot IgM: 2/3 bands positive (23, 41 kDa)

Western blot IgG: 3/10 bands positive

Interpretation: Positive for early Lyme

Understanding Lyme Testing:

Two-tier testing required:

1. EIA or IFA screening
2. If positive/equivocal → Western blot

IgM criteria: 2 of 3 bands (23, 39, 41 kDa) IgG criteria: 5 of 10 specific bands

But There's More - Coinfection Screen:

Anaplasma phagocytophilum PCR: POSITIVE

Babesia microti PCR: Negative

Ehrlichia PCR: Negative

Powassan virus: Not tested

Dual Tick-Borne Infection

Anaplasmosis findings:

CBC: WBC 3,200, Platelets 89,000

Transaminases: AST 124, ALT 98

Blood smear: Morulae in neutrophils seen

Modified Treatment for Coinfection:

For Lyme + Anaplasmosis:

- Doxycycline 100 mg PO BID x14 days

- Covers both infections

- Monitor CBC and liver enzymes

The Geographic Expansion Problem

Tick-borne diseases spreading:

- Lyme: Northeast → Midwest, Mid-Atlantic

- Anaplasmosis: Similar distribution

- Babesiosis: More limited but expanding

- Powassan: Rare but severe

Follow-up Challenges:

Week 4 post-treatment:

- Symptoms resolved

- Repeat Lyme serology still positive (expected)

- IgG now 6/10 bands (seroconversion)

Serology remains positive for years - don't retest.

Six Months Later:

Rachel returns with fatigue, arthralgia: "Is my Lyme back?"

Evaluation for Post-Treatment Lyme Disease Syndrome:

- Repeat serology not helpful (stays positive)

267

- PCR blood: Negative

- Synovial fluid PCR: Negative

- Likely PTLDS, not active infection

- Antibiotics won't help

Case 13: The Silent Epidemic

Routine Screening: "I'm here for my annual check-up"

Michael, 24, MSM (men who have sex with men), asymptomatic, requests routine HIV screening as part of regular healthcare.

Initial Screening:

HIV 1/2 antigen/antibody (4th generation): Reactive

Supplemental testing initiated

The Confirmation Algorithm:

HIV-1/HIV-2 antibody differentiation assay:

- HIV-1: Positive

- HIV-2: Negative

HIV-1 RNA quantitative: 125,000 copies/mL

CD4 count: 298 cells/μL (18%)

CD4/CD8 ratio: 0.4

Acute HIV Infection Identified

Timeline reconstruction:

- Negative HIV test 4 months ago

- Recent acute retroviral syndrome 6 weeks ago

  o Attributed to "flu"

  o Fever, rash, lymphadenopathy

  o Resolved spontaneously

Currently in early chronic phase.

Baseline Resistance Testing:

HIV genotype:

- Subtype B

- NRTI mutations: None

- NNRTI mutations: None

- PI mutations: None

- INSTI mutations: None

Transmitted resistance: None detected

Additional Baseline Labs:

HLA-B*5701: Negative (can use abacavir)

Hepatitis B: Susceptible (needs vaccination)

Hepatitis C: Negative

Syphilis: Negative

Gonorrhea/Chlamydia: Negative

CrCl: 110 mL/min

G6PD: Normal

Treatment Initiation:

Start immediately (current guidelines):

- Bictegravir/tenofovir alafenamide/emtricitabine

- Single tablet daily

- Excellent resistance barrier

The Rapid Start Protocol:

Same-day ART initiation:

- Improves retention in care

- Reduces transmission risk

- Better clinical outcomes

Labs can be pending except:

- Pregnancy test (affects regimen choice)

- CrCl if using TDF

- HBV status (flare risk)

Week 4 Follow-up:

HIV RNA: 8,400 copies/mL (1.5 log drop)

CD4: 342 cells/µL

Adherence: 100% by pharmacy refill

Tolerating well

Reaching Undetectable:

Week 12:

HIV RNA: <20 copies/mL (undetectable)

CD4: 445 cells/µL

U=U counseling provided

Undetectable = Untransmittable

- Revolutionary for prevention
- Reduces stigma
- Requires consistent adherence

Long-term Monitoring:

Every 3-6 months:

- HIV RNA (maintain suppression)
- CD4 (until >250 x2)
- Comprehensive metabolic panel
- STI screening if at risk

Case 14: The Grandfather's Persistent Cough

TB Clinic Referral: "His skin test turned positive during green card application"

Vijay, 68, emigrated from India 6 months ago. Required TB screening showed:

- Tuberculin skin test: 18 mm induration
- Chest X-ray: Apical scarring
- No symptoms initially

Now developing cough and night sweats.

Evaluating Latent vs Active TB:

Sputum AFB smears x3: Negative

Sputum cultures: Pending

QuantiFERON-Gold: Positive (>10 IU/mL)

CT chest: Tree-in-bud opacities suggesting active disease

Sputum Culture at 3 Weeks:

MGIT signal positive

AFB seen on smear from broth

PCR: M. tuberculosis complex

Drug susceptibility pending

The India Connection - Concern for Drug Resistance:

India has high rates of drug-resistant TB:

- 2.8% of new cases are MDR-TB

- 12% of retreatment cases

Risk factors in Vijay:

- Previous TB treatment in India (1995)

- Incomplete records

- From high MDR region (Mumbai)

Molecular Rapid Testing:

Xpert MTB/RIF Ultra:

- MTB detected

- Rifampin resistance NOT detected

Line probe assay:

- Isoniazid resistance detected (katG mutation)

- Rifampin sensitive confirmed

Isoniazid Monoresistant TB

Treatment modification required:

- Rifampin 600 mg daily

- Pyrazinamide 1500 mg daily

- Ethambutol 1200 mg daily

- Levofloxacin 750 mg daily

- Duration: 6-9 months

Contact Investigation Critical:

Household contacts:

- Wife: TST 14 mm, CXR normal → Latent TB

- Son: TST 0 mm, QuantiFERON negative

- Daughter-in-law: TST 6 mm, pregnant, CXR deferred

- Grandchildren (2): TST 0 mm

Wife started on latent TB treatment:

- Rifampin daily x4 months (INH resistance in source)

Cultural Competency in TB Care:

Challenges with Vijay:

- Stigma about TB diagnosis

- Concerns about deportation (unfounded)

- Ayurvedic medicine interactions

- Fasting during religious holidays

- DOT (directly observed therapy) acceptance

Solutions:

- Video DOT via smartphone

- Cultural liaison involvement

- Extended family education

- Flexible dosing around fasting

Treatment Outcome:

Month 2: Culture conversion Month 6: Treatment completion Month 12: Remained disease-free

---

Case 15: The Respiratory Panel Puzzle

Pediatric ICU: "She's on ECMO, and we still don't know what's causing this"

Emily, 4 years old, admitted with severe respiratory failure. Started as "cold" 5 days ago, rapidly progressed to ARDS requiring ECMO support.

Initial Viral Testing:

Rapid influenza A/B: Negative

Rapid RSV: Negative

SARS-CoV-2 PCR: Negative

Blood cultures: No growth

Endotracheal aspirate: Normal flora

Comprehensive Respiratory Pathogen Panel:

BioFire FilmArray Respiratory Panel 2.1:

Viruses detected:

- Human metapneumovirus: POSITIVE

- Rhinovirus/Enterovirus: POSITIVE

- Coronavirus HKU1: POSITIVE

All others negative (influenza, RSV, parainfluenza, adenovirus)

Triple Viral Infection - But Which Is the Culprit?

Interpreting multiple positives:

- Could be sequential infections

- Could be co-infection

- Rhinovirus might be colonization

Quantitative Testing Helps:

Metapneumovirus viral load: 8.2 log copies/mL (very high)

Rhinovirus load: 3.1 log copies/mL (low)

Coronavirus load: 4.5 log copies/mL (moderate)

Primary pathogen likely metapneumovirus

Looking for Bacterial Superinfection:

Procalcitonin: 14.2 ng/mL (suggests bacterial)

Endotracheal aspirate repeated:

- Streptococcus pneumoniae 10^6 CFU/mL

- Haemophilus influenzae 10^5 CFU/mL

Bacterial superinfection confirmed

The Immunity Question:

Why so severe in a healthy child?

Immunology workup:

- IgG, IgA, IgM: Normal

- Lymphocyte subsets: Normal

- CH50, C3, C4: Normal

- Vaccine titers: Protective

No immunodeficiency found

Treatment Complexity:

Viral infection treatment:

- Ribavirin considered (limited evidence)

- Primarily supportive care

- IVIG given (immunomodulatory)

Bacterial coverage:

- Ceftriaxone + azithromycin

- Based on local antibiogram

The ECMO Challenge:

Drug pharmacokinetics altered on ECMO:

- Increased volume of distribution

- Drug sequestration in circuit

- Altered clearance

Antibiotic dosing adjusted:

- Higher doses needed

274

- More frequent monitoring

- Therapeutic drug monitoring when available

Week 2 - Slow Improvement:

Viral loads decreasing:

- Metapneumovirus: 5.1 log (down from 8.2)

- Others clearing

Bacterial cultures: Negative

Inflammatory markers improving

ECMO Decannulation Day 16:

Successfully weaned off ECMO Extubated day 20 Significant lung injury remains

Three-Month Follow-up:

Persistent effects:

- Reduced exercise tolerance

- Reactive airway disease

- Supplemental oxygen weaned

- Pulmonary function testing pending

This case illustrates modern respiratory diagnostics:

- Multiplex PCR identifies multiple pathogens

- Quantitative testing suggests primary agent

- Bacterial superinfection common

- Severe disease even with normal immunity

Mastering Microbiology Diagnostics

These fifteen cases show you the full spectrum of clinical microbiology. From Marcus's fastidious *Capnocytophaga* that took 76 hours to grow, to Emily's triple viral infection detected in 45 minutes by molecular testing. Each case demonstrated that microbiology isn't just about growing bugs on plates – it's about understanding pathogen behavior, resistance patterns, and host-pathogen interactions.

Speed Versus Accuracy Trade-offs:

You've seen how different situations demand different approaches. Jennifer's meningitis required immediate empiric therapy based on a Gram stain, while Robert's TB could wait weeks for susceptibility testing. Brandon's gonorrhea was diagnosed in hours by NAAT but still needed culture for susceptibility testing. The art lies in knowing when to act on preliminary results and when to wait for confirmation.

Resistance Pattern Recognition:

From Patricia's ESBL *E. coli* to Margaret's KPC-producing *Klebsiella*, antibiotic resistance shaped every treatment decision. You learned that "sensitive" doesn't always mean effective (like James's MRSA with vancomycin MIC of 2.0), and that resistance can develop during therapy (Margaret's colistin resistance). Each resistance mechanism – ESBL, KPC, VRE, MRSA – requires specific detection methods and treatment strategies.

Molecular Diagnostics Revolution:

These cases showed how molecular testing has transformed microbiology. Xpert MTB/RIF diagnosed Robert's TB in 2 hours versus 3 weeks for culture. Multiplex PCR revealed Emily's triple viral infection. Molecular typing linked Jennifer's meningitis to a college outbreak. But you also learned the limitations – PCR detects dead organisms, can't determine susceptibility for all drugs, and colonization looks the same as infection.

Public Health Integration:

Microbiology connects individual patients to population health. Jennifer's meningitis triggered contact prophylaxis for dozens. Sandra's typhoid initiated an international investigation. Michael's HIV diagnosis led to partner notification. Every positive TB test starts a contact investigation. The lab doesn't just diagnose individual infections – it protects communities.

The Human Side of Microbiology:

Behind every culture is a person whose life depends on getting it right. Carol's *C. diff* meant isolation from her grandchildren. Vijay's TB diagnosis carried cultural stigma. Brandon's recurrent STIs prompted difficult conversations about prevention. David's aspergillosis threatened his stem cell transplant success.

Modern clinical microbiology requires integrating traditional culture techniques with molecular diagnostics, understanding local resistance patterns while recognizing emerging threats, and balancing individual patient needs with public health obligations. Each specimen tells a story – not just of what's growing, but of where it came from, how it got there, and what it means for treatment.

Most importantly, these cases teach that negative cultures don't mean no infection, positive cultures don't always mean pathogen, and the difference between colonization and infection can be life-saving to recognize. That's the real art of clinical microbiology – knowing not just what's growing, but what it means.

Chapter 6: Molecular Diagnostics and Genetics

Case 6.1: Inherited Bleeding Disorder Genetic Confirmation

Clinical Presentation: A 28-year-old male presents to hematology clinic with lifelong history of easy bruising and prolonged bleeding after minor trauma. His maternal grandfather and maternal uncle had similar bleeding tendencies. Recent dental extraction required multiple visits for persistent oozing. He is planning to start a family and seeks genetic counseling.

Initial Laboratory Findings:

- PT: 12.5 seconds (normal: 11-13.5)
- aPTT: 58 seconds (normal: 25-35) **PROLONGED**
- Platelets: 245,000/μL (normal)
- Factor VIII activity: 8% (normal: 50-150%) **SEVERELY DECREASED**
- vWF antigen: Normal
- vWF activity: Normal

Diagnostic Reasoning Questions:

1. What is the most likely diagnosis based on family history and coagulation studies?
2. Why is molecular confirmation important for this patient?
3. What types of genetic variants cause this disorder?
4. How would you counsel this patient regarding inheritance patterns?

Sequential Test Results:

Molecular Testing Ordered: F8 gene sequencing (hemophilia A panel)

Results:

- Variant detected: c.5096G>A (p.Arg1699His) in F8 gene (intron 22 inversion testing negative)
- Classification: Pathogenic variant
- Zygosity: Hemizygous (X-linked)
- Predicted effect: Severe hemophilia A
- Parental testing recommended for carrier identification

Carrier Testing Results (Mother):

- Heterozygous carrier of same F8 variant
- Factor VIII activity: 45% (lower end of normal for carrier state)

Final Diagnosis: Severe Hemophilia A (F8 gene pathogenic variant)

Teaching Points:

1. **X-linked Recessive Inheritance:** Males are affected; females are carriers. All daughters of affected males will be carriers.
2. **Genotype-Phenotype Correlation:** Factor VIII levels <1% = severe; 1-5% = moderate; 5-40% = mild hemophilia A
3. **Clinical Significance:** Molecular confirmation enables accurate genetic counseling, prenatal diagnosis options, and family screening
4. **Variant Types:** Most common severe hemophilia A mutations include intron 22 inversion (~45%), intron 1 inversion (~5%), and point mutations/deletions
5. **Inhibitor Risk:** Certain mutations carry higher risk for developing inhibitory antibodies to factor VIII replacement therapy
6. **Reproductive Options:** Preimplantation genetic diagnosis, prenatal testing, and family planning counseling
7. **Carrier Detection:** Female relatives should be offered carrier testing; carriers may have reduced factor VIII levels and increased bleeding risk during surgery/childbirth

Related Cases: Hemophilia B (Factor IX deficiency), von Willebrand disease variants, acquired hemophilia with inhibitors

---

Case 6.2: Cancer Molecular Profiling for Targeted Therapy

Clinical Presentation: A 62-year-old female non-smoker presents with persistent cough and weight loss. Chest CT reveals a 4.5 cm right upper lobe mass with mediastinal lymphadenopathy. CT-guided biopsy performed.

Initial Laboratory Findings:

- Histopathology: Adenocarcinoma of lung, moderately differentiated
- Tumor staging: T2N2M0 (Stage IIIA)
- PD-L1 immunohistochemistry: Tumor proportion score 15%
- Adequate tissue available for molecular testing

Diagnostic Reasoning Questions:

1. Why is molecular profiling essential for this patient before treatment decisions?
2. Which molecular targets should be tested in lung adenocarcinoma?
3. How do molecular findings influence treatment selection?
4. What is the difference between driver mutations and resistance mutations?

Sequential Test Results:

Next-Generation Sequencing (NGS) Solid Tumor Panel Ordered

Results:

- **EGFR exon 19 deletion detected:** c.2235_2249del15 (p.Glu746_Ala750del)
- Variant allele frequency: 42%
- Classification: Pathogenic, actionable mutation

- **Additional findings:**
  - TP53 mutation: c.743G>A (p.Arg248Gln) - VAF 38%
  - TMB (Tumor Mutational Burden): 4 mutations/Mb (low)
  - MSI (Microsatellite Instability): Stable

No variants detected in:

- ALK rearrangements
- ROS1 rearrangements
- BRAF V600E
- KRAS mutations
- MET exon 14 skipping
- RET rearrangements
- NTRK fusions
- HER2 mutations

Final Diagnosis: Stage IIIA Lung Adenocarcinoma with EGFR Exon 19 Deletion (Targetable Driver Mutation)

Treatment Implications:

- First-line therapy: EGFR tyrosine kinase inhibitor (osimertinib preferred)
- Expected response rate: 70-80%
- Median progression-free survival: 18-20 months
- Resistance monitoring plan: Liquid biopsy for T790M mutation at progression

Teaching Points:

1. **Driver Mutations:** EGFR exon 19 deletions and L858R point mutations account for 85% of EGFR-mutant lung cancers; highly responsive to EGFR TKIs
2. **Targetable Alterations:** NCCN guidelines recommend testing for EGFR, ALK, ROS1, BRAF, NTRK, MET, RET, KRAS G12C, and emerging targets
3. **Mutually Exclusive Mutations:** Driver mutations (EGFR, ALK, ROS1) are typically mutually exclusive; presence of multiple drivers is rare
4. **Resistance Mechanisms:** T790M mutation emerges in ~60% of patients progressing on 1st/2nd generation EGFR TKIs; detected through repeat biopsy or liquid biopsy
5. **PD-L1 and TMB:** Low TMB and moderate PD-L1 suggest limited benefit from immunotherapy alone; TKI is superior first-line choice
6. **Specimen Requirements:** Minimum 20% tumor content and adequate DNA yield required for comprehensive NGS panels
7. **Turnaround Time:** NGS results typically available in 7-14 days; critical for treatment planning
8. **Co-Mutations:** TP53 co-mutations are common in EGFR-mutant cancers and may influence prognosis but not treatment selection

Related Cases: ALK-rearranged lung cancer, KRAS G12C-mutant cancer with specific inhibitor, acquired resistance mutations, liquid biopsy monitoring

Case 6.3: Prenatal Genetic Screening

Clinical Presentation: A 35-year-old G2P1 woman at 12 weeks gestation presents for routine prenatal care. First pregnancy was uncomplicated with healthy child. Family history significant for mother's brother with Down syndrome. Patient desires comprehensive prenatal screening.

Initial Laboratory Findings:

- First trimester combined screening:
    - Maternal age: 35 years (advanced maternal age)
    - NT (Nuchal Translucency): 3.2 mm (elevated; normal <3.0 mm)
    - Free β-hCG: 2.1 MoM (elevated)
    - PAPP-A: 0.4 MoM (decreased)
    - Risk assessment: 1 in 45 for trisomy 21 (HIGH RISK)
    - Risk for trisomy 18: 1 in 380
    - Risk for trisomy 13: 1 in 1200

Diagnostic Reasoning Questions:

1. What do these screening results indicate?
2. What is the difference between screening and diagnostic testing?
3. What are the next appropriate steps?
4. How should cell-free DNA testing be interpreted?

Sequential Test Results:

Non-Invasive Prenatal Testing (NIPT) - Cell-Free DNA Screening Ordered

Results:

- Fetal fraction: 8.5% (adequate; >4% required)
- **Trisomy 21 (Down syndrome): POSITIVE (High probability)**
- Trisomy 18: Negative
- Trisomy 13: Negative
- Sex chromosome aneuploidies: No abnormalities detected
- Fetal sex: Male
- Microdeletion panel: No deletions detected

Genetic Counseling Session: Patient counseled that NIPT is screening, not diagnostic. Positive predictive value for trisomy 21 at age 35 is ~90%. Offered diagnostic confirmation.

Patient opts for diagnostic testing: Chorionic Villus Sampling (CVS) at 13 weeks

Cytogenetic Analysis (CVS) Results:

- Karyotype: 47,XY,+21 (confirmed in 20 metaphase cells)
- **Confirmed Diagnosis: Trisomy 21 (Down syndrome)**
- No evidence of mosaicism

- No structural chromosomal abnormalities

Chromosomal Microarray Analysis (CMA):

- Additional testing reveals complete trisomy 21
- No clinically significant copy number variants
- Consistent with standard trisomy 21

Final Diagnosis: Fetal Trisomy 21 (Down Syndrome) - Non-mosaic, Non-disjunction Type

Teaching Points:

1. **Screening vs. Diagnostic Testing:** NIPT/serum screening are screening tests (high sensitivity/specificity but not 100%); karyotype/CMA are diagnostic
2. **Fetal Fraction Requirements:** NIPT requires adequate fetal DNA fraction ($\geq$4%); low fetal fraction may require repeat or alternative testing
3. **Positive Predictive Value:** PPV for NIPT varies with maternal age and baseline risk; false positives occur due to confined placental mosaicism, vanishing twin, maternal factors
4. **Diagnostic Confirmation:** All positive NIPT results should be confirmed with diagnostic testing (CVS or amniocentesis) before making major decisions
5. **Advanced Maternal Age:** Risk of trisomy 21: age 35 = 1/350; age 40 = 1/100; age 45 = 1/30
6. **Non-Disjunction Types:** 95% of trisomy 21 cases are due to maternal meiotic non-disjunction; 4% are translocations; 1% are mosaic
7. **Recurrence Risk:** For standard trisomy 21, recurrence risk is ~1% above age-related risk; for translocation carriers, risk is much higher (5-100% depending on type)
8. **Genetic Counseling:** Essential for discussing diagnostic accuracy, implications, management options, and support resources

Related Cases: Trisomy 18 (Edwards syndrome), trisomy 13 (Patau syndrome), sex chromosome aneuploidies (Turner, Klinefelter), confined placental mosaicism

---

Case 6.4: Pharmacogenomic Testing for Drug Metabolism

Clinical Presentation: A 45-year-old male with newly diagnosed major depressive disorder is started on citalopram 20 mg daily. After 6 weeks at therapeutic dose, patient reports no improvement in symptoms. Previous trial of sertraline also showed poor response. Patient requests genetic testing to guide medication selection. Family history notable for mother requiring multiple antidepressant trials.

Initial Laboratory Findings:

- Depression screening (PHQ-9): Score 19 (moderately severe depression)
- No improvement after 6 weeks of citalopram therapy
- Drug compliance confirmed via patient interview and pharmacy records
- Therapeutic drug monitoring: Citalopram level 50 ng/mL (expected therapeutic range: 50-110 ng/mL)
- Patient is on no other medications

Diagnostic Reasoning Questions:

1. Why might this patient not be responding to standard SSRI therapy?
2. Which pharmacogenomic markers affect antidepressant metabolism?
3. How do CYP450 polymorphisms affect drug levels and response?
4. How should pharmacogenomic results guide prescribing?

Sequential Test Results:

Pharmacogenomic Panel Ordered: CYP450 Genotyping (Psychiatry Panel)

Genetic Results:

CYP2D6 Genotype: *4/*4 (Homozygous)

- Phenotype: **Poor Metabolizer (PM)**
- Activity Score: 0
- Frequency: 5-10% of Caucasian population

CYP2C19 Genotype: *1/*17

- Phenotype: **Rapid Metabolizer (RM)**
- Activity Score: 1.5
- Frequency: 18-25% of population

CYP2C9 Genotype: *1/*1

- Phenotype: Normal Metabolizer (NM)
- Activity Score: 2.0

Additional Pharmacogenes:

- SLCO1B1: *1/*1 (normal)
- VKORC1: -1639 G/A (intermediate warfarin sensitivity)
- TPMT: *1/*1 (normal thiopurine metabolism)

Clinical Pharmacist Interpretation:

For Current Medication (Citalopram):

- Metabolized primarily by CYP2C19 (with minor CYP2D6 contribution)
- Patient's CYP2C19 rapid metabolizer status: Drug levels may be LOWER than expected
- Recommendation: Likely underexposure; may need higher dose OR alternative drug

Medication Recommendations Based on Genotype:

AVOID or Use with Caution (due to CYP2D6 PM status):

- Tricyclic antidepressants (amitriptyline, nortriptyline): Risk of TOXICITY
- Venlafaxine: Reduced conversion to active metabolite
- Codeine: No analgesic effect (prodrug requires CYP2D6)
- Tramadol: Reduced efficacy

PREFERRED Options:

- Sertraline: Minimal CYP2D6 metabolism
- Escitalopram with dose adjustment: May increase to 30 mg
- Mirtazapine: Not dependent on CYP2D6
- Bupropion: Alternative mechanism, less affected

Adjusted Treatment Plan: Switch to mirtazapine 15 mg nightly (CYP2D6-independent metabolism)

Follow-Up at 6 Weeks:

- PHQ-9 score: 7 (minimal depression) - **Significant improvement**
- Side effects: Minimal sedation, well-tolerated
- Patient reports this is first antidepressant that has helped

Final Diagnosis: Major Depressive Disorder with Pharmacogenomic-Guided Treatment Optimization (CYP2D6 Poor Metabolizer, CYP2C19 Rapid Metabolizer)

Teaching Points:

1. **CYP2D6 Polymorphisms:** Highly polymorphic gene; PM (no activity), IM (reduced), NM (normal), UM (increased); affects 25% of commonly prescribed drugs
2. **Poor Metabolizer Phenotype:** Increased drug levels and side effects for drugs metabolized by that enzyme; REDUCED efficacy for prodrugs (codeine, tramadol, clopidogrel)
3. **CYP2C19 Variability:** Affects clopidogrel activation, SSRI metabolism, PPI metabolism; rapid metabolizers may have subtherapeutic levels
4. **Clinical Implementation:** FDA labels include pharmacogenomic information for >200 drugs; CPIC guidelines provide dosing recommendations
5. **Phenoconversion:** Drug interactions can change phenotype (CYP2D6 inhibitors like fluoxetine, paroxetine convert NM→PM functionally)
6. **Cost-Effectiveness:** Prevents trial-and-error prescribing, reduces adverse events, improves outcomes in certain therapeutic areas
7. **Limitations:** Genotype doesn't account for drug interactions, organ function, compliance, or non-genetic factors affecting response
8. **Testing Platforms:** Genotyping (specific alleles) vs. phenotyping (measure enzyme activity); genotyping is standard for PGx

Related Cases: Clopidogrel non-responder (CYP2C19 PM), warfarin dosing (CYP2C9 and VKORC1), thiopurine toxicity (TPMT deficiency), codeine toxicity in UM

Case 6.5: Familial Hypercholesterolemia

Clinical Presentation: A 32-year-old male presents for cardiovascular risk assessment. Father had myocardial infarction at age 42 and currently on high-dose statins. Patient is asymptomatic but concerned about family history. Physical exam reveals bilateral corneal arcus and tendon xanthomas on Achilles tendons.

Initial Laboratory Findings:

- Total cholesterol: 385 mg/dL (desirable <200)
- LDL cholesterol: 310 mg/dL (optimal <100) **SEVERELY ELEVATED**
- HDL cholesterol: 48 mg/dL (normal)
- Triglycerides: 135 mg/dL (normal)
- Fasting glucose: 92 mg/dL (normal)
- TSH: 2.1 mIU/L (normal - excludes hypothyroidism)
- Creatinine: 0.9 mg/dL (normal - excludes nephrotic syndrome)

Diagnostic Reasoning Questions:

1. What clinical features suggest familial hypercholesterolemia (FH)?
2. What is the Dutch Lipid Clinic Network Score for FH diagnosis?
3. Which genes are associated with FH?
4. Why is genetic testing important for this patient and family?

Dutch Lipid Clinic Network Criteria Score:

- LDL >330 mg/dL: 8 points
- Tendon xanthomas: 6 points
- Corneal arcus before age 45: 4 points
- Family history of premature CHD in 1st degree relative: 2 points
- **Total: 20 points = Definite FH (>8 points)**

Sequential Test Results:

Genetic Testing: Familial Hypercholesterolemia Panel Ordered

Genes Tested: LDLR, APOB, PCSK9, LDLRAP1, APOE

Molecular Results:

- **LDLR gene: c.1646G>A (p.Gly549Asp)**
- Zygosity: **Heterozygous**
- Classification: **Pathogenic variant**
- Variant type: Missense mutation affecting LDL receptor binding domain
- Functional effect: ~50% reduction in LDL receptor activity
- Inheritance: Autosomal dominant

No pathogenic variants in:

- APOB (apolipoprotein B-100)
- PCSK9 (gain-of-function mutations)
- LDLRAP1 (recessive FH)

Family Cascade Screening Initiated:

Father (age 55):

- Same LDLR variant detected (heterozygous)
- LDL: 295 mg/dL
- History of MI at age 42

Brother (age 29):

- LDLR variant NOT detected
- LDL: 105 mg/dL (normal)

Sister (age 35):

- Same LDLR variant detected (heterozygous)
- LDL: 278 mg/dL
- Previously undiagnosed

Patient's Children:

- 50% risk of inheriting variant
- Screening recommended starting age 2-10 years

Final Diagnosis: Heterozygous Familial Hypercholesterolemia (HeFH) due to LDLR Pathogenic Variant

Treatment Plan:

- High-intensity statin (atorvastatin 80 mg or rosuvastatin 40 mg)
- Ezetimibe 10 mg
- Target LDL <70 mg/dL (high cardiovascular risk)
- If target not met: consider PCSK9 inhibitor (alirocumab or evolocumab)
- Lifestyle modifications
- Coronary artery calcium score for risk stratification

Teaching Points:

1. **Genetic Basis:** LDLR mutations (90%), APOB mutations (5%), PCSK9 gain-of-function mutations (1%); autosomal dominant inheritance
2. **Prevalence:** 1 in 250 for heterozygous FH; 1 in 160,000-300,000 for homozygous FH
3. **Phenotypic Features:** Severely elevated LDL from birth, tendon xanthomas, corneal arcus, premature cardiovascular disease
4. **Homozygous FH:** Extremely rare; LDL >500 mg/dL; CVD in childhood; requires aggressive therapy (apheresis, PCSK9 inhibitors)

5. **Cascade Screening:** Identifying one FH case enables testing of 5-10 relatives on average; improves detection and early treatment
6. **Cardiovascular Risk:** Untreated HeFH: 50% risk of fatal/non-fatal CHD by age 50 in men, age 60 in women
7. **Treatment Efficacy:** Early statin therapy reduces CVD risk by 80%; genetic diagnosis ensures compliance and intensive treatment
8. **Genetic Counseling:** 50% chance of passing to each child; prenatal diagnosis available; preimplantation genetic diagnosis option

Related Cases: Homozygous FH, sitosterolemia, polygenic hypercholesterolemia, APOB p.Arg3527Gln mutation, PCSK9 loss-of-function variants (protective)

Case 6.6: Hereditary Cancer Syndrome

Clinical Presentation: A 38-year-old woman is diagnosed with invasive ductal carcinoma of the right breast (ER+, PR+, HER2-negative). Strong family history: mother diagnosed with ovarian cancer at age 52, maternal aunt with breast cancer at age 45, maternal grandmother with breast cancer at age 48. Patient has two young daughters and is concerned about hereditary risk.

Initial Laboratory Findings:

- Tumor pathology: Invasive ductal carcinoma, Grade 2, Stage IIA (T2N0M0)
- ER: 90% positive
- PR: 75% positive
- HER2: Negative (IHC 1+)
- Ki-67: 18%

Family Pedigree Analysis:

- Three generation pedigree shows autosomal dominant pattern
- Multiple breast and ovarian cancers on maternal side
- Early age of onset (<50 years)
- Ashkenazi Jewish ancestry noted

Diagnostic Reasoning Questions:

1. What features suggest hereditary breast and ovarian cancer syndrome (HBOC)?
2. Which genes should be tested?
3. How do BRCA1 vs BRCA2 mutations differ in cancer risk?
4. What are the implications for the patient and family members?

Sequential Test Results:

Hereditary Cancer Panel: Multi-Gene NGS Testing

Genes Tested: BRCA1, BRCA2, PALB2, CHEK2, ATM, TP53, PTEN, CDH1, STK11, MLH1, MSH2, MSH6, PMS2, EPCAM, and others

Molecular Results:

BRCA1 gene: c.68_69delAG (p.Glu23ValfsX17)

- Zygosity: Heterozygous
- Classification: **PATHOGENIC**
- Variant type: Frameshift deletion (founder mutation in Ashkenazi Jewish population: 185delAG)
- Frequency: ~1% in Ashkenazi Jews; rare in general population
- Inheritance: Autosomal dominant

All other genes: No pathogenic or likely pathogenic variants detected

Variants of Uncertain Significance (VUS):

- CHEK2: c.1100T>C (p.Ile367Thr) - VUS; insufficient evidence for pathogenicity
- Clinical management should NOT be based on VUS

Cancer Risk Assessment with BRCA1 Mutation:

Lifetime Risks (up to age 80):

- Breast cancer: 55-72% (vs 12% general population)
- Contralateral breast cancer: 40-60%
- Ovarian cancer: 39-44% (vs 1.3% general population)
- Pancreatic cancer: Slightly increased
- Melanoma: Slightly increased

Family Testing Results:

Mother (ovarian cancer survivor):

- Same BRCA1 mutation detected
- Source of inherited mutation confirmed

Sister (age 42, unaffected):

- BRCA1 mutation detected
- Initiates enhanced surveillance

Daughter 1 (age 16):

- Genetic testing deferred until age 18-25 per guidelines
- 50% inheritance risk

Daughter 2 (age 12):

- Testing deferred until age 18-25
- 50% inheritance risk

Final Diagnosis: Hereditary Breast and Ovarian Cancer Syndrome (HBOC) due to BRCA1 Founder Mutation (185delAG)

Management Implications:

For Index Patient:

- **Surgical options:** Consider bilateral mastectomy (prophylactic contralateral mastectomy reduces risk by 90%)
- Risk-reducing salpingo-oophorectomy (RRSO) at age 40 or completion of childbearing
- Enhanced surveillance if retains ovaries: pelvic ultrasound + CA-125 every 6 months
- Chemoprevention: Consider tamoxifen/raloxifene

For Unaffected Carriers:

- Breast MRI annually starting age 25-30
- Mammography + MRI alternating every 6 months starting age 30
- Clinical breast exam every 6-12 months
- Consider risk-reducing mastectomy
- Risk-reducing salpingo-oophorectomy by age 35-40

For Male Relatives with Mutation:

- Increased risk of breast cancer (1-5%), prostate cancer, pancreatic cancer
- Annual clinical breast exam, prostate screening

Teaching Points:

1. **BRCA1 vs BRCA2:** BRCA1 has higher ovarian cancer risk, earlier onset, more triple-negative breast cancers; BRCA2 has male breast cancer, higher pancreatic cancer risk
2. **Founder Mutations:** Three Ashkenazi Jewish founder mutations (185delAG and 5382insC in BRCA1; 6174delT in BRCA2) account for most HBOC in this population
3. **Autosomal Dominant Inheritance:** 50% transmission to each child regardless of sex; male carriers can transmit to children
4. **Variable Penetrance:** Not all mutation carriers develop cancer; modifying genetic and environmental factors influence individual risk
5. **Tumor Characteristics:** BRCA1 tumors often triple-negative (ER-, PR-, HER2-); BRCA2 tumors often ER-positive
6. **Therapeutic Implications:** BRCA-mutated cancers sensitive to PARP inhibitors (olaparib, talazoparib) and platinum chemotherapy
7. **Genetic Discrimination:** Federal law (GINA) prohibits health insurance and employment discrimination; does NOT cover life, disability, or long-term care insurance
8. **VUS Management:** Variants of uncertain significance should NOT guide clinical management; may be reclassified as more data emerges

Related Cases: Lynch syndrome (hereditary colon cancer), Li-Fraumeni syndrome (TP53), Cowden syndrome (PTEN), hereditary diffuse gastric cancer (CDH1)

Case 6.7: Mitochondrial Disease

Clinical Presentation: A 14-year-old previously healthy girl develops progressive exercise intolerance, muscle weakness, and recurrent episodes of severe headache with vomiting. Episodes are triggered by physical exertion. Recent school screening reveals short stature (5th percentile) and hearing difficulties. Neurological exam shows mild ptosis and proximal muscle weakness. Mother reports similar, milder symptoms in adolescence.

Initial Laboratory Findings:

- **Serum lactate (fasting):** 4.5 mmol/L (normal <2.0) **ELEVATED**
- **Serum lactate (post-exercise):** 9.2 mmol/L **MARKEDLY ELEVATED**
- Pyruvate: 0.25 mmol/L (elevated; normal <0.10)
- Lactate/pyruvate ratio: 18 (elevated; normal <20)
- Creatine kinase: 450 U/L (mildly elevated; normal <200)
- Ammonia: Normal
- Blood glucose: Normal
- Complete blood count: Mild macrocytic anemia (MCV 102 fL)

Diagnostic Reasoning Questions:

1. What features suggest mitochondrial disease?
2. Why is lactate elevated at rest and post-exercise?
3. What is the difference between nuclear and mitochondrial DNA mutations?
4. How does heteroplasmy affect disease severity?

Sequential Test Results:

Brain MRI with Spectroscopy:

- Bilateral basal ganglia T2 hyperintensities
- Lactate peak on MR spectroscopy (suggests mitochondrial dysfunction)
- Findings consistent with mitochondrial encephalomyopathy

Muscle Biopsy Performed:

- Modified Gomori trichrome stain: **Ragged red fibers present** (abnormal mitochondrial accumulation)
- Succinate dehydrogenase (SDH) stain: Increased staining
- Cytochrome c oxidase (COX) stain: COX-deficient fibers
- Electron microscopy: Abnormal mitochondria with paracrystalline inclusions
- Biochemical analysis: Respiratory chain Complex I activity 35% of control (severely reduced)

Molecular Genetic Testing: Mitochondrial DNA Sequencing

Results:

Mitochondrial DNA (mtDNA) Mutation:

- **m.3243A>G variant in MT-TL1 gene (tRNA-Leu)**
- Classification: **PATHOGENIC**
- **Heteroplasmy level (blood): 42%** (mixture of mutant and wild-type mtDNA)
- **Heteroplasmy level (muscle): 68%** (higher in affected tissue)

Associated Syndrome: MELAS (Mitochondrial Encephalomyopathy, Lactic Acidosis, and Stroke-like episodes)

Additional mtDNA Analysis:

- No large-scale mtDNA deletions detected
- No other pathogenic point mutations

Family Testing:

Mother:

- Same m.3243A>G mutation detected
- Heteroplasmy level (blood): 28% (lower than daughter)
- Symptoms: Mild exercise intolerance, migraine history, hearing loss
- **Maternal inheritance confirmed**

Maternal Grandmother:

- Same mutation detected
- Heteroplasmy level: 15%
- Symptoms: Late-onset diabetes, hearing loss

Brother (age 11):

- Same mutation detected
- Heteroplasmy level: 35%
- Currently asymptomatic but at risk

Final Diagnosis: MELAS Syndrome (Mitochondrial Encephalomyopathy, Lactic Acidosis, and Stroke-like Episodes) due to m.3243A>G Mitochondrial DNA Mutation

Clinical Features of MELAS:

- Stroke-like episodes before age 40
- Seizures and/or dementia
- Mitochondrial myopathy (ragged red fibers)
- Lactic acidosis
- Additional features: diabetes, hearing loss, cardiac involvement, short stature

Management:

- Mitochondrial "cocktail": Coenzyme Q10, L-carnitine, creatine, B vitamins

- Avoid: Valproic acid (mitochondrial toxin), aminoglycosides (hearing loss)
- Stroke prophylaxis: L-arginine during acute episodes
- Multidisciplinary care: neurology, genetics, cardiology, endocrinology
- Monitor: Cardiac function, hearing, vision, endocrine function, growth

Teaching Points:

1. **Maternal Inheritance:** Mitochondrial DNA is inherited exclusively from mother; all maternal offspring at risk
2. **Heteroplasmy:** Mixture of mutant and normal mtDNA; higher mutation load correlates with more severe disease
3. **Threshold Effect:** Symptoms appear when mutant mtDNA exceeds tissue-specific threshold (typically 60-90%)
4. **Tissue Variability:** Mutation load varies between tissues; muscle/CNS typically most affected due to high energy demands
5. **Common Mutations:** m.3243A>G (MELAS), m.8344A>G (MERRF), large-scale deletions (Kearns-Sayre syndrome), m.8993T>G (NARP/Leigh)
6. **Nuclear vs Mitochondrial:** Nuclear mutations follow Mendelian inheritance; mtDNA mutations show maternal inheritance and heteroplasmy
7. **Prenatal Prediction:** Difficult due to bottleneck effect (random shift in heteroplasmy between generations)
8. **Multisystem Involvement:** Mitochondrial diseases affect high-energy tissues: brain, muscle, heart, kidneys, eyes, ears, endocrine system

Related Cases: Leigh syndrome, MERRF (myoclonic epilepsy with ragged red fibers), Kearns-Sayre syndrome, Leber hereditary optic neuropathy (LHON)

Case 6.8: Cystic Fibrosis Carrier Screening

Clinical Presentation: A 28-year-old woman and her 30-year-old husband present for preconception genetic counseling. The woman's first cousin (maternal side) has cystic fibrosis. The couple is of mixed European ancestry and desires carrier screening before attempting pregnancy. Both partners are healthy with no pulmonary or gastrointestinal symptoms.

Initial Laboratory Findings:

- Both partners: Healthy, no clinical features of CF
- No history of recurrent respiratory infections, pancreatic insufficiency, or infertility
- Family history: Woman's maternal aunt is obligate CF carrier (has affected child)

Diagnostic Reasoning Questions:

1. What is the carrier frequency for cystic fibrosis in different populations?
2. What is the inheritance pattern and what are the risks for this couple?
3. Which CFTR mutations should be included in screening panels?
4. What are the limitations of CF carrier screening?

Sequential Test Results:

Cystic Fibrosis Carrier Screening: CFTR Gene Analysis

Female Partner Results:

- **CFTR gene: c.1521_1523delCTT (p.Phe508del or F508del)**
- Zygosity: Heterozygous
- Classification: **PATHOGENIC** - Most common CF-causing mutation
- **Carrier status: POSITIVE**
- Allele frequency: ~70% of CF chromosomes in Northern European populations

Male Partner Results:

- **No pathogenic variants detected in CFTR gene**
- Panel tested: ACMG/ACOG recommended 23-mutation panel + extended panel (>400 variants)
- Residual risk of being carrier: ~1/240 (reduced from 1/25 pre-test risk for Northern European ancestry)

Risk Assessment for Offspring:

Current scenario:

- Female: Confirmed carrier (F508del)
- Male: Negative screening but residual carrier risk ~1/240

Risk calculations:

- Risk of affected child: $(1) \times (1/240) \times (1/4) =$ **1/960** (~0.1%)
- If male partner were confirmed carrier: 1/4 = 25% affected
- If male partner not a carrier: 0% affected

Genetic Counseling Discussion:

Option 1: Proceed with pregnancy

- Low but not zero risk (~1/960)
- Consider expanded CFTR sequencing for male partner

Option 2: Extended CFTR sequencing for male partner

- Full gene sequencing + deletion/duplication analysis
- Detects >99% of mutations
- Further reduces residual risk

Couple opts for extended sequencing:

Male Partner - Extended CFTR Analysis:

- Full gene sequencing (all 27 exons)
- Large deletion/duplication analysis
- **Result: c.3718-2477C>T (5T variant in intron 8)**
- Classification: **VARIANT OF VARIABLE CLINICAL SIGNIFICANCE**
- Associated with: CFTR-related disorders (CBAVD - congenital bilateral absence of vas deferens) more than classic CF
- Impact: Mild/variable disease; depends on other CFTR variant present

Revised Risk Assessment:

Female partner: F508del (severe mutation) Male partner: 5T variant (mild variant)

If both variants inherited:

- Likely phenotype: Mild CF or CFTR-related metabolic syndrome (CRMS)
- Risk of classic CF: Very low
- Risk of CFTR-related disorder: Possible
- Risk calculation: 25% chance of inheriting both variants

Couple counseled about:

1. Phenotypic variability with F508del/5T genotype
2. Most individuals with this combination have mild or no symptoms
3. Options: Proceed with pregnancy with prenatal diagnosis, PGT-M (preimplantation genetic testing), consider alternative reproductive options

Final Diagnosis: Female Partner: Cystic Fibrosis Carrier (F508del/normal) Male Partner: 5T Variant (variable penetrance, CFTR-related)

Management Plan:

- Couple decides to proceed with pregnancy
- Prenatal diagnosis offered: CVS or amniocentesis with CFTR mutation analysis
- Newborn screening will detect CF if present
- Genetic counseling provided regarding 25% chance of both variants

Teaching Points:

1. **Inheritance Pattern:** Autosomal recessive; both parents must be carriers for affected child (25% risk each pregnancy)
2. **Carrier Frequencies:** Northern European 1/25; Ashkenazi Jewish 1/24; Hispanic 1/46; African American 1/61; Asian American 1/90
3. **F508del Mutation:** Most common (70% of CF chromosomes); causes severe phenotype with pancreatic insufficiency
4. **CFTR Mutations:** >2000 mutations identified; ACMG/ACOG panel includes 23 most common mutations (detects ~90% of carriers in general population)
5. **Residual Risk:** Negative screening doesn't eliminate carrier risk; residual risk depends on ethnicity and panel used

6. **Genotype-Phenotype Correlation:** Severe mutations (F508del, G542X, W1282X) → classic CF; mild mutations (R117H, 5T) → milder disease or CFTR-related disorders
7. **5T Variant:** Polymorphism in intron 8 affecting splicing; 5T (vs 7T or 9T) reduces normal CFTR protein; associated with CBAVD in males, mild/atypical CF
8. **CFTR Modulator Therapies:** New treatments (ivacaftor, lumacaftor, elexacaftor-tezacaftor-ivacaftor) target specific mutations; genotype determines eligibility
9. **Reproductive Options:** Prenatal diagnosis, preimplantation genetic testing (PGT-M), adoption, donor gametes

Related Cases: Carrier screening for other recessive disorders (Tay-Sachs, sickle cell, thalassemia), expanded carrier screening panels, CFTR-related disorders (CBAVD, chronic pancreatitis)

Chapter 7: Urinalysis and Body Fluid Analysis

Case 7.1: Nephrotic Syndrome Workup

Clinical Presentation: A 45-year-old man presents with progressive leg swelling over 3 weeks, facial puffiness in the mornings, and foamy urine. He has a 10-year history of type 2 diabetes mellitus with suboptimal glycemic control (HbA1c typically 8-9%). Recent 15-pound weight gain. Denies hematuria, dysuria, or flank pain.

Physical Examination:

- BP: 148/92 mmHg
- Periorbital edema
- 3+ pitting edema bilateral lower extremities to mid-thigh
- Abdominal examination: No ascites appreciated

Initial Laboratory Findings:

- Serum creatinine: 1.4 mg/dL (baseline 0.9 mg/dL) - **ELEVATED**
- BUN: 28 mg/dL
- Serum albumin: 2.1 g/dL (normal 3.5-5.0) **SEVERELY LOW**
- Total cholesterol: 340 mg/dL (markedly elevated)
- LDL: 245 mg/dL
- Triglycerides: 385 mg/dL

Diagnostic Reasoning Questions:

1. What is the classic tetrad of nephrotic syndrome?
2. How does nephrotic syndrome differ from nephritic syndrome?
3. What urinalysis findings confirm nephrotic range proteinuria?
4. What is the significance of examining urine sediment?

Sequential Test Results:

Urinalysis (Random Spot Urine):

Physical Characteristics:

- Color: Yellow
- Clarity: Slightly cloudy
- Specific gravity: 1.020

Chemical Analysis (Dipstick):

- pH: 6.0

- **Protein: 4+ (≥300 mg/dL) MARKEDLY ELEVATED**
- Glucose: Negative
- Ketones: Negative
- Blood: Trace
- Leukocyte esterase: Negative
- Nitrites: Negative
- Bilirubin: Negative
- Urobilinogen: Normal

Microscopic Examination:

- **RBCs: 5-10/hpf** (mildly increased; normal <3)
- WBCs: 0-2/hpf (normal)
- Epithelial cells: Few
- **Oval fat bodies: Present** (lipid-laden renal tubular epithelial cells)
- **Fatty casts: Present** (pathognomonic for nephrotic syndrome)
- Hyaline casts: 2-5/lpf
- **Waxy casts: Occasional** (suggests chronic kidney disease)
- Crystals: None
- Bacteria: None
- **Maltese cross pattern under polarized light: Positive** (cholesterol esters in oval fat bodies)

Quantitative Urine Protein Studies:

24-Hour Urine Collection:

- Total volume: 1800 mL
- **Total protein: 8.5 grams/24 hours** (normal <150 mg/day) **NEPHROTIC RANGE**
- Urine creatinine: 1.2 g/24 hours (adequate collection)

Spot Urine Protein/Creatinine Ratio:

- **Protein/creatinine ratio: 7.8 mg protein/mg creatinine** (normal <0.2)
- Confirms nephrotic range proteinuria (>3.5 g/day or ratio >3.5)

Urine Albumin/Creatinine Ratio (Random Spot):

- **ACR: 6800 mg/g** (severely increased albuminuria; normal <30 mg/g)

Urine Protein Electrophoresis:

- **Pattern: Selective proteinuria (predominantly albumin ~90%)**
- Minimal excretion of larger proteins (IgG, alpha-2-macroglobulin)
- Consistent with glomerular proteinuria

Additional Diagnostic Tests:

Serology:

- ANA: Negative (excludes lupus nephritis)
- Anti-dsDNA: Negative
- Complement C3: Normal (excludes complement-mediated GN)
- Complement C4: Normal
- Hepatitis B surface antigen: Negative
- Hepatitis C antibody: Negative
- HIV: Negative

Renal Ultrasound:

- Right kidney: 11.2 cm (normal size)
- Left kidney: 10.8 cm
- Increased echogenicity bilaterally (suggests chronic changes)
- No hydronephrosis or masses

Final Diagnosis: Nephrotic Syndrome, likely secondary to Diabetic Nephropathy (Diabetic Kidney Disease)

Nephrotic Syndrome Tetrad (All Present):

1. √ Massive proteinuria (>3.5 g/day)
2. √ Hypoalbuminemia (<3.0 g/dL)
3. √ Edema
4. √ Hyperlipidemia

Teaching Points:

1. **Nephrotic vs Nephritic:** Nephrotic = protein, edema, hypoalbuminemia, lipiduria; Nephritic = hematuria, RBC casts, HTN, oliguria, renal insufficiency
2. **Oval Fat Bodies:** Renal tubular epithelial cells with reabsorbed lipoproteins; appear as refractile droplets
3. **Maltese Cross Pattern:** Cholesterol esters under polarized light create characteristic appearance; pathognomonic for lipiduria
4. **Fatty Casts:** Tubular casts containing lipid droplets; specific for nephrotic syndrome
5. **Selective vs Non-Selective Proteinuria:** Selective (mostly albumin) suggests minimal change disease; non-selective (all proteins) suggests more severe glomerular damage
6. **Diabetic Nephropathy:** Most common cause of nephrotic syndrome in adults; progression: microalbuminuria → macroalbuminuria → nephrotic syndrome → ESRD
7. **Complications:** Hypercoagulable state (loss of antithrombin III), infections (loss of immunoglobulins), vitamin D deficiency, acute kidney injury
8. **24-Hour vs Spot Urine:** Spot protein/creatinine ratio correlates with 24-hour collection; more convenient and adequate for monitoring

Related Cases: Minimal change disease, focal segmental glomerulosclerosis (FSGS), membranous nephropathy, lupus nephritis, amyloidosis

Case 7.2: Acute Glomerulonephritis

Clinical Presentation: A 12-year-old boy presents with cola-colored urine for 2 days, facial puffiness, and decreased urine output. Two weeks ago, he had a sore throat treated symptomatically. Physical exam reveals periorbital edema, BP 145/95 mmHg (elevated for age), and trace pretibial edema.

Initial Laboratory Findings:

- Serum creatinine: 1.8 mg/dL (elevated; normal for age 0.3-0.7)
- BUN: 42 mg/dL (elevated)
- Serum albumin: 3.2 g/dL (low-normal)

Diagnostic Reasoning Questions:

1. What features suggest acute glomerulonephritis?
2. What are the characteristic urinalysis findings?
3. How do RBC casts form and what is their significance?
4. What is the differential diagnosis for acute GN in a child?

Sequential Test Results:

Urinalysis:

Physical Characteristics:

- **Color: Brown/cola-colored** (suggests hematuria)
- Clarity: Cloudy
- Specific gravity: 1.025 (concentrated)

Chemical Analysis:

- pH: 6.5
- **Protein: 3+ (~100-300 mg/dL) POSITIVE**
- Glucose: Negative
- Ketones: Negative
- **Blood: 3+ STRONGLY POSITIVE**
- Leukocyte esterase: 1+
- Nitrites: Negative

Microscopic Examination:

- **RBCs: >100/hpf, too numerous to count MARKEDLY ELEVATED**
- **RBC morphology: Dysmorphic RBCs >80%** (irregular, blebs, acanthocytes)
- **RBC casts: 5-10/lpf PATHOGNOMONIC FOR GLOMERULONEPHRITIS**
- WBCs: 10-20/hpf
- **WBC casts: Occasional**
- **Granular casts: 3-8/lpf** (muddy brown)
- Hyaline casts: Numerous

- Epithelial cells: Few
- No crystals or bacteria

Phase Contrast Microscopy (Specialized):

- **Dysmorphic RBCs: 85%** (confirms glomerular origin of bleeding)
- Acanthocytes (Mickey Mouse cells): Present
- RBC fragmentation: Present

Quantitative Studies:

24-Hour Urine:

- Protein: 1.8 g/24 hours (sub-nephrotic range)
- Creatinine clearance: 42 mL/min/1.73m² (reduced; normal >90)

Additional Serologic Tests:

Complement Levels:

- **C3: 45 mg/dL** (low; normal 90-180) **HYPOCOMPLEMENTEMIA**
- C4: 28 mg/dL (normal)
- Pattern: Low C3, normal C4 (suggests post-infectious GN)

Streptococcal Serology:

- **Anti-streptolysin O (ASO) titer: 620 Todd units** (elevated; normal <200)
- **Anti-DNase B: 480 units** (elevated; normal <170)
- Confirms recent Group A Streptococcal infection

Other Serology:

- ANA: Negative (excludes SLE)
- ANCA: Negative (excludes vasculitis)
- Anti-GBM antibody: Negative (excludes Goodpasture syndrome)

Throat Culture:

- No Group A Streptococcus isolated (infection was 2 weeks ago)

Renal Ultrasound:

- Both kidneys normal size with increased echogenicity
- No masses or obstruction

Final Diagnosis: Acute Post-Streptococcal Glomerulonephritis (APSGN)

Classic Triad Present:

1. ✓ Hematuria (macroscopic - cola-colored urine)
2. ✓ Hypertension (BP 145/95)
3. ✓ Edema (periorbital and pretibial)

Teaching Points:

1. **RBC Casts:** Form when RBCs pass through damaged glomeruli and become trapped in tubular protein matrix; PATHOGNOMONIC for glomerulonephritis
2. **Dysmorphic RBCs:** Irregular shape, blebs, membrane irregularities from passage through damaged glomerular basement membrane; >40% dysmorphic suggests glomerular hematuria
3. **Acanthocytes (G1 cells):** Specific type of dysmorphic RBC with vesicle-like protrusions; highly specific for glomerular bleeding
4. **Phase Contrast Microscopy:** Improves detection of RBC morphology; distinguishes glomerular from non-glomerular hematuria
5. **Cola-Colored Urine:** Caused by oxidation of hemoglobin in acidic urine; distinguishes from bright red urine (lower urinary tract bleeding)
6. **Hypocomplementemia:** Low C3 with normal C4 suggests alternate complement pathway activation (APSGN, MPGN); low C3 AND C4 suggests classical pathway (SLE)
7. **APSGN Timeline:** Pharyngitis → 1-2 week latency → acute GN; skin infection → 3-6 week latency
8. **Prognosis:** Children >95% complete recovery; adults higher risk of chronic kidney disease
9. **Management:** Supportive care, salt/fluid restriction, antihypertensives; no antibiotics indicated (infection already resolved)

Related Cases: IgA nephropathy, lupus nephritis, Goodpasture syndrome, ANCA-associated vasculitis, Henoch-Schönlein purpura

---

Case 7.3: Diabetic Nephropathy

Clinical Presentation: A 52-year-old woman with 15-year history of type 2 diabetes presents for routine follow-up. She has been on metformin and insulin but admits poor glycemic control. Recent HbA1c: 9.2%. Also has hypertension and hyperlipidemia. Denies urinary symptoms. Retinal exam by ophthalmology shows diabetic retinopathy.

Physical Examination:

- BP: 152/88 mmHg
- No edema
- Fundoscopic exam: Diabetic retinopathy with microaneurysms

Initial Laboratory Findings:

- Serum creatinine: 1.3 mg/dL (baseline 0.8 mg/dL 3 years ago)
- eGFR: 48 mL/min/1.73m² (Stage 3 CKD)
- Serum albumin: 3.8 g/dL (normal)
- HbA1c: 9.2% (poor control)

Diagnostic Reasoning Questions:

1. What are the stages of diabetic kidney disease progression?
2. How is microalbuminuria detected and what is its significance?
3. What urinalysis findings are expected in diabetic nephropathy?
4. Why is urine albumin/creatinine ratio preferred over dipstick?

Sequential Test Results:

Standard Urinalysis:

Physical Characteristics:

- Color: Yellow
- Clarity: Clear
- Specific gravity: 1.015

Chemical Analysis:

- pH: 6.0
- **Protein: 1+ (~30 mg/dL) TRACE POSITIVE**
- Glucose: 2+ (250 mg/dL) - reflects hyperglycemia
- Ketones: Negative
- Blood: Negative
- Leukocyte esterase: Negative
- Nitrites: Negative

Microscopic Examination:

- RBCs: 0-2/hpf (normal)
- WBCs: 0-3/hpf (normal)
- Epithelial cells: Few
- **Hyaline casts: 5-10/lpf** (increased)
- **Waxy casts: 1-2/lpf** (suggests chronic kidney disease)
- No RBC casts, granular casts minimal
- Crystals: None
- Bacteria: None

Quantitative Urine Albumin Testing:

First Morning Spot Urine Albumin/Creatinine Ratio (ACR):

- **ACR: 285 mg/g creatinine MODERATELY INCREASED ALBUMINURIA**
- Urine albumin: 85 mg/dL
- Urine creatinine: 30 mg/dL

Classification:

- Normal: <30 mg/g
- Microalbuminuria (A2): 30-300 mg/g ← **PATIENT IS HERE**
- Macroalbuminuria (A3): >300 mg/g

Repeat ACR (2 weeks later to confirm):

- ACR: 310 mg/g (confirms persistent albuminuria)

Three-Month Follow-Up ACR (after initiating ACE inhibitor):

- ACR: 195 mg/g (decreased but still elevated)

24-Hour Urine Studies:

- Total protein: 420 mg/24 hours (elevated; normal <150)
- Albumin: 380 mg/24 hours
- Creatinine clearance: 52 mL/min

Additional Testing:

Urine Protein Electrophoresis:

- Pattern: Predominantly albumin (>95%)
- Minimal globulins
- Consistent with glomerular proteinuria (diabetic nephropathy)

Other Causes Excluded:

- Urine culture: Negative (excludes UTI)
- No recent exercise or fever
- No urinary tract obstruction on imaging

Diabetic Kidney Disease Staging:

KDIGO Classification:

- **eGFR category:** G3a (45-59 mL/min/1.73m²)
- **Albuminuria category:** A2-A3 (30-300+ mg/g)
- **Risk category:** High risk for progression to ESRD and cardiovascular events

Stages of Diabetic Nephropathy (Mogensen):

1. Stage 1: Hyperfiltration (eGFR >90, no albuminuria)
2. Stage 2: Silent stage (eGFR >90, no albuminuria, structural changes)
3. **Stage 3: Microalbuminuria (30-300 mg/g) ← PATIENT IS HERE**
4. Stage 4: Macroalbuminuria (>300 mg/g, overt nephropathy)
5. Stage 5: ESRD (dialysis-dependent)

Final Diagnosis: Diabetic Kidney Disease (Diabetic Nephropathy), Stage 3 - Moderately Increased Albuminuria with eGFR 48 mL/min

Management Initiated:

- ACE inhibitor (lisinopril 10 mg daily) - reduces albuminuria and slows progression
- Improved glycemic control (target HbA1c <7%)
- Blood pressure control (target <130/80)
- SGLT2 inhibitor added (empagliflozin) - renoprotective
- Monitor ACR every 3-6 months
- Monitor eGFR and potassium
- Diabetic retinopathy care (microvascular complications often coexist)

Teaching Points:

1. **Microalbuminuria:** Earliest clinical sign of diabetic nephropathy; indicates glomerular damage; albumin 30-300 mg/g creatinine
2. **ACR vs Dipstick:** Dipstick detects protein at ~30 mg/dL (insensitive for microalbuminuria); ACR detects lower levels and corrects for urine concentration
3. **Spot vs 24-Hour:** Spot ACR correlates well with 24-hour collection; more convenient; first morning void preferred (reduces variability)
4. **Transient Albuminuria:** Can be caused by exercise, fever, UTI, heart failure, uncontrolled hyperglycemia; confirm with repeat testing
5. **Natural History:** 20-40% of diabetics develop nephropathy; progression microalbuminuria → macroalbuminuria → declining eGFR → ESRD over 5-15 years
6. **Hyaline Casts:** Non-specific; formed from Tamm-Horsfall protein; seen in concentrated urine, proteinuria, and chronic kidney disease
7. **Waxy Casts:** Wide casts with smooth, waxy appearance; indicate chronic kidney disease with tubular atrophy
8. **Renoprotection:** ACE-I/ARB slow progression even in normotensive patients; SGLT2 inhibitors provide additional benefit
9. **Screening Recommendations:** Annual ACR screening for all diabetics starting at diagnosis (Type 2) or 5 years after diagnosis (Type 1)

Related Cases: Hypertensive nephrosclerosis, nephrotic syndrome from diabetic nephropathy, contrast-induced nephropathy in diabetic, uremic syndrome

---

Case 7.4: Rhabdomyolysis

Clinical Presentation: A 28-year-old male bodybuilder presents to ED with severe muscle pain, weakness, and dark urine for 2 days. Three days ago, he completed an intense "CrossFit challenge" after taking a pre-workout supplement. He reports decreased urine output. No recent trauma or falls.

Physical Examination:

- Vital signs stable
- Severe tenderness bilateral thighs, calves, and upper arms

303

- Muscle swelling noted
- No compartment syndrome signs

Initial Laboratory Findings:

- **Serum creatine kinase (CK): 85,000 U/L** (normal <200) **MARKEDLY ELEVATED**
- Serum creatinine: 2.8 mg/dL (elevated; baseline 1.0)
- BUN: 38 mg/dL
- **Potassium: 6.2 mEq/L** (hyperkalemia - from muscle breakdown)
- Phosphorus: 6.8 mg/dL (elevated)
- Calcium: 7.2 mg/dL (hypocalcemia - calcium precipitation in damaged muscle)
- AST: 450 U/L (elevated - released from muscle)
- ALT: 85 U/L (normal - helps distinguish from liver disease)
- LDH: 1200 U/L (markedly elevated)

Diagnostic Reasoning Questions:

1. What is rhabdomyolysis and what causes it?
2. How does myoglobin appear in urine and what are the urinalysis findings?
3. Why is the urine dipstick positive for blood without RBCs on microscopy?
4. What are the complications of rhabdomyolysis?

Sequential Test Results:

Urinalysis:

Physical Characteristics:

- **Color: Dark brown/tea-colored** (myoglobinuria)
- Clarity: Clear
- Specific gravity: 1.025

Chemical Analysis:

- pH: 5.5 (acidic - contributes to myoglobin precipitation)
- Protein: 1+ (~30-100 mg/dL)
- Glucose: Negative
- Ketones: Negative
- **Blood: 3+ (large) STRONGLY POSITIVE ON DIPSTICK**
- Leukocyte esterase: Negative
- Nitrites: Negative

Microscopic Examination:

- **RBCs: 0-2/hpf DISCREPANCY - dipstick positive but microscopy negative!**
- WBCs: 0-3/hpf (normal)
- Epithelial cells: Few
- **Pigmented granular casts (muddy brown): 5-10/lpf** (myoglobin casts)
- Hyaline casts: Occasional

- **No RBC casts** (excludes glomerulonephritis)
- Crystals: Occasional urate crystals
- Bacteria: None

Key Finding: Blood-positive dipstick WITHOUT RBCs on microscopy = MYOGLOBINURIA or HEMOGLOBINURIA

Confirmatory Testing:

Serum Myoglobin:

- **Serum myoglobin: 3500 ng/mL** (normal <90) **MARKEDLY ELEVATED**

Urine Myoglobin:

- **Urine myoglobin: Positive** (qualitative test)
- Darkens further on standing

Serum Haptoglobin:

- Normal (excludes intravascular hemolysis as cause of hemoglobinuria)

Distinguishing Myoglobinuria from Hemoglobinuria:

Finding	Myoglobinuria	Hemoglobinuria
Serum CK	Markedly elevated	Normal or mildly elevated
Serum myoglobin	Elevated	Normal
Serum haptoglobin	Normal	Decreased (binds free Hb)
Plasma color	Clear	Pink/red (free Hb)
Clinical context	Muscle injury	Hemolysis

Additional Testing:

Urine Electrolytes:

- Urine sodium: 55 mEq/L
- FENa (fractional excretion of sodium): 2.5% (suggests ATN)

Renal Ultrasound:

- Normal-sized kidneys
- No hydronephrosis
- Increased echogenicity (acute kidney injury)

Follow-Up Labs (24 hours after aggressive IV hydration):

- CK: 62,000 U/L (decreasing)
- Creatinine: 2.2 mg/dL (improving)
- Potassium: 4.8 mEq/L (corrected)
- Urine output: Increasing

Final Diagnosis: Severe Rhabdomyolysis with Myoglobinuria and Acute Kidney Injury (Myoglobinuric ATN)

Rhabdomyolysis Triad:

1. ✓ Muscle pain/weakness
2. ✓ Elevated CK (>1,000 U/L; often >5,000)
3. ✓ Myoglobinuria (tea-colored urine)

Causes of Rhabdomyolysis (This Case: Exertional):

- Exertional: Extreme exercise, especially in untrained individuals
- Trauma: Crush injury, compartment syndrome
- Drugs: Statins, cocaine, amphetamines
- Toxins: Alcohol
- Infections: Influenza, COVID-19
- Metabolic: Electrolyte abnormalities, hypothyroidism
- Genetic: McArdle disease, carnitine palmitoyltransferase II deficiency

Management:

- **Aggressive IV fluid resuscitation** (goal urine output 200-300 mL/hr)
- Alkalinize urine (sodium bicarbonate) - prevents myoglobin precipitation in tubules
- Monitor for complications: hyperkalemia, hypocalcemia (early), hypercalcemia (late), compartment syndrome
- Dialysis if severe AKI or life-threatening hyperkalemia

Teaching Points:

1. **Dipstick Blood Without RBCs:** Dipstick detects heme (in Hb, myoglobin, or RBCs); positive dipstick with few/no RBCs = myoglobinuria or hemoglobinuria
2. **Myoglobin Clearance:** Myoglobin cleared rapidly from serum (2-6 hours); if presentation delayed, serum myoglobin may be normal while CK remains elevated
3. **CK Elevation:** CK >5,000 U/L strongly suggests rhabdomyolysis; CK >15,000-20,000 associated with AKI risk
4. **Myoglobin Nephrotoxicity:** Myoglobin precipitates in acidic urine, forms casts, causes direct tubular toxicity and vasoconstriction → ATN
5. **Pigmented Casts:** Dark, muddy brown granular casts containing myoglobin; suggestive of myoglobinuric ATN
6. **Electrolyte Abnormalities:** Hyperkalemia (muscle release), hyperphosphatemia, hypocalcemia (early - precipitation), hypercalcemia (late - mobilization)
7. **AST >> ALT:** AST released from muscle; AST:ALT ratio >3 suggests muscle source rather than liver

8. **Urine pH:** Acidic urine promotes myoglobin cast formation; alkalinization (pH >6.5) may be protective
9. **Compartment Syndrome:** Complication of severe rhabdomyolysis; requires urgent fasciotomy

Related Cases: Hemoglobinuria from intravascular hemolysis, acute tubular necrosis from other causes, compartment syndrome, exertional heatstroke

---

Case 7.5: Pleural Effusion Analysis

Clinical Presentation: A 68-year-old man with history of congestive heart failure (CHF) presents with progressive dyspnea and right-sided chest pain for 1 week. He has had CHF exacerbations in the past, but this episode seems different with unilateral symptoms and pleuritic pain. Low-grade fever (100.8°F) for 2 days.

Physical Examination:

- BP: 128/76, HR: 92, RR: 22, Temp: 100.8°F
- Decreased breath sounds right base
- Dullness to percussion right lower chest
- No JVD, no peripheral edema (on diuretics)

Imaging:

- **Chest X-ray:** Large right-sided pleural effusion, blunting costophrenic angle
- **Ultrasound:** Confirms moderate-to-large effusion, no septations or loculations

Diagnostic Reasoning Questions:

1. What are Light's criteria for distinguishing transudate vs exudate?
2. What cell count/differential findings help determine etiology?
3. When should pleural fluid pH and glucose be measured?
4. How do different diseases affect pleural fluid characteristics?

Procedure: Thoracentesis performed under ultrasound guidance. 1000 mL cloudy yellow fluid removed.

Sequential Test Results:

Pleural Fluid Analysis:

Physical Characteristics:

- **Appearance: Cloudy, turbid yellow**
- Odor: None (foul odor would suggest anaerobic empyema)
- Clotting: No (heparin added to specimen)

Cell Count and Differential:

- **Nucleated cell count: 12,500 cells/μL ELEVATED**
- **Neutrophils: 85% MARKEDLY ELEVATED** (suggests bacterial infection)
- Lymphocytes: 10%
- Monocytes/macrophages: 5%
- Eosinophils: <1%
- Mesothelial cells: Rare
- **RBC count: 8,000/μL** (mildly elevated; suggests minor bleeding)

Chemistry:

- **Total protein (pleural): 4.8 g/dL**
- Serum protein: 6.5 g/dL
- Pleural/serum protein ratio: **4.8/6.5 = 0.74** (>0.5 suggests exudate)
- **LDH (pleural): 580 U/L**
- Serum LDH: 210 U/L
- Pleural/serum LDH ratio: **580/210 = 2.76** (>0.6 suggests exudate)
- Pleural LDH >2/3 upper limit normal serum LDH (>220) = **YES**
- **Glucose: 32 mg/dL VERY LOW** (normal >60; <60 suggests infection, rheumatoid, malignancy)
- **pH: 7.15 LOW** (normal 7.60-7.64; <7.20 suggests complicated parapneumonic effusion/empyema)

Light's Criteria Applied (Exudate if ≥1 of 3 criteria met):

1. √ Pleural/serum protein ratio >0.5 (0.74) → **POSITIVE**
2. √ Pleural/serum LDH ratio >0.6 (2.76) → **POSITIVE**
3. √ Pleural LDH >2/3 upper limit of normal (580 > 220) → **POSITIVE**

Diagnosis: EXUDATE (all 3 criteria positive)

Microbiology:

- **Gram stain: Numerous WBCs, gram-positive cocci in chains**
- **Culture: Streptococcus pneumoniae (heavy growth)**
- Sensitivity: Sensitive to penicillin, ceftriaxone
- **Anaerobic culture: Negative**
- **AFB smear: Negative**
- **Fungal culture: Pending (negative at 4 weeks)**

Cytology:

- Abundant neutrophils
- Reactive mesothelial cells
- **No malignant cells seen**

Additional Testing:

- Pleural fluid ADA (adenosine deaminase): 18 U/L (normal; <40 makes TB unlikely)
- Pleural fluid amylase: Normal (excludes esophageal rupture, pancreatitis)

Final Diagnosis: Complicated Parapneumonic Effusion (Empyema Stage 2) due to *Streptococcus pneumoniae*

Classification of Parapneumonic Effusions:

- **Uncomplicated:** pH >7.20, glucose >60, negative culture, sterile
- **Complicated:** pH <7.20, glucose <60, positive Gram stain/culture, requires drainage ← **PATIENT HERE**
- **Empyema:** Frank pus (thick, purulent), positive culture

Management:

- IV antibiotics (ceftriaxone)
- Chest tube placement for drainage (pH <7.20 indicates need)
- Consider intrapleural fibrinolytics if loculated
- Follow-up imaging to ensure resolution

Teaching Points:

1. **Light's Criteria:** 98% sensitive for exudates; identifies effusions needing further workup; occasionally misclassifies diuretic-treated transudates as exudates
2. **Transudate Causes:** CHF, cirrhosis, nephrotic syndrome, hypoalbuminemia
3. **Exudate Causes:** Infection (parapneumonic, TB, empyema), malignancy, PE, collagen vascular disease, pancreatitis
4. **Neutrophil Predominance:** Suggests acute bacterial infection or pulmonary embolism
5. **Lymphocyte Predominance (>50%):** Suggests TB, malignancy, sarcoidosis, or chronic effusion
6. **Eosinophil Predominance (>10%):** Suggests air/blood in pleural space, drugs, parasites, asbestos
7. **Low Glucose (<60 mg/dL):** Suggests empyema, TB, rheumatoid pleuritis, malignancy, lupus
8. **Low pH (<7.30):** Indicates complicated parapneumonic effusion requiring drainage; pH <7.20 = absolute indication for chest tube
9. **Elevated ADA (>40 U/L):** Suggestive of tuberculous pleuritis (sensitivity 90-100%)
10. **RBC Count:** <10,000/µL usually insignificant; >100,000/µL suggests trauma, malignancy, PE, or vascular injury

Related Cases: Empyema, tuberculous pleuritis, malignant effusion, chylothorax, hemothorax

---

Case 7.6: Ascitic Fluid Evaluation

Clinical Presentation: A 56-year-old man with history of alcoholic cirrhosis presents with increasing abdominal distention and discomfort for 2 weeks. He has had prior ascites managed with diuretics. Today, he developed fever (101.2°F) and diffuse abdominal pain. He denies nausea, vomiting, or diarrhea.

Physical Examination:

- Temp: 101.2°F, BP: 108/68, HR: 102
- Icteric sclera
- Distended abdomen with shifting dullness, fluid wave positive

- **Diffuse abdominal tenderness** (new finding)
- No rebound or guarding
- Spider angiomas, palmar erythema

Initial Laboratory Findings:

- WBC: 12,500/μL (elevated)
- Platelets: 85,000/μL (thrombocytopenia - chronic liver disease)
- Total bilirubin: 3.8 mg/dL
- Albumin: 2.4 g/dL
- PT-INR: 1.8

Diagnostic Reasoning Questions:

1. What is spontaneous bacterial peritonitis (SBP) and who is at risk?
2. What ascitic fluid findings diagnose SBP?
3. How is SAAG (serum-ascites albumin gradient) used to determine etiology?
4. When should ascites fluid cultures be obtained?

Procedure: Diagnostic and therapeutic paracentesis performed. 4 liters straw-colored fluid removed.

Sequential Test Results:

Ascitic Fluid Analysis:

Physical Characteristics:

- **Appearance: Cloudy, slightly turbid yellow**
- Clotting: No
- Odor: None

Cell Count and Differential:

- **Nucleated cell count: 850 cells/μL ELEVATED**
- **Absolute neutrophil count (PMN): 520 cells/μL ELEVATED (>250 = SBP)**
- Lymphocytes: 280 cells/μL (33%)
- Monocytes/macrophages: 50 cells/μL
- **RBC count: 1,200/μL** (slightly bloody - traumatic tap vs. disease)

Critical Diagnostic Criterion: PMN >250 cells/μL = Spontaneous Bacterial Peritonitis

Chemistry:

Serum-Ascites Albumin Gradient (SAAG):

- Serum albumin: 2.4 g/dL
- Ascitic fluid albumin: 0.8 g/dL
- **SAAG = 2.4 - 0.8 = 1.6 g/dL HIGH GRADIENT (≥1.1)**

310

SAAG Interpretation:

- **SAAG ≥1.1 g/dL:** Portal hypertension (97% accurate) → cirrhosis, CHF, Budd-Chiari
- SAAG <1.1 g/dL: Non-portal hypertension causes → peritoneal carcinomatosis, TB peritonitis, pancreatitis

Other Chemistry:

- **Total protein (ascites): 1.2 g/dL LOW** (<2.5 in cirrhotic ascites)
- LDH (ascites): 85 U/L (normal for ascites)
- Glucose: 75 mg/dL (normal)
- Amylase: Normal (excludes pancreatic ascites)

Microbiology:

Gram Stain:

- Few WBCs seen
- **No organisms visualized** (Gram stain often negative in SBP due to low bacterial count)

Cultures (inoculated at bedside into blood culture bottles):

- **Aerobic bottle: Positive (Escherichia coli identified at 24 hours)**
- Sensitivity: Sensitive to ceftriaxone, piperacillin-tazobactam
- **Anaerobic bottle: No growth**
- **AFB culture: Negative**
- **Fungal culture: No growth**

Cytology:

- Reactive mesothelial cells
- Neutrophils and lymphocytes
- **No malignant cells identified**

Additional Testing:

- Ascites ADA: 12 U/L (normal; <40 makes TB peritonitis unlikely)
- Triglycerides: 28 mg/dL (normal; <50 excludes chylous ascites)
- Bilirubin (ascites): 0.8 mg/dL (lower than serum; excludes bowel perforation)

Ascites-to-Serum Bilirubin Ratio: 0.8/3.8 = 0.21 (<1.0 excludes bowel perforation)

Follow-Up Paracentesis (48 hours after antibiotics):

- PMN count: 120 cells/μL (decreased - treatment response)
- Culture: Negative

Final Diagnosis:

1. **Spontaneous Bacterial Peritonitis (SBP) due to *E. coli***
2. Cirrhotic Ascites (high SAAG, low protein)
3. Alcoholic Cirrhosis with Decompensation

SBP Diagnostic Criteria (Met):

1. √ PMN >250 cells/μL in ascites
2. √ Positive culture (E. coli)
3. √ No evidence of secondary peritonitis (surgical cause)

Management:

- **Empiric IV ceftriaxone 2g daily** (started immediately)
- **Albumin infusion** (1.5 g/kg on day 1, then 1 g/kg on day 3) - reduces renal dysfunction and mortality
- Secondary prophylaxis: Norfloxacin 400 mg daily (or double-strength TMP-SMX) to prevent recurrence
- Repeat paracentesis at 48 hours if not improving

Teaching Points:

1. **SBP Diagnosis:** PMN ≥250 cells/μL with positive culture OR PMN ≥250 with negative culture (culture-negative SBP); treat both
2. **Bedside Inoculation:** Inoculating blood culture bottles at bedside increases culture yield to 80% (vs 50% in lab)
3. **SAAG:** More accurate than transudate/exudate classification for ascites; reflects portal pressure
4. **High SAAG (≥1.1):** Cirrhosis (81%), cardiac ascites, Budd-Chiari, massive liver metastases
5. **Low SAAG (<1.1):** Peritoneal carcinomatosis, TB peritonitis, pancreatic/biliary ascites, nephrotic syndrome, serositis
6. **Low Protein Ascites (<1 g/dL):** Increased SBP risk; consider prophylactic antibiotics in high-risk patients
7. **Secondary Peritonitis:** Should be suspected if: PMN >10,000, protein >1 g/dL, glucose <50, LDH > upper limit normal serum, multiple organisms on culture
8. **Neutrocytic Ascites:** PMN ≥250 but negative culture; treat as SBP (likely prior antibiotics or low bacterial load)
9. **Bloody Ascites:** RBC >50,000/μL suggests malignancy, traumatic tap, or hepatocellular carcinoma
10. **TB Peritonitis:** Lymphocyte-predominant (>70%), elevated ADA (>39 U/L), low SAAG; requires peritoneal biopsy

Related Cases: Secondary bacterial peritonitis (bowel perforation), tuberculous peritonitis, malignant ascites (peritoneal carcinomatosis), pancreatic ascites, chylous ascites

Chapter 8: Toxicology and Therapeutic Drug Monitoring

Case 8.1: Acetaminophen Overdose Management

Clinical Presentation: A 19-year-old female is brought to the ED by friends 6 hours after reportedly ingesting "a whole bottle" of acetaminophen (Tylenol) in a suicide attempt. She took approximately 15 grams (thirty 500mg tablets). Currently, she complains of nausea and abdominal pain but appears relatively well. No altered mental status. Friends report she has been depressed after a breakup.

Physical Examination:

- Vital signs: BP 118/72, HR 88, RR 16, Temp 98.6°F
- Alert and oriented x3
- Mild epigastric tenderness
- No jaundice (too early)
- Neurologically intact

Initial Laboratory Findings:

- **Time of ingestion: 6 hours ago** (critical for Rumack-Matthew nomogram)
- Basic metabolic panel: Normal
- Liver enzymes (AST/ALT): Normal (too early for hepatotoxicity)
- PT/INR: 1.0 (normal)

Diagnostic Reasoning Questions:

1. Why is timing of ingestion critical in acetaminophen overdose?
2. How is the Rumack-Matthew nomogram used for risk stratification?
3. What is the mechanism of acetaminophen hepatotoxicity?
4. When should N-acetylcysteine (NAC) be initiated?

Sequential Test Results:

Serum Acetaminophen Level (4 hours post-ingestion):

- **Acetaminophen: 185 µg/mL** at 4 hours post-ingestion
- Plotted on Rumack-Matthew nomogram

Rumack-Matthew Nomogram Interpretation:

- Toxic threshold at 4 hours: 150 µg/mL
- Patient level: 185 µg/mL **ABOVE treatment line**
- **Risk: Probable hepatotoxicity without treatment**
- **Action: Immediate NAC (N-acetylcysteine) therapy indicated**

Additional Baseline Labs:

- AST: 32 U/L (normal)
- ALT: 28 U/L (normal)
- Total bilirubin: 0.6 mg/dL (normal)
- Creatinine: 0.8 mg/dL (normal)
- Salicylate level: Negative (rule out co-ingestion)
- Urine drug screen: Negative

Treatment Initiated:

- **NAC (Acetadote) IV protocol started within 8 hours of ingestion**
- Loading dose: 150 mg/kg over 1 hour
- Maintenance: 50 mg/kg over 4 hours, then 100 mg/kg over 16 hours

Serial Monitoring:

12 Hours Post-Ingestion:

- Acetaminophen: 95 µg/mL (declining)
- AST: 42 U/L (mild elevation beginning)
- ALT: 38 U/L

24 Hours Post-Ingestion:

- Acetaminophen: 15 µg/mL
- AST: 285 U/L (**elevated - early hepatotoxicity**)
- ALT: 320 U/L
- INR: 1.2 (minimally elevated)
- Total bilirubin: 1.1 mg/dL

48 Hours Post-Ingestion:

- AST: 180 U/L (improving)
- ALT: 240 U/L (improving)
- INR: 1.1
- Creatinine: 0.9 mg/dL (stable)

72 Hours Post-Ingestion:

- AST: 95 U/L (near baseline)
- ALT: 150 U/L (continuing to improve)
- INR: 1.0
- Patient asymptomatic

Final Diagnosis: Acute Acetaminophen Overdose with Mild Hepatotoxicity (Successfully Treated with NAC)

Acetaminophen Metabolism and Toxicity:

1. **Therapeutic doses:** 90% conjugated to glucuronide/sulfate (non-toxic); 5-10% metabolized by CYP2E1 to NAPQI (toxic metabolite)
2. **Toxic doses:** NAPQI production exceeds glutathione stores → hepatocyte necrosis
3. **NAC mechanism:** Replenishes glutathione, prevents NAPQI-induced damage

Teaching Points:

1. **Rumack-Matthew Nomogram:** Used for single acute ingestion; plots serum level vs. time; only valid 4-24 hours post-ingestion; levels above treatment line require NAC
2. **Timing Critical:** NAC most effective within 8 hours; efficacy decreases significantly after 8 hours; still beneficial up to 24-36 hours
3. **Four Stages of Toxicity:** Stage 1 (0-24h): nausea, vomiting, anorexia; Stage 2 (24-72h): RUQ pain, elevated AST/ALT; Stage 3 (72-96h): peak hepatotoxicity, jaundice, coagulopathy; Stage 4 (>5 days): recovery or fulminant hepatic failure
4. **NAC Indications:** Acetaminophen >150 μg/mL at 4h OR >75 μg/mL at 8h OR any detectable level with elevated AST/ALT OR unknown time with any level >10 μg/mL
5. **King's College Criteria:** Predict need for transplant: pH <7.3 OR (INR >6.5 AND creatinine >3.4 AND grade III-IV encephalopathy)
6. **Extended Release:** Different kinetics; may need to measure level at 4h AND 8h post-ingestion
7. **Chronic Overdose:** No nomogram; treat based on clinical presentation and transaminases
8. **Co-Ingestions:** Always check salicylate level; evaluate for other toxins

Related Cases: Salicylate overdose, toxic alcohol ingestion, drug-induced liver injury, fulminant hepatic failure

---

Case 8.2: Therapeutic Drug Monitoring - Digoxin Toxicity

Clinical Presentation: An 82-year-old woman with atrial fibrillation on chronic digoxin therapy presents with 3 days of nausea, vomiting, fatigue, and confusion. Family reports she has been increasingly confused and "seeing yellow halos around lights." She recently started furosemide for ankle swelling. Takes multiple medications including digoxin 0.25 mg daily.

Physical Examination:

- BP 108/64, HR 48 (bradycardia), irregularly irregular
- Confused, oriented only to person
- Cardiac exam: irregular rhythm, no murmurs
- Yellow-green visual disturbance reported (xanthopsia)

Initial Laboratory Findings:

- Potassium: 2.9 mEq/L **LOW** (diuretic effect)
- Creatinine: 1.8 mg/dL (baseline 1.2; **acute kidney injury**)
- Magnesium: 1.4 mg/dL (low)

Diagnostic Reasoning Questions:

1. What factors increase risk of digoxin toxicity?
2. When should digoxin levels be measured?
3. How do electrolyte abnormalities affect digoxin toxicity?
4. What are the indications for digoxin-specific antibody fragments?

Sequential Test Results:

ECG Findings:

- Heart rate: 48 bpm
- **Atrial fibrillation with slow ventricular response**
- **Frequent PVCs, bigeminy pattern** (classic digoxin toxicity)
- **ST depression with "scooped" appearance** (digitalis effect)
- No AV block (yet)

Digoxin Level:

- **Sample timing: 18 hours after last dose** (appropriate - trough level)
- **Digoxin level: 3.8 ng/mL TOXIC** (therapeutic 0.5-2.0 ng/mL for AFib)
- Previous level 6 months ago: 1.2 ng/mL (therapeutic)

Factors Contributing to Toxicity:

1. **Hypokalemia (2.9 mEq/L):** Enhances digoxin binding to Na-K-ATPase
2. **Acute kidney injury (Cr 1.8):** Reduced renal clearance (digoxin 70% renally excreted)
3. **Hypomagnesemia (1.4):** Increases digoxin toxicity
4. **Advanced age:** Reduced volume of distribution, reduced clearance
5. **Recent diuretic:** Caused electrolyte depletion

Additional Labs:

- Troponin: Normal (excludes MI)
- TSH: Normal (excludes thyroid as cause of bradycardia)
- BNP: Elevated (chronic heart failure)

Calculation of Renal Function:

- Cockcroft-Gault CrCl: 28 mL/min (severe renal impairment)
- Digoxin clearance directly proportional to CrCl
- **Digoxin dose should be reduced to 0.125 mg every other day**

Management Initiated:

- **STOP digoxin immediately**
- **Aggressive potassium repletion:** Target K+ 4.0-5.0 mEq/L
- Magnesium supplementation

- IV fluids for renal function
- Continuous cardiac monitoring
- **Digoxin-specific antibody fragments (DigiFab) NOT given** (no life-threatening arrhythmias)

DigiFab Indications (Life-Threatening):

- Ventricular arrhythmias refractory to treatment
- Symptomatic bradycardia unresponsive to atropine
- Potassium >5.5 mEq/L in acute overdose
- Ingestion >10 mg in adults
- Hemodynamic instability

Serial Monitoring:

12 Hours After Stopping Digoxin:

- Potassium: 3.6 mEq/L (improving with repletion)
- HR: 55 bpm
- Mental status: Slightly improved
- PVCs less frequent

24 Hours:

- Digoxin level: 2.8 ng/mL (declining, half-life ~36-48 hours)
- Potassium: 4.1 mEq/L (normalized)
- Magnesium: 1.9 mg/dL (normalized)
- HR: 62 bpm
- Mental status: Clear
- Visual disturbances resolving

48 Hours:

- Digoxin level: 1.9 ng/mL (therapeutic range)
- Creatinine: 1.4 mg/dL (improving)
- Symptoms resolved

Final Diagnosis: Digoxin Toxicity due to Drug Accumulation (Acute Kidney Injury + Hypokalemia from Diuretic Therapy)

Discharge Plan:

- Digoxin reduced to 0.125 mg every other day
- Monitor potassium and magnesium closely
- Follow renal function
- Next digoxin level in 1 week
- Patient/family education on toxicity signs

Teaching Points:

1. **Timing of Levels:** Measure trough level (>6 hours post-dose, ideally 12-24 hours); levels drawn too early falsely elevated due to distribution phase
2. **Narrow Therapeutic Index:** Therapeutic 0.5-2.0 ng/mL; toxic >2.0 ng/mL; but toxicity can occur at therapeutic levels with hypokalemia
3. **Clinical Manifestations:** GI (nausea, vomiting, anorexia); CNS (confusion, weakness, xanthopsia); Cardiac (ANY arrhythmia - PVCs, heart block, atrial tachycardia with block)
4. **Electrolyte Effects:** Hypokalemia potentiates toxicity; hyperkalemia in acute overdose suggests severe toxicity; hypomagnesemia increases risk
5. **Renal Dosing:** Essential; digoxin 70% renally cleared; CrCl <50 requires dose reduction
6. **Drug Interactions:** Amiodarone, verapamil, quinidine, clarithromycin, spironolactone all increase digoxin levels
7. **Half-Life:** 36-48 hours in normal renal function; longer in renal impairment; takes 5-7 days to reach steady state
8. **DigiFab Dosing:** Based on amount ingested OR serum level; binds digoxin 1:1; renders digoxin inactive; causes falsely elevated digoxin levels for days
9. **Fab Fragments vs Whole Antibody:** Fab fragments (DigiFab, Digibind) are smaller, less immunogenic, faster acting than whole antibodies

Related Cases: Lithium toxicity, phenytoin toxicity, vancomycin monitoring, aminoglycoside toxicity

Case 8.3: Heavy Metal Poisoning - Lead Toxicity

Clinical Presentation: A 3-year-old boy living in an old apartment building is brought to clinic by his mother for developmental concerns and behavioral problems. He has become increasingly irritable, has decreased appetite, and complains of intermittent abdominal pain for 2 months. His speech development has plateaued. The apartment was built in 1950 and has peeling paint. Older sibling also lives in home and is asymptomatic.

Physical Examination:

- Irritable, poorly interactive
- Appears pale
- Abdomen soft, mild diffuse tenderness
- Neurologic: Developmentally delayed for age
- No focal deficits

Initial Laboratory Findings:

- **Hemoglobin: 9.2 g/dL** (anemia; normal 11-13 for age)
- **MCV: 72 fL** (microcytic; normal 75-87)
- Ferritin: 45 ng/mL (low-normal)
- Reticulocyte count: 1.8% (appropriately elevated)

Diagnostic Reasoning Questions:

1. What clinical features suggest lead poisoning in children?
2. How is lead toxicity diagnosed and what are the action levels?

3. What peripheral blood smear findings are characteristic?
4. When is chelation therapy indicated?

Sequential Test Results:

Blood Lead Level (BLL):

- **Venous blood lead: 38 µg/dL ELEVATED** (reference <5 µg/dL)
- CDC classification: Level IV (35-44 µg/dL) - requires case management, chelation consideration

CDC Blood Lead Level Classifications:

- <5 µg/dL: Reference level (no action)
- 5-14 µg/dL: Level I - retest, education
- 15-24 µg/dL: Level II - environmental investigation
- 25-44 µg/dL: Level III - chelation consideration
- **35-44 µg/dL: Level IV ← PATIENT HERE**
- ≥45 µg/dL: Level V - medical emergency, immediate chelation
- ≥70 µg/dL: Encephalopathy risk

Peripheral Blood Smear:

- **Basophilic stippling of RBCs** (classic finding - ribosomes due to inhibited heme synthesis)
- Microcytic, hypochromic RBCs
- Anisocytosis
- Target cells occasional

Iron Studies (to exclude iron deficiency as sole cause):

- Serum iron: 55 µg/dL (low-normal)
- TIBC: 380 µg/dL (elevated)
- Transferrin saturation: 14% (low)
- **Concurrent iron deficiency present** (common with lead poisoning)

Additional Testing:

Erythrocyte Protoporphyrin (EP) or Zinc Protoporphyrin (ZPP):

- **ZPP: 185 µg/dL** (elevated; normal <35)
- Mechanism: Lead inhibits ferrochelatase → protoporphyrin accumulates instead of forming heme

Abdominal X-ray:

- **Radio-opaque material in bowel** (lead paint chips visible)
- Bowel prep and whole bowel irrigation considered

24-Hour Urine Lead (not routine but obtained):

- Urine lead: 42 µg/24h (elevated)

Environmental Investigation:

- **Home inspection: Peeling lead-based paint confirmed**
- Soil samples: Elevated lead in yard
- Water testing: Within acceptable limits
- **Sibling screening:** Blood lead 12 µg/dL (also elevated but lower)

Neurodevelopmental Testing:

- Formal assessment shows mild developmental delays
- IQ testing: Lower than expected for age

Final Diagnosis: Childhood Lead Poisoning (Blood Lead 38 µg/dL) with Lead-Induced Anemia and Neurodevelopmental Effects

Source: Environmental exposure from deteriorating lead-based paint in old housing

Management:

Medical:

- **Oral chelation therapy: Succimer (DMSA) 10 mg/kg TID x 5 days, then BID x 14 days**
- Iron supplementation (treat concurrent iron deficiency)
- Nutritional counseling (adequate calcium, iron, vitamin C reduce absorption)
- Repeat BLL weekly during chelation, then monthly

Environmental:

- **Child temporarily relocated from contaminated home**
- Lead abatement required before return
- Environmental health department involved
- Family education on lead hazards

Chelation Indications:

- BLL ≥45 µg/dL: Immediate chelation
- BLL 35-44 µg/dL: Chelation if symptomatic OR not declining with environmental intervention
- BLL 25-34 µg/dL: Environmental intervention, consider chelation if not improving
- **Patient qualifies due to BLL 38 + symptoms + documented exposure**

Chelation Agents:

- **Succimer (DMSA):** Oral, for BLL 25-45 µg/dL
- **CaNa2-EDTA:** IV/IM, for BLL 45-69 µg/dL
- **BAL (dimercaprol) + CaNa2-EDTA:** For BLL ≥70 or encephalopathy

Follow-Up (Post-Chelation):

1 Week After Completing Chelation:

- BLL: 22 μg/dL (decreased but still elevated)
- Hemoglobin: 10.1 g/dL (improving)

1 Month:

- BLL: 15 μg/dL (continuing to decline)
- Home remediation completed
- Family allowed to return

3 Months:

- BLL: 7 μg/dL (approaching normal)
- Hemoglobin: 11.5 g/dL (normalized)
- Behavior improving
- Developmental intervention ongoing

Teaching Points:

1. **Sources of Lead:** Old paint (pre-1978), contaminated soil, imported pottery, certain cosmetics, occupational exposure, contaminated water
2. **Mechanism of Toxicity:** Inhibits δ-aminolevulinic acid dehydratase and ferrochelatase → impaired heme synthesis; damages CNS, kidneys, GI tract
3. **Clinical Manifestations:** Children - developmental delays, behavioral problems, learning disabilities, abdominal pain, anemia; Adults - neuropathy, nephropathy, hypertension, reproductive effects
4. **Screening:** All children at age 1 and 2 years in high-risk areas; Medicaid-eligible children; children in old housing
5. **Basophilic Stippling:** RNA remnants (ribosomes) in RBCs; seen in lead poisoning, thalassemia, other causes; not specific but suggestive
6. **ZPP/EP Ratio:** Elevated in lead poisoning and iron deficiency; ZPP:heme ratio >100 μg/dL suggests toxicity
7. **Chelation Complications:** Rebound phenomenon (BLL rises after chelation due to redistribution from bone); may need repeat courses
8. **Irreversible Effects:** Neurodevelopmental damage in children may be permanent; early intervention crucial
9. **Pregnancy Considerations:** Lead crosses placenta; mobilized from maternal bone stores; screen pregnant women in high-risk situations

Related Cases: Iron deficiency anemia, mercury poisoning, arsenic toxicity, occupational heavy metal exposure

Case 8.4: Alcohol Withdrawal Syndrome

Clinical Presentation: A 54-year-old homeless man is admitted for pneumonia. He reports drinking "a pint of vodka daily" for 20 years. Last drink was 18 hours ago. Currently complaining of tremors, sweating, anxiety, and "feeling like bugs are crawling on me." Nursing staff reports he is agitated and confused.

Physical Examination:

- BP 168/98 (hypertensive), HR 118 (tachycardia), Temp 100.2°F, RR 24
- Diaphoretic, tremulous
- Disoriented to time and place
- **Coarse tremor of hands**
- Hyperreflexia
- Auditory and visual hallucinations ("seeing spiders")

Initial Laboratory Findings:

- WBC: 14,500/μL (pneumonia)
- Platelets: 125,000/μL (mild thrombocytopenia - chronic alcohol)
- AST: 185 U/L (elevated)
- ALT: 78 U/L
- AST:ALT ratio: 2.4:1 (suggests alcoholic liver disease)
- GGT: 420 U/L (markedly elevated)
- Albumin: 3.1 g/dL (low)
- Magnesium: 1.3 mg/dL (low)
- Phosphate: 2.1 mg/dL (low)
- Glucose: 92 mg/dL

Diagnostic Reasoning Questions:

1. What are the stages and timeline of alcohol withdrawal?
2. How is Clinical Institute Withdrawal Assessment (CIWA-Ar) used?
3. What laboratory tests suggest chronic alcohol use?
4. Why are thiamine and other vitamins critical in alcohol withdrawal?

Sequential Test Results:

Toxicology Screening:

Blood Alcohol Level (BAL):

- **Ethanol: <10 mg/dL** (essentially zero - patient in withdrawal)
- Last drink 18 hours ago

Urine Drug Screen:

- Ethyl glucuronide (EtG): Positive (confirms recent alcohol use up to 80 hours)

- Ethyl sulfate (EtS): Positive
- Other drugs: Negative

Carbohydrate-Deficient Transferrin (CDT):

- **CDT: 8.5%** (elevated; normal <1.7%)
- Marker of chronic heavy alcohol consumption (>60 g/day for ≥2 weeks)
- Sensitivity: 70%; Specificity: 90%

Mean Corpuscular Volume (MCV):

- **MCV: 103 fL** (macrocytosis - chronic alcohol effect on bone marrow)

Liver Function Tests:

- AST: 185 U/L (ALT 78 U/L) - **AST > ALT ratio >2:1** classic for alcoholic liver disease
- GGT: 420 U/L (very sensitive for alcohol use; elevated in 70-80% of heavy drinkers)
- Alkaline phosphatase: 145 U/L (mildly elevated)
- Total bilirubin: 2.2 mg/dL (elevated)
- INR: 1.4 (mild coagulopathy)

Clinical Institute Withdrawal Assessment (CIWA-Ar) Score:

Initial Assessment (18 hours post-last drink):

- Nausea/vomiting: 3
- Tremor: 4
- Paroxysmal sweats: 5
- Anxiety: 5
- Agitation: 4
- Tactile disturbances: 4
- Auditory disturbances: 3
- Visual disturbances: 4
- Headache: 3
- Orientation: 3 (disoriented to time/place)
- **Total CIWA-Ar: 38 SEVERE WITHDRAWAL**

CIWA-Ar Scoring:

- <10: Mild withdrawal
- 10-15: Moderate withdrawal
- **>15: Severe withdrawal** (patient at risk for seizures, DTs)

Management Initiated:

Immediate Treatment:

- **Benzodiazepines:** Lorazepam 2 mg IV q15min PRN for CIWA >15

- **Symptom-triggered protocol:** CIWA assessed q1-2h
- **Thiamine 100 mg IV BEFORE glucose** (prevent Wernicke's encephalopathy)
- Folic acid 1 mg daily
- Multivitamin
- Magnesium sulfate 2 g IV
- Phosphate repletion
- IV fluids (D5NS)

Seizure Prophylaxis Consideration:

- History of prior DTs or seizures? Yes (per patient)
- **Scheduled benzodiazepines added** (lorazepam 2 mg q6h)

Serial CIWA-Ar Monitoring:

24 Hours (6 hours after admission):

- CIWA: 28 (improving with treatment)
- HR: 102, BP: 152/88
- Total lorazepam given: 16 mg

36 Hours:

- CIWA: 18 (still elevated)
- Patient more oriented, less agitated
- Hallucinations decreased
- Total lorazepam: 24 mg

48 Hours (Critical Window for Delirium Tremens):

- CIWA: 12 (moderate)
- Vital signs stabilizing
- No seizure activity
- Total lorazepam: 32 mg

72 Hours:

- CIWA: 8 (mild)
- Tremor minimal
- Oriented x3
- Benzodiazepine taper begun

Final Diagnosis:

1. Severe Alcohol Withdrawal Syndrome (CIWA 38)
2. Alcoholic Liver Disease (AST >> ALT, elevated GGT, macrocytosis)
3. Alcohol Use Disorder, Severe
4. Community-Acquired Pneumonia (admission diagnosis)

Alcohol Withdrawal Timeline:

- **6-12 hours:** Tremulousness, anxiety, GI upset, diaphoresis, tachycardia
- **12-24 hours:** Hallucinations (visual, auditory, tactile)
- **24-48 hours: Seizures** (generalized tonic-clonic) - **CRITICAL PERIOD**
- **48-72 hours: Delirium tremens (DTs)** - confusion, autonomic instability, severe agitation (5-15% mortality if untreated)

Teaching Points:

1. **CIWA-Ar Protocol:** Validated 10-item scale; guides symptom-triggered benzodiazepine dosing; more effective than fixed-dose protocols; reduces total benzodiazepine use and hospitalization length
2. **Thiamine First:** Give IV thiamine BEFORE glucose to prevent precipitating Wernicke's encephalopathy (glucose increases thiamine demand)
3. **Benzodiazepine Selection:** Lorazepam (intermediate-acting, no active metabolites, IM/IV available) preferred in liver disease; chlordiazepoxide/diazepam (long-acting) preferred in normal liver function
4. **AST:ALT Ratio >2:1:** Classic for alcoholic hepatitis; AST rarely >300-400 U/L in pure alcoholic liver disease (vs viral/drug-induced can be >1000)
5. **GGT:** Sensitive (not specific) marker of alcohol use; elevated in 70-80% of heavy drinkers; also elevated in obesity, diabetes, some medications
6. **CDT (Carbohydrate-Deficient Transferrin):** Specific marker of chronic heavy drinking; elevated with >60 g/day alcohol for ≥2 weeks; returns to normal 2-4 weeks after abstinence
7. **Phosphate/Magnesium Depletion:** Common in alcoholics; repletion prevents arrhythmias, seizures, rhabdomyolysis
8. **Delirium Tremens:** Medical emergency; 5-15% mortality without treatment; <1% with treatment; ICU monitoring may be needed
9. **Seizure Management:** Brief, self-limited; benzodiazepines first-line; avoid phenytoin (less effective in alcohol withdrawal seizures)

Related Cases: Wernicke-Korsakoff syndrome, benzodiazepine withdrawal, alcoholic ketoacidosis, hepatic encephalopathy

---

Case 8.5: Urine Drug Screen Interpretation - Workplace Testing

Clinical Presentation: A 32-year-old truck driver undergoes routine pre-employment drug screening as required by Department of Transportation (DOT) regulations. He reports no illicit drug use. Takes ibuprofen for chronic back pain and recently completed a course of amoxicillin for sinusitis. Consumed a poppy seed bagel this morning. He is concerned about test accuracy.

Background:

- Denies illicit drug use
- Takes ibuprofen 600 mg TID
- Recently finished amoxicillin
- Ate poppy seed bagel 2 hours before collection

- No prescription opioids or controlled substances

Diagnostic Reasoning Questions:

1. What is the difference between screening and confirmatory drug testing?
2. What substances are included in standard DOT drug panels?
3. What causes false-positive and false-negative results?
4. What is the role of Medical Review Officer (MRO)?

Sequential Test Results:

Urine Collection (Observed Collection per DOT Protocol):

- Temperature: 96°F (acceptable range 90-100°F within 4 minutes)
- pH: 6.0 (normal; <3 or >11 suggests adulteration)
- Specific gravity: 1.020 (normal; <1.003 or >1.025 flagged)
- Creatinine: 85 mg/dL (normal; <20 mg/dL suggests dilution)
- Color: Yellow (normal)
- **Specimen validity tests: PASS** (no adulteration detected)

Initial Immunoassay Screening (Point-of-Care Dipstick):

DOT 5-Panel Drug Screen:

- Marijuana (THC): **NEGATIVE** (cutoff 50 ng/mL)
- Cocaine: **NEGATIVE** (cutoff 150 ng/mL)
- Amphetamines: **NEGATIVE** (cutoff 500 ng/mL)
- Opiates: **PRESUMPTIVE POSITIVE** (cutoff 2000 ng/mL)
- Phencyclidine (PCP): **NEGATIVE** (cutoff 25 ng/mL)

Preliminary Result: POSITIVE for opiates

Immunoassay Limitations:

- **Cross-reactivity:** Ibuprofen can cause false-positive for marijuana (rare)
- **Poppy seeds:** Contain morphine/codeine → can cause positive opiate screen
- **Other causes:** Quinolone antibiotics (false-positive opiates), SSRI (false-positive amphetamines)

Reflex to Confirmatory Testing (per DOT Protocol):

Gas Chromatography-Mass Spectrometry (GC-MS) Confirmation:

Opiates Panel (Confirmation cutoffs - higher than screening):

- **Morphine: 2,500 ng/mL** (cutoff 2,000 ng/mL) **POSITIVE**
- **Codeine: 380 ng/mL** (cutoff 2,000 ng/mL) **NEGATIVE**
- 6-Monoacetylmorphine (6-MAM): **NOT DETECTED** (heroin metabolite; cutoff 10 ng/mL)
- Hydrocodone: **NOT DETECTED**

- Hydromorphone: **NOT DETECTED**
- Oxycodone: **NOT DETECTED**

Pattern Analysis:

- **Morphine > Codeine** (ratio >2:1)
- **No 6-MAM** (excludes heroin use)
- **Pattern consistent with poppy seed ingestion** (morphine without 6-MAM)

Medical Review Officer (MRO) Evaluation:

- Patient interviewed
- No prescription opioids verified
- Reports poppy seed consumption
- **MRO interpretation: Positive test attributed to poppy seed ingestion**
- **Final result: NEGATIVE (test cancelled due to legitimate explanation)**

Additional Testing Performed (Research Purposes):

Extended Panel - Non-DOT Substances:

- Benzodiazepines: Negative
- Barbiturates: Negative
- Methadone: Negative
- Propoxyphene: Negative
- Fentanyl: **Negative** (not detected on standard screens)
- Buprenorphine: Negative
- Synthetic cannabinoids: Negative (not detected on THC screens)
- Bath salts (synthetic cathinones): Negative (not detected on amphetamine screens)

Adulterant Testing (Specimen Validity):

- Nitrites: Negative
- Glutaraldehyde: Negative
- Pyridinium chlorochromate (PCC): Negative
- Oxidants: Negative
- pH: Normal
- Specific gravity: Normal
- Creatinine: Normal

Final Diagnosis: False-Positive Urine Opiate Screen due to Poppy Seed Ingestion (Test Cancelled by MRO)

Chain of Custody:

- Proper collection, labeling, sealing documented
- Tamper-evident seals intact
- All transfers documented
- Legal defensibility maintained

Teaching Points:

1. **Screening vs. Confirmation:** Immunoassay screening = high sensitivity, low specificity, faster, cheaper; GC-MS/LC-MS confirmation = high specificity, definitive, slower, expensive
2. **Cutoff Levels:** Screening cutoffs lower to maximize detection; confirmation cutoffs higher to minimize false positives; prevents detection of passive exposure
3. **DOT 5-Panel:** Marijuana, cocaine, amphetamines, opiates, PCP; does NOT include benzodiazepines, synthetic opioids (fentanyl), alcohol
4. **False Positives:** Poppy seeds (opiates); ibuprofen (marijuana - rare); quinolones (opiates); SSRI/bupropion (amphetamines); dextromethorphan (PCP)
5. **False Negatives:** Dilution, adulteration, substitution; synthetic cannabinoids ("spice") don't cross-react with THC; fentanyl not detected on opiate screens
6. **6-MAM (6-Monoacetylmorphine):** Specific heroin metabolite; only present for 2-8 hours; definitive proof of heroin use
7. **Poppy Seed Defense:** Legitimate; can cause morphine/codeine detection up to 2,500-3,000 ng/mL; morphine:codeine ratio >2:1; no 6-MAM
8. **MRO Role:** Licensed physician who reviews lab results, interviews donor, determines if legitimate medical explanation exists, makes final determination
9. **Detection Windows:** Marijuana 3-30 days (longer for chronic users); cocaine 2-4 days; opiates 2-4 days; amphetamines 2-4 days; alcohol 6-12 hours (up to 80 hours for EtG)
10. **Specimen Validity:** Tests for dilution (creatinine, specific gravity), substitution (temperature), adulteration (oxidants, pH); ensures authentic sample

Related Cases: Positive test for prescription medication, synthetic drug detection, adulterated specimen, alcohol testing (EtG/EtS)

Case 8.6: Neonatal Abstinence Syndrome (NAS)

Clinical Presentation: A term newborn male (39 weeks gestation) is born to a 28-year-old mother with history of opioid use disorder on methadone maintenance therapy (80 mg daily) during pregnancy. Mother engaged in prenatal care and compliant with methadone program. Baby appears initially well at delivery but at 24 hours of life develops irritability, tremors, and feeding difficulty.

Birth History:

- Birth weight: 2,680 grams (appropriate for gestational age, lower end)
- Apgar scores: 8 at 1 minute, 9 at 5 minutes
- No resuscitation required
- Maternal prenatal labs: HIV negative, HBsAg negative, RPR negative, GBS positive (treated)

Physical Examination (24 Hours of Life):

- Irritable, high-pitched cry
- **Tremors when disturbed**
- Increased muscle tone
- **Frequent sneezing and yawning**
- Mottled skin

- Feeding poorly, regurgitation
- Loose stools
- Tachypnea (RR 68)

Diagnostic Reasoning Questions:

1. What is neonatal abstinence syndrome and which substances cause it?
2. How is NAS assessed and scored?
3. What are the differences between opioid, SSRI, and benzodiazepine withdrawal in neonates?
4. When is pharmacologic treatment indicated?

Sequential Test Results:

Maternal and Neonatal Drug Testing:

Maternal Urine (at delivery):

- Methadone: **POSITIVE** (prescribed)
- Opiates: **POSITIVE** (methadone metabolites)
- Cocaine, amphetamines, THC: Negative
- Benzodiazepines: Negative

Neonatal Meconium Drug Testing (sent at birth):

- **Methadone: POSITIVE** (confirms in-utero exposure)
- EDDP (methadone metabolite): Positive
- Other opiates: Negative
- Cocaine: Negative
- Amphetamines: Negative
- Cannabinoids: Negative

Neonatal Urine Drug Screen:

- Methadone: Positive
- Consistent with maternal methadone use

Why Meconium Testing?

- Detects drug exposure during 2nd and 3rd trimesters
- More sensitive than urine (detects 3-5 times more exposures)
- Longer detection window than urine or umbilical cord

Finnegan Neonatal Abstinence Scoring System:

Assessment at 24 Hours (scoring q3-4h):

Central Nervous System:

- High-pitched cry: 2 points
- Continuous high-pitched cry: 0 (intermittent)
- Sleeps <1 hour after feeding: 3 points
- Sleeps <2 hours: 2 points
- Hyperactive Moro reflex: 2 points
- Tremors (disturbed): 1 point
- Tremors (undisturbed): 3 points
- Increased muscle tone: 2 points
- Myoclonic jerks: 0
- Generalized seizures: 0

Metabolic/Vasomotor/Respiratory:

- Sweating: 1 point
- Fever 37.2-38.3°C: 1 point
- Frequent yawning: 1 point
- Mottling: 1 point
- Nasal stuffiness: 1 point
- Sneezing: 1 point
- Respiratory rate >60: 1 point

Gastrointestinal:

- Excessive sucking: 1 point
- Poor feeding: 2 points
- Regurgitation: 2 points
- Loose stools: 2 points

Total Finnegan Score: 25 SEVERE NAS (>12 indicates need for treatment consideration)

Scoring Interpretation:

- <8: Minimal withdrawal, supportive care
- 8-12: Moderate withdrawal, increased monitoring
- **>12: Severe withdrawal** - pharmacologic treatment if 3 consecutive scores >12 or 2 consecutive >16

Serial Finnegan Scores:

36 Hours:

- Finnegan: 16 (worsening)
- Supportive care continued: rooming-in, demand feeding, swaddling, reduced stimulation

48 Hours:

- Finnegan: 18 (continued elevation)
- **Decision: Initiate pharmacologic treatment**

Treatment Initiated:

Morphine Sulfate Oral Solution:

- Initial dose: 0.04 mg/kg/dose q3-4h
- Titrated based on Finnegan scores
- Goal: Scores <8

Alternative Treatments (Not Used in This Case):

- Methadone (alternative first-line)
- Phenobarbital (adjunctive or for polysubstance)
- Clonidine (adjunctive, for autonomic symptoms)

Laboratory Monitoring:

Baseline Labs:

- CBC: Normal (Hgb 16.2 g/dL, WBC 12,000/μL)
- Glucose: 68 mg/dL (low-normal)
- Calcium: 9.8 mg/dL (normal)
- Magnesium: 2.0 mg/dL (normal)
- Electrolytes: Normal

After Treatment Initiation:

72 Hours (24h on morphine):

- Finnegan: 10 (improving)
- Morphine dose: 0.05 mg/kg q3h

96 Hours:

- Finnegan: 8 (stabilized)
- Feeding improved
- Less irritable

1 Week:

- Finnegan: 6-8 (controlled)
- Begin morphine wean (10-20% reduction q24-48h)

2 Weeks:

- Continued slow wean
- Finnegan scores remain <8

3 Weeks:

- Morphine successfully discontinued
- Finnegan scores 4-6 off medication
- Baby feeding well, gaining weight
- **Discharged home with mother**

Final Diagnosis: Neonatal Abstinence Syndrome (NAS) due to In-Utero Methadone Exposure - Successfully Treated

Long-Term Considerations:

- Developmental follow-up
- Maternal substance use disorder treatment continuation
- Family support services
- Child protective services involvement (varies by jurisdiction)

Teaching Points:

1. **NAS Causes:** Opioids (methadone, buprenorphine, heroin, prescription opioids) most common; also SSRIs, benzodiazepines, barbiturates, alcohol
2. **Onset Timing:** Opioids: 24-72 hours (methadone/buprenorphine may be delayed to 72-96h due to long half-life); shorter-acting opioids (heroin) may present within 24h
3. **Finnegan Score:** Most widely used assessment tool; scores q3-4h; guides treatment initiation and weaning
4. **Meconium vs Urine:** Meconium detects 2nd/3rd trimester exposure (ethanol, opioids, cocaine, cannabinoids); urine detects recent exposure (last few days)
5. **Non-Pharmacologic Interventions:** Rooming-in with mother, breastfeeding (if safe - no contraindications like HIV), swaddling, demand feeding, low-stimulation environment
6. **Pharmacologic Treatment:** Morphine or methadone first-line for opioid NAS; phenobarbital for polysubstance or adjunctive; clonidine for autonomic symptoms
7. **Treatment Threshold:** Usually 3 consecutive scores >12 OR 2 consecutive >16; varies by protocol
8. **Duration:** Average treatment 3-4 weeks; methadone/buprenorphine exposure may require longer treatment than illicit opioids
9. **Breastfeeding:** Generally encouraged if mother on stable methadone/buprenorphine, no illicit drugs, no contraindications (HIV); reduces NAS severity
10. **Long-Term Outcomes:** Some studies show developmental and behavioral concerns; early intervention improves outcomes

Related Cases: Fetal alcohol syndrome, prenatal cocaine exposure, SSRI discontinuation syndrome in newborns, benzodiazepine withdrawal in neonates

Chapter 9: Immunology and Serology

Case 9.1: Systemic Lupus Erythematosus (SLE)

Clinical Presentation: A 28-year-old African American woman presents with 3 months of fatigue, joint pain in hands and knees, intermittent low-grade fevers, and a facial rash that worsens with sun exposure. She also reports oral ulcers and hair loss. Recently developed swelling in her legs. Family history: Mother has rheumatoid arthritis.

Physical Examination:

- BP 148/92 (elevated), Temp 100.2°F
- **Malar rash** (butterfly distribution across cheeks and nasal bridge, sparing nasolabial folds)
- Oral ulcers on buccal mucosa
- Diffuse alopecia
- Synovitis in MCP and PIP joints bilaterally (non-erosive)
- 2+ pitting edema lower extremities

Initial Laboratory Findings:

- WBC: 3,200/µL (leukopenia)
- Hemoglobin: 9.8 g/dL (anemia)
- Platelets: 95,000/µL (thrombocytopenia) - **Pancytopenia**
- ESR: 78 mm/hr (markedly elevated)
- CRP: 2.1 mg/dL (mildly elevated - often low in SLE)
- Creatinine: 1.4 mg/dL (elevated)
- Urinalysis: 3+ protein, RBCs 20-30/hpf, RBC casts present

Diagnostic Reasoning Questions:

1. What are the SLICC/ACR classification criteria for SLE?
2. Which autoantibodies are specific vs. sensitive for SLE?
3. How do complement levels help assess SLE activity?
4. What is the significance of anti-dsDNA antibodies?

Sequential Test Results:

Autoantibody Panel:

ANA (Antinuclear Antibody) - Initial Screening:

- **ANA titer: 1:1280 STRONGLY POSITIVE** (normal <1:80)
- **Pattern: Homogeneous** (suggests anti-dsDNA or anti-histone antibodies)
- Sensitivity for SLE: 95-98%

ANA Patterns and Significance:

- Homogeneous: dsDNA, histones (SLE, drug-induced lupus)
- Speckled: Sm, RNP, Ro, La (SLE, Sjögren's, MCTD)
- Nucleolar: Scl-70, RNA polymerase (scleroderma)
- Centromere: Anti-centromere (limited scleroderma/CREST)

Extractable Nuclear Antigen (ENA) Panel:

- **Anti-dsDNA (double-stranded DNA): 285 IU/mL STRONGLY POSITIVE** (normal <30)
  - Specific for SLE (95-98% specificity)
  - Correlates with disease activity and lupus nephritis
- **Anti-Smith (Sm): POSITIVE** (high specificity 98% for SLE, low sensitivity 30%)
- Anti-RNP: Negative
- **Anti-Ro/SSA: POSITIVE** (associated with photosensitivity, neonatal lupus, congenital heart block)
- Anti-La/SSB: Negative
- Anti-histone: Negative (would suggest drug-induced lupus)

Additional Autoantibodies:

- **Anti-cardiolipin antibodies (IgG): 48 GPL units** (elevated; normal <20) - **Antiphospholipid syndrome**
- **Lupus anticoagulant: POSITIVE**
- Beta-2 glycoprotein I antibodies (IgG): Positive
- Anti-ribosomal P: Negative (if positive, associated with neuropsychiatric lupus)

Complement Levels:

- **C3: 42 mg/dL LOW** (normal 90-180)
- **C4: 8 mg/dL LOW** (normal 10-40)
- **Total hemolytic complement (CH50): 15 U/mL LOW** (normal 30-75)
- Interpretation: Hypocomplementemia indicates active disease, immune complex formation

Direct Coombs Test (DAT):

- **Positive** (IgG) - autoimmune hemolytic anemia component

Urinary Studies:

24-Hour Urine:

- **Total protein: 3.8 g/24h NEPHROTIC RANGE** (normal <150 mg)
- Creatinine clearance: 58 mL/min (reduced)

Spot Urine Protein/Creatinine Ratio:

- 3.5 mg/mg (confirms nephrotic-range proteinuria)

Renal Biopsy Performed:

- **Histology: Class IV lupus nephritis** (diffuse proliferative glomerulonephritis)
- Immunofluorescence: "Full house" pattern (IgG, IgM, IgA, C3, C1q deposits) - **pathognomonic for lupus nephritis**
- Electron microscopy: Subendothelial and mesangial deposits

Final Diagnosis: Systemic Lupus Erythematosus (SLE) with:

1. Class IV Lupus Nephritis
2. Autoimmune Hemolytic Anemia
3. Secondary Antiphospholipid Syndrome

SLICC Criteria Met (Need 4 of 11 Clinical + Immunologic, OR lupus nephritis + ANA or anti-dsDNA):

Clinical Criteria (7/11):

1. ✓ Acute cutaneous lupus (malar rash)
2. ✓ Non-scarring alopecia
3. ✓ Oral ulcers
4. ✓ Non-erosive arthritis
5. ✓ Renal (proteinuria, RBC casts)
6. ✓ Hematologic (leukopenia, thrombocytopenia, hemolytic anemia)
7. ✓ Hypertension, edema

Immunologic Criteria (5/6):

1. ✓ ANA positive
2. ✓ Anti-dsDNA positive
3. ✓ Anti-Sm positive
4. ✓ Antiphospholipid antibodies positive
5. ✓ Low complement (C3, C4)
6. ✓ Direct Coombs positive

Treatment Initiated:

- High-dose corticosteroids (prednisone 1 mg/kg/day)
- Mycophenolate mofetil (induction therapy for lupus nephritis)
- Hydroxychloroquine 400 mg daily (maintenance, reduces flares)
- ACE inhibitor for blood pressure and proteinuria
- Anticoagulation consideration for antiphospholipid syndrome
- Sunscreen, sun avoidance
- Calcium/vitamin D supplementation

Monitoring:

- Anti-dsDNA and complement levels (track disease activity)
- Urinalysis and urine protein (monitor nephritis response)
- CBC (watch for cytopenias)
- Creatinine (renal function)

Teaching Points:

1. **Anti-dsDNA:** High specificity for SLE (95-98%); correlates with disease activity; high titers associated with lupus nephritis
2. **Anti-Smith:** Most specific antibody for SLE (98%) but low sensitivity (30%); does NOT correlate with disease activity
3. **Low Complement:** C3 and C4 consumption indicates active disease, immune complex formation; useful for monitoring
4. **Antiphospholipid Syndrome:** Can be primary or secondary (to SLE); requires ≥2 positive tests 12 weeks apart; associated with thrombosis, pregnancy loss
5. **Lupus Nephritis Classes:** Class I-II (minimal/mesangial); Class III-IV (focal/diffuse proliferative - most severe); Class V (membranous); Class VI (sclerotic)
6. **"Full House" IF Pattern:** IgG, IgM, IgA, C3, C1q deposition; highly specific for lupus nephritis
7. **Drug-Induced Lupus:** Anti-histone antibodies positive; drugs include hydralazine, procainamide, isoniazid, minocycline; resolves with drug discontinuation
8. **ANA Patterns:** Homogeneous (dsDNA, histones); Speckled (Sm, RNP, Ro, La); Nucleolar (scleroderma); Centromere (limited scleroderma)

Related Cases: Drug-induced lupus, mixed connective tissue disease, Sjögren's syndrome, antiphospholipid syndrome

---

Case 9.2: Rheumatoid Arthritis vs. Other Arthropathies

Clinical Presentation: A 52-year-old woman presents with 4 months of progressive joint pain and stiffness in her hands, wrists, and feet. Morning stiffness lasts >2 hours and improves with activity. She reports fatigue and has noticed swelling in her finger joints. Denies rash, oral ulcers, or Raynaud's phenomenon. No family history of autoimmune disease.

Physical Examination:

- Symmetric swelling and tenderness of MCPs, PIPs bilaterally
- Wrists tender with limited range of motion
- MTPs tender bilaterally
- **Swan neck deformities** beginning in 3rd and 4th digits (PIP hyperextension, DIP flexion)
- **Subcutaneous nodules** on extensor surface of elbows (rheumatoid nodules)
- No skin changes, no tophi

Initial Laboratory Findings:

- WBC: 10,200/µL (normal)
- Hemoglobin: 10.8 g/dL (anemia of chronic disease)
- Platelets: 445,000/µL (thrombocytosis - reactive)

336

- **ESR: 62 mm/hr** (elevated)
- **CRP: 4.8 mg/dL** (markedly elevated)
- Creatinine: 0.9 mg/dL (normal)

Imaging:

- Hand X-rays: Periarticular osteopenia, marginal erosions at MCPs and PIPs, joint space narrowing
- No chondrocalcinosis

Diagnostic Reasoning Questions:

1. What serologic tests distinguish rheumatoid arthritis from other arthropathies?
2. What is the significance of anti-CCP antibodies vs. rheumatoid factor?
3. How do you differentiate RA from psoriatic arthritis, gout, and lupus arthritis?
4. What are the 2010 ACR/EULAR classification criteria for RA?

Sequential Test Results:

Rheumatoid Factor (RF):

- **RF (IgM): 285 IU/mL POSITIVE** (normal <14)
- Elevated RF present in:
  - Rheumatoid arthritis: 70-80%
  - Sjögren's syndrome: 60-70%
  - SLE: 15-35%
  - Chronic infections (hepatitis C, endocarditis): 15-65%
  - Healthy elderly: 10-25%
- **Specificity for RA: Only 85%** (not highly specific)

Anti-Cyclic Citrullinated Peptide (Anti-CCP) Antibodies:

- **Anti-CCP (IgG): 340 U/mL STRONGLY POSITIVE** (normal <20)
- **Specificity for RA: 95-98%** (much more specific than RF)
- Sensitivity: 60-70%
- Present in early RA, even before symptoms
- Associated with more erosive, severe disease
- **Best single test for RA diagnosis**

Additional Autoantibodies (to Exclude Other Diagnoses):

- ANA: 1:80 (low titer, borderline; not significant)
- Anti-dsDNA: Negative (excludes SLE)
- Anti-CCP negative in other arthropathies (helps differentiate from lupus, psoriatic arthritis)

Acute Phase Reactants:

- ESR: 62 mm/hr (elevated - tracks inflammation)
- CRP: 4.8 mg/dL (elevated - more specific than ESR)

- Both useful for monitoring disease activity and treatment response

Synovial Fluid Analysis (MCP Joint Aspiration):

- Appearance: Cloudy, yellow
- WBC: 18,000 cells/μL (inflammatory; 2,000-50,000)
- Neutrophils: 75%
- **No crystals** (excludes gout, pseudogout)
- Gram stain: Negative (excludes septic arthritis)
- Culture: No growth

Synovial Fluid Classification:

- Normal: <200 WBC, <25% PMN
- Non-inflammatory: 200-2,000 WBC (osteoarthritis)
- **Inflammatory: 2,000-50,000 WBC, >50% PMN** (RA, lupus, psoriatic arthritis)
- Septic: >50,000 WBC, >75% PMN

Additional Testing to Exclude Other Diagnoses:

Uric Acid:

- Serum uric acid: 4.8 mg/dL (normal; excludes gout)

HLA-B27:

- Negative (excludes ankylosing spondylitis, reactive arthritis)

Complement Levels:

- C3, C4: Normal (lupus would have low complement)

Imaging:

- **X-rays: Symmetric joint involvement, erosions at margins** (classic RA)
- **No DIP involvement** (would suggest psoriatic arthritis or osteoarthritis)
- **No sacroiliitis** (would suggest ankylosing spondylitis)

Final Diagnosis: Seropositive Rheumatoid Arthritis (RF-positive, Anti-CCP-positive) with Erosive Disease

2010 ACR/EULAR Classification Criteria (Score ≥6/10 = RA):

1. **Joint involvement:** MCPs, PIPs, wrists, MTPs = 5 points (2-10 small joints)
2. **Serology:** RF high-positive + Anti-CCP high-positive = 3 points
3. **Acute phase reactants:** ESR and CRP elevated = 1 point
4. **Duration:** >6 weeks = 1 point **Total: 10/10 points → Definite RA**

Comparison with Other Arthropathies:

Feature	RA	Psoriatic Arthritis	SLE	Gout
Anti-CCP	**Positive**	Negative	Negative	Negative
RF	Positive 70%	Negative usually	Positive 15-35%	Negative
Joint pattern	Symmetric, small joints	Asymmetric, DIP often	Non-erosive	Monoarticular, 1st MTP
Erosions	Yes, marginal	Yes, "pencil-in-cup"	No	Tophi, punched-out
Extra-articular	Nodules, lung	Psoriasis, nail pits	Malar rash, renal	Tophi, kidney stones
Synovial fluid	Inflammatory	Inflammatory	Inflammatory	Urate crystals

Treatment Initiated:

- **Methotrexate 15 mg weekly** (DMARD, first-line)
- Folic acid 1 mg daily (reduce MTX toxicity)
- **Prednisone 10 mg daily** (bridge therapy, taper)
- NSAIDs for symptom relief
- Hydroxychloroquine may be added (combination DMARD)
- If inadequate response: Add biologic (TNF-inhibitor, rituximab, etc.)

Teaching Points:

1. **Anti-CCP Antibodies:** Most specific test for RA (95-98%); present early in disease course; predicts erosive disease; more specific than RF
2. **Rheumatoid Factor:** Sensitive (70-80%) but less specific (85%); positive in many conditions (Sjögren's, SLE, chronic infections, healthy elderly)
3. **Seronegative RA:** 20-30% of RA patients are RF and anti-CCP negative; diagnosed by clinical criteria and exclusion
4. **Erosive vs Non-Erosive:** RA causes marginal erosions; SLE typically non-erosive; psoriatic arthritis causes "pencil-in-cup" deformities
5. **DIP Involvement:** Rare in RA (if present, consider psoriatic arthritis or osteoarthritis); RA typically spares DIPs
6. **Symmetry:** RA classically symmetric; psoriatic arthritis and reactive arthritis often asymmetric
7. **Rheumatoid Nodules:** Present in 20-30% of RA patients; associated with RF-positive disease, worse prognosis; found on extensor surfaces
8. **Anemia of Chronic Disease:** Common in RA; normocytic or microcytic; low serum iron, low TIBC, normal/high ferritin

Related Cases: Psoriatic arthritis, ankylosing spondylitis, gout, lupus arthritis, seronegative RA

Case 9.3: ANCA-Associated Vasculitis

Clinical Presentation: A 58-year-old man presents with 2 months of fatigue, weight loss (15 lbs), sinusitis with bloody nasal discharge, and progressive shortness of breath. Recently developed hematuria and leg weakness. He has had recurrent sinusitis for years, previously attributed to allergies.

Physical Examination:

- BP 168/98, HR 92, RR 22, Temp 100.8°F
- **Saddle nose deformity** (nasal septum perforation)
- Crusting and ulceration in nasal passages
- Lungs: Bilateral crackles
- Skin: Palpable purpura on lower extremities
- Neurologic: Foot drop on right (mononeuritis multiplex)

Initial Laboratory Findings:

- WBC: 14,500/µL (leukocytosis)
- Hemoglobin: 9.2 g/dL (anemia)
- Platelets: 485,000/µL (thrombocytosis)
- **Creatinine: 3.2 mg/dL ELEVATED** (baseline 1.0)
- BUN: 58 mg/dL
- **Urinalysis: 3+ blood, 2+ protein, RBCs >100/hpf, RBC casts present**
- ESR: 98 mm/hr (markedly elevated)
- CRP: 8.5 mg/dL (markedly elevated)

Imaging:

- **Chest X-ray:** Bilateral nodules and cavitary lesions
- **CT chest:** Multiple pulmonary nodules, some with cavitation
- **CT sinuses:** Chronic sinusitis, bony destruction

Diagnostic Reasoning Questions:

1. What are the different ANCA patterns and their clinical associations?
2. How do you differentiate granulomatosis with polyangiitis (GPA) from other vasculitides?
3. What is the significance of PR3-ANCA vs MPO-ANCA?
4. When is tissue biopsy necessary for diagnosis?

Sequential Test Results:

ANCA (Anti-Neutrophil Cytoplasmic Antibodies) Testing:

Indirect Immunofluorescence (IIF):

- **c-ANCA (cytoplasmic pattern): POSITIVE, titer 1:320**
- p-ANCA (perinuclear pattern): Negative

- c-ANCA highly suggestive of GPA (granulomatosis with polyangiitis, formerly Wegener's)

Antigen-Specific ELISA (Confirmatory):

- **Anti-PR3 (proteinase 3): STRONGLY POSITIVE, 185 U/mL** (normal <20)
- Anti-MPO (myeloperoxidase): Negative
-

ANCA Pattern Interpretation:

Pattern	Antigen	Associated Disease	Specificity
c-ANCA	**PR3**	**GPA (Wegener's)**	**90%**
p-ANCA	MPO	MPA, EGPA, drug-induced	50-70%
Atypical p-ANCA	Other	IBD, autoimmune hepatitis	Low

Additional Autoantibodies (to Exclude Other Diagnoses):

- ANA: Negative
- Anti-dsDNA: Negative (excludes SLE)
- Anti-GBM (anti-glomerular basement membrane): Negative (excludes Goodpasture syndrome)
- RF: Negative
- Complement C3, C4: Normal (vasculitis typically normocomplementemic; low in immune complex diseases like SLE)

Renal Function Studies:

- eGFR: 18 mL/min/1.73m² (Stage 4 CKD, acute on chronic)
- 24-hour urine protein: 2.8 g/24h

Renal Biopsy:

- **Pauci-immune necrotizing crescentic glomerulonephritis**
- Crescent formation in 60% of glomeruli
- **No immune complex deposits on immunofluorescence** (pauci-immune)
- Consistent with ANCA-associated vasculitis

Lung Biopsy (Transbronchial):

- **Necrotizing granulomatous inflammation**
- Vasculitis of small and medium vessels
- Geographic necrosis
- Multinucleated giant cells
- Consistent with GPA

Nasal Biopsy:

- Chronic inflammation with granulomas

- Vasculitis
- Necrosis

Final Diagnosis: Granulomatosis with Polyangiitis (GPA, formerly Wegener's Granulomatosis) - PR3-ANCA Positive

Classic Triad of GPA:

1. ✓ **Upper respiratory tract involvement** (sinusitis, nasal ulcers, saddle nose)
2. ✓ **Pulmonary involvement** (nodules, cavitary lesions, alveolar hemorrhage)
3. ✓ **Glomerulonephritis** (rapidly progressive, crescentic)

Additional Features Present:

- Mononeuritis multiplex (peripheral nerve involvement)
- Palpable purpura (skin vasculitis)
- Constitutional symptoms

Differential Diagnosis of ANCA-Associated Vasculitis:

1. GPA (Granulomatosis with Polyangiitis):

- c-ANCA (PR3) in 90%
- Upper/lower respiratory tract + kidney
- Necrotizing granulomas

2. MPA (Microscopic Polyangiitis):

- p-ANCA (MPO) in 50-75%
- Pulmonary-renal syndrome
- NO granulomas
- Small vessel vasculitis

3. EGPA (Eosinophilic Granulomatosis with Polyangiitis, formerly Churg-Strauss):

- p-ANCA (MPO) in 40%
- Asthma, eosinophilia, sinusitis
- Peripheral neuropathy common

Treatment Initiated:

Induction (Remission Induction):

- **High-dose corticosteroids:** Methylprednisolone 1 g IV daily x 3 days, then prednisone 1 mg/kg/day
- **Cyclophosphamide 2 mg/kg/day** (or rituximab 375 mg/m² weekly x 4)
- **Plasmapheresis** (for severe renal involvement with creatinine >4 or pulmonary hemorrhage)

Maintenance (after remission):

- Azathioprine or methotrexate
- Low-dose prednisone taper
- Rituximab alternative

Prophylaxis:

- PCP prophylaxis (TMP-SMX) due to immunosuppression
- Calcium and vitamin D
- Osteoporosis prevention

Monitoring:

- Serial ANCA titers (rising titers may predict relapse)
- Creatinine, urinalysis
- Chest imaging
- CBC (cyclophosphamide myelosuppression)

Follow-Up (3 Months):

- Creatinine: 1.8 mg/dL (improved)
- PR3-ANCA: 45 U/mL (decreased, clinical improvement)
- Urinalysis: Trace blood, no casts
- Chest X-ray: Nodules resolving
- Sinusitis improved

Teaching Points:

1. **c-ANCA/PR3:** 90% specific for GPA; may be negative in limited disease; titer correlates with disease activity
2. **p-ANCA/MPO:** Associated with MPA (50-75%), EGPA (40%), drug-induced vasculitis (hydralazine, levamisole), and non-vasculitic conditions (IBD, autoimmune hepatitis)
3. **Pauci-Immune GN:** Glomerulonephritis with minimal/absent immune deposits on IF; characteristic of ANCA-associated vasculitis
4. **Rapidly Progressive GN:** Crescent formation on biopsy; urgent treatment required to preserve renal function; can lead to ESRD in weeks
5. **GPA vs MPA:** Both ANCA-positive vasculitides; GPA has granulomas and upper respiratory involvement; MPA does NOT have granulomas
6. **Limited vs Generalized GPA:** Limited = upper/lower respiratory without renal; Generalized = multi-organ including kidney
7. **Relapse Risk:** 50% relapse within 5 years; rising ANCA titers may predict relapse but treat based on clinical findings
8. **Differential of Pulmonary-Renal Syndrome:** ANCA vasculitis, Goodpasture syndrome (anti-GBM), SLE, cryoglobulinemia

Related Cases: Microscopic polyangiitis, eosinophilic granulomatosis with polyangiitis, Goodpasture syndrome, polyarteritis nodosa

Case 9.4: Complement Deficiency

Clinical Presentation: A 22-year-old previously healthy man presents to ED with sudden-onset fever (103°F), severe headache, neck stiffness, and altered mental status for 6 hours. This is his **third episode of bacterial meningitis** in 4 years. Previous episodes were *Neisseria meningitidis* serogroup C (2 years ago) and serogroup B (6 months ago), both successfully treated. Family history notable for cousin who died of meningococcal sepsis at age 18.

Physical Examination:

- Temp 103.2°F, BP 102/68, HR 125, RR 24
- Altered mental status, lethargic
- **Nuchal rigidity, positive Kernig's and Brudzinski's signs**
- Petechial rash on trunk and extremities
- No other focal findings

Initial Laboratory Findings:

- WBC: 22,000/μL with left shift
- Platelets: 95,000/μL (thrombocytopenia)
- Creatinine: 1.2 mg/dL

Lumbar Puncture:

- Opening pressure: Elevated
- **CSF: 5,200 WBC/μL (95% neutrophils)**
- Protein: 380 mg/dL (elevated)
- Glucose: 18 mg/dL (low; serum glucose 105)
- **Gram stain: Gram-negative diplococci**
- **Culture: *Neisseria meningitidis* serogroup Y**

Diagnostic Reasoning Questions:

1. What complement deficiencies predispose to recurrent Neisseria infections?
2. How is the complement system evaluated?
3. What is the difference between classical, alternative, and terminal pathway deficiencies?
4. What other immunodeficiencies cause recurrent bacterial infections?

Sequential Test Results:

Complement Function Studies:

Total Hemolytic Complement (CH50):

- **CH50: Undetectable (<1 U/mL)** (normal 30-75 U/mL)

344

- Measures **classical complement pathway** (C1-C9)
- Undetectable CH50 indicates deficiency in classical or terminal pathway

Alternative Pathway (AH50):

- **AH50: Undetectable** (normal 40-100%)
- Measures alternative pathway (factor B, factor D, properdin, C3, C5-C9)

Individual Complement Component Levels:

Early Components (Classical Pathway):

- C1q: Normal
- C4: Normal
- C2: Normal

Central Component:

- **C3: Normal** (critical junction of all pathways)

Terminal Components (Membrane Attack Complex):

- **C5: Undetectable <1 mg/dL** (normal 55-120)
- **C6: Normal**
- **C7: Normal**
- **C8: Normal**
- **C9: Normal**

Interpretation:

- **Isolated C5 deficiency**
- Terminal pathway dysfunction (cannot form membrane attack complex C5b-9)
- Unable to lyse encapsulated bacteria (especially Neisseria)

Genetic Testing:

- **C5 gene sequencing:** Homozygous mutation identified (c.754C>T, p.Arg252*)
- Nonsense mutation causing premature stop codon
- **Autosomal recessive inheritance**

Family Screening:

- Parents: Heterozygous carriers (C5 levels 50% of normal, asymptomatic)
- Sibling: Carrier status
- Cousin (deceased from meningococcal sepsis): Likely had same deficiency

Functional Complement Assay:

- **Inability to form membrane attack complex** (MAC, C5b-9)
- Bacteria not lysed in presence of patient serum
- Normal complement-mediated opsonization (C3b intact)

Additional Immunologic Workup:

Immunoglobulin Levels:

- IgG, IgA, IgM: Normal (excludes hypogammaglobulinemia)

Lymphocyte Subsets:

- CD4, CD8, B cells, NK cells: Normal

Vaccine Response Testing:

- **Antibody response to meningococcal vaccine:** Normal
- **Antibody response to pneumococcal vaccine:** Normal
- Patient can mount antibody responses (not antibody deficiency)

Final Diagnosis: Hereditary C5 Complement Deficiency (Terminal Complement Pathway Deficiency) with Recurrent Neisseria Meningitidis Infections

Clinical Consequences of Complement Deficiencies:

Deficiency	Pathway Affected	Clinical Manifestations
C1, C2, C4	Classical	SLE-like illness, infections (less common)
C3	All pathways	Severe recurrent pyogenic infections
C5, C6, C7, C8, C9	**Terminal (MAC)**	**Recurrent Neisseria infections**
Factor H, I	Alternative	Atypical HUS, infections
Properdin	Alternative	Severe meningococcal disease (X-linked)
C1 inhibitor	Regulation	Hereditary angioedema

Management:

Acute Treatment:

- IV antibiotics (ceftriaxone) for current meningitis
- Supportive care

Long-Term Prevention:

- **Meningococcal vaccination:**
  - **MenACWY vaccine** (conjugate): Already given, boosters every 5 years
  - **MenB vaccine** (Bexsero, Trumenba): Two-dose series
  - **Vaccination ESSENTIAL** but does not provide 100% protection

- **Prophylactic antibiotics:** Consider daily penicillin or amoxicillin (controversial)
- **Patient education:** Seek immediate medical care for fever, headache, rash
- **Medical alert bracelet:** Identifying complement deficiency
- **Avoid travel to endemic areas** during outbreaks

Eculizumab Consideration:

- C5 inhibitor (blocks C5 cleavage, prevents MAC formation)
- Approved for paroxysmal nocturnal hemoglobinuria (PNH), atypical HUS
- Paradoxically, eculizumab **INCREASES meningococcal infection risk** (iatrogenic C5 deficiency)
- **NOT indicated** for hereditary C5 deficiency

Genetic Counseling:

- Autosomal recessive inheritance
- 25% recurrence risk for future offspring
- Carrier testing available for family members

Teaching Points:

1. **Terminal Complement Deficiency:** C5, C6, C7, C8, C9 deficiencies cause inability to form membrane attack complex (MAC); predispose to **recurrent Neisseria infections** (meningitidis, gonorrhoeae)
2. **CH50 vs AH50:** CH50 screens classical pathway (C1-C9); AH50 screens alternative pathway; both abnormal in terminal deficiencies since they share C5-C9
3. **C3 Deficiency:** Most severe; affects all three pathways; recurrent severe pyogenic infections (S. pneumoniae, H. influenzae, S. aureus)
4. **Classical Pathway Deficiency (C1, C2, C4):** SLE-like autoimmune disease more common than infections; impaired immune complex clearance
5. **Properdin Deficiency:** X-linked; increased risk of **fulminant meningococcal disease**; high mortality
6. **Meningococcal Vaccine:** Does NOT provide complete protection; reduces but does not eliminate risk; multiple serogroups exist
7. **Recurrent Neisseria:** Always evaluate for complement deficiency or asplenia/hyposplenia
8. **Functional vs Quantitative:** Terminal complement levels may be normal but function impaired; CH50/AH50 assess functional activity

Related Cases: Properdin deficiency, C3 deficiency, asplenia with recurrent encapsulated bacteria, antibody deficiency

---

Case 9.5: Primary Immunodeficiency - Common Variable Immunodeficiency (CVID)

Clinical Presentation: A 28-year-old woman presents with her 6th episode of pneumonia in 3 years. She has also had recurrent sinusitis, bronchitis, and two episodes of gastroenteritis requiring hospitalization. She reports chronic diarrhea and recent weight loss (12 lbs over 6 months). Childhood was unremarkable, but infections began in her early 20s. No family history of immunodeficiency.

Physical Examination:

- Appears chronically ill
- Lungs: Crackles right lower lobe
- Abdomen: Mild diffuse tenderness
- **No palpable lymph nodes, no splenomegaly** (absence suggests antibody deficiency rather than lymphoproliferative)
- No skin abnormalities, no eczema

Initial Laboratory Findings:

- WBC: 6,800/μL (normal)
- Hemoglobin: 10.2 g/dL (anemia)
- Platelets: 185,000/μL
- **Sputum culture: *Haemophilus influenzae***

Imaging:

- Chest X-ray: Right lower lobe consolidation (current pneumonia) + **bronchiectasis** bilateral lower lobes (chronic changes from recurrent infections)

Diagnostic Reasoning Questions:

1. What clinical features suggest antibody deficiency?
2. How is CVID diagnosed and how does it differ from other antibody deficiencies?
3. What is the role of vaccine response testing?
4. What are the complications and associated conditions of CVID?

Sequential Test Results:

Quantitative Immunoglobulin Levels:

Initial Testing:

- **IgG: 285 mg/dL SEVERELY LOW** (normal 700-1,600 mg/dL)
- **IgA: <7 mg/dL UNDETECTABLE** (normal 70-400 mg/dL)
- **IgM: 18 mg/dL LOW** (normal 40-230 mg/dL)

Immunoglobulin Subclasses:

- IgG1: Low
- IgG2: Low
- IgG3: Low
- IgG4: Low
- **All IgG subclasses decreased** (panhypogammaglobulinemia)

B Cell and T Cell Evaluation:

Flow Cytometry (Lymphocyte Subsets):

- Total lymphocytes: 1,800/µL (normal)
- **CD19+ B cells: 180/µL (10%) NORMAL OR SLIGHTLY LOW** (normal 5-20%)
- CD3+ T cells: 1,260/µL (70%) - normal
- CD4+ T cells: 680/µL - normal
- CD8+ T cells: 450/µL - normal
- CD4:CD8 ratio: 1.5 - normal
- NK cells: Normal

Key Finding: B cells are PRESENT (distinguishes CVID from X-linked agammaglobulinemia where B cells are absent)

Memory B Cell Analysis:

- **Switched memory B cells (CD27+IgD-): Severely reduced**
- Unswitched memory B cells: Present but reduced
- Indicates impaired B cell differentiation and class switching

Vaccine Response Testing (Specific Antibody Deficiency Assessment):

Pre-Vaccination Titers:

- **Pneumococcal antibodies:** Protective levels to 0/23 serotypes tested (should respond to >50% in normal individuals)
- **Tetanus antibody:** <0.1 IU/mL (non-protective; normal >0.15)

Post-Vaccination (4 weeks after pneumococcal vaccine and tetanus booster):

- **Pneumococcal antibodies:** NO response (protective to 1/23 serotypes only)
- **Tetanus antibody:** 0.08 IU/mL (inadequate response)
- **Impaired vaccine response confirms antibody deficiency**

Additional Diagnostic Testing:

Complement Levels:

- C3, C4: Normal (excludes complement deficiency)

HIV Testing:

- HIV antibody/antigen: Negative (secondary immunodeficiency excluded)

Genetic Testing:

- **Mutation screening:** No mutations in BTK (excludes X-linked agammaglobulinemia)
- No mutations in AID, UNG, CD40, CD40L genes
- **Most CVID cases have no identified genetic mutation** (polygenic/multifactorial)

GI Workup (for chronic diarrhea):

Upper Endoscopy with Biopsy:

- **Nodular lymphoid hyperplasia** in duodenum
- Villous atrophy (resembles celiac disease)
- Increased intraepithelial lymphocytes
- **Giardia lamblia cysts identified**

Stool Studies:

- **Giardia antigen: Positive**
- No other pathogens

Final Diagnosis: Common Variable Immunodeficiency (CVID) with:

1. Recurrent Sinopulmonary Infections
2. Bronchiectasis (chronic lung disease)
3. Giardiasis (opportunistic GI infection)
4. Nodular Lymphoid Hyperplasia

CVID Diagnostic Criteria (All Required):

1. ✓ **Marked decrease in IgG** (>2 SD below mean)
2. ✓ **Marked decrease in IgA and/or IgM**
3. ✓ **Poor/absent antibody response to vaccines**
4. ✓ **Onset after age 2 years** (excludes transient hypogammaglobulinemia of infancy)
5. ✓ **Exclusion of other causes:** HIV, medications, malignancy, X-linked agammaglobulinemia

Comparison of Antibody Deficiencies:

Disorder	IgG	IgA	IgM	B Cells	Age of Onset	Genetics
CVID	Low	Low	Low/Normal	Present	>2 years	Usually unknown
XLA	Very low	Very low	Very low	Absent	<1 year	BTK mutation (X-linked)
Selective IgA def	Normal	Absent	Normal	Present	Variable	Often asymptomatic
IgG subclass def	Normal total, subclass low	Normal	Normal	Present	Variable	Variable

Treatment Initiated:

Immunoglobulin Replacement Therapy (IRT):

- **IVIG (IV immunoglobulin) or SCIG (subcutaneous):** 400-600 mg/kg every 3-4 weeks

- **Target trough IgG level: >500-600 mg/dL** (prevents infections)
- Lifelong therapy required

Antimicrobial Therapy:

- Metronidazole for *Giardia*
- Amoxicillin for current pneumonia
- **Prophylactic antibiotics** may be considered if recurrent infections despite IVIG

Monitoring:

- **Trough IgG levels** before each IVIG infusion (adjust dose to maintain target)
- Monitor for complications: autoimmunity, lymphoma, granulomatous disease
- Regular pulmonary function tests (monitor bronchiectasis)
- Surveillance for malignancy

Complications of CVID:

1. **Infections:** Sinopulmonary (most common), GI (*Giardia*, *Campylobacter*), opportunistic
2. **Autoimmunity:** ITP, AIHA, inflammatory arthritis, vitiligo (20-30%)
3. **Granulomatous disease:** Lung, liver, spleen, lymph nodes (10-20%)
4. **Malignancy:** Lymphoma (5-8% lifetime risk), gastric cancer
5. **Chronic lung disease:** Bronchiectasis, interstitial lung disease
6. **GI disease:** Nodular lymphoid hyperplasia, celiac-like enteropathy, inflammatory bowel disease

Follow-Up (6 Months on IVIG):

- IgG trough level: 680 mg/dL (therapeutic)
- **No new infections** (sinopulmonary infection rate dramatically reduced)
- Weight gain, diarrhea resolved
- Repeat endoscopy: *Giardia* cleared, villous architecture improved

Teaching Points:

1. **CVID Definition:** Hypogammaglobulinemia (low IgG + IgA/IgM) with impaired vaccine response; B cells present but dysfunctional
2. **Age of Onset:** After age 2 (distinguishes from transient hypogammaglobulinemia of infancy and X-linked agammaglobulinemia)
3. **B Cells Present:** Key feature distinguishing CVID from XLA (X-linked agammaglobulinemia where B cells absent due to BTK mutation)
4. **Vaccine Response:** Essential for diagnosis; patients cannot generate protective antibodies to protein or polysaccharide antigens
5. **Bronchiectasis:** Chronic complication of recurrent sinopulmonary infections; prevention with IVIG critical
6. **Encapsulated Bacteria:** *S. pneumoniae*, *H. influenzae* most common pathogens; antibodies are primary defense
7. **GI Manifestations:** *Giardia* infections common; nodular lymphoid hyperplasia characteristic; celiac-like disease

8. **IVIG Therapy:** Prevents infections, improves quality of life; does NOT correct underlying B cell dysfunction
9. **CVID vs Selective IgA Deficiency:** Most common primary immunodeficiency is selective IgA deficiency (1:700); usually asymptomatic; no treatment

Related Cases: X-linked agammaglobulinemia, selective IgA deficiency, IgG subclass deficiency, specific antibody deficiency

---

Case 9.6: Celiac Disease Screening

Clinical Presentation: A 32-year-old woman presents with 8 months of chronic diarrhea (4-6 watery stools daily), abdominal bloating, fatigue, and unintentional 18-pound weight loss. She also reports intermittent mouth sores and an intensely itchy rash on her elbows and knees. Her sister was recently diagnosed with celiac disease. She has been eating a normal diet including bread and pasta.

Physical Examination:

- BMI: 18.5 (underweight)
- Appears pale, fatigued
- **Dermatitis herpetiformis:** Grouped vesicles and excoriations on extensor surfaces of elbows and knees
- Abdominal exam: Distended, diffusely tender, increased bowel sounds
- **Angular cheilitis** (mouth corners)

Initial Laboratory Findings:

- Hemoglobin: 9.8 g/dL (anemia)
- **MCV: 76 fL** (microcytic - iron deficiency)
- Albumin: 3.0 g/dL (low)
- **Ferritin: 8 ng/mL** (very low; normal 12-150)
- **Vitamin D: 12 ng/mL** (deficient; normal >30)
- Calcium: 8.2 mg/dL (low)
- **Elevated transaminases:** AST 68, ALT 72

Diagnostic Reasoning Questions:

1. What are the serologic tests for celiac disease and their sensitivity/specificity?
2. Why must patients continue gluten-containing diet during testing?
3. How is celiac disease confirmed?
4. What are the associated conditions and complications of celiac disease?

Sequential Test Results:

Celiac Serology Panel (Patient on Gluten-Containing Diet):

Tissue Transglutaminase Antibodies (tTG-IgA):

- **tTG-IgA: 156 U/mL STRONGLY POSITIVE** (normal <20 U/mL)
- **Most sensitive and specific test for celiac disease**
- Sensitivity: 95-98%; Specificity: 95-97%

Endomysial Antibodies (EMA-IgA):

- **EMA-IgA: POSITIVE, titer 1:160**
- Highly specific for celiac disease (98-100% specificity)
- More expensive, operator-dependent (immunofluorescence)
- Used as confirmatory test

Deamidated Gliadin Peptide Antibodies (DGP):

- DGP-IgA: Positive
- DGP-IgG: Positive
- Useful in children <2 years and IgA-deficient patients

Total IgA Level:

- **Total IgA: 245 mg/dL NORMAL** (important to measure!)
- If IgA-deficient (1-3% of celiac patients), IgA-based tests falsely negative
- **Must check total IgA** when ordering celiac panel

HLA Typing (Genetic Susceptibility):

- **HLA-DQ2: POSITIVE** (present in 90-95% of celiac patients)
- HLA-DQ8: Negative (present in 5-10%)
- **Negative HLA-DQ2 and DQ8 has 99% negative predictive value** (essentially excludes celiac)
- Positive HLA does NOT diagnose celiac (30-40% of general population has these genes)

Confirmatory Testing:

Upper Endoscopy with Small Bowel Biopsies (Duodenum):

Histopathology (Marsh Classification):

- **Marsh 3b:** Subtotal villous atrophy
- **Increased intraepithelial lymphocytes (IEL):** >25 per 100 enterocytes (normal <25)
- **Crypt hyperplasia:** Elongated crypts
- **Villous atrophy:** Villus:crypt ratio <2:1 (normal >3:1)
- **Confirms celiac disease diagnosis**

Marsh-Oberhuber Classification:

- Marsh 0: Normal
- Marsh 1: Increased IEL (>25)
- Marsh 2: Crypt hyperplasia
- Marsh 3a: Partial villous atrophy

- **Marsh 3b: Subtotal villous atrophy ← PATIENT**
- Marsh 3c: Total villous atrophy

Additional Testing:

Nutritional Deficiencies (Secondary to Malabsorption):

- **Iron deficiency anemia:** Present (microcytic anemia, low ferritin)
- **Vitamin D deficiency:** 12 ng/mL
- **Folate:** 2.8 ng/mL (low; normal >5)
- **Vitamin B12:** 285 pg/mL (low-normal)
- **Bone density (DEXA scan):** Osteopenia (T-score -1.8)

Thyroid Function:

- TSH: 4.8 mIU/L (high-normal)
- Anti-TPO antibodies: Positive
- **Subclinical hypothyroidism/Hashimoto's** (common association)

Final Diagnosis: Celiac Disease (Confirmed by Serology and Biopsy) with:

1. Dermatitis Herpetiformis (skin manifestation of celiac)
2. Iron Deficiency Anemia
3. Vitamin D Deficiency
4. Subclinical Hypothyroidism (Hashimoto's thyroiditis)
5. Elevated Transaminases (celiac hepatitis)

Associated Conditions with Celiac Disease:

- Type 1 diabetes (5-10%)
- **Hashimoto's thyroiditis** (10-15%)
- Selective IgA deficiency (2-3%)
- Down syndrome
- Turner syndrome
- Dermatitis herpetiformis
- First-degree relatives (10-15% risk)

Treatment:

Strict Lifelong Gluten-Free Diet:

- Eliminate wheat, barley, rye
- <20 ppm gluten in food products
- Oats may be tolerated (ensure gluten-free oats)
- Nutritionist consultation

Nutritional Supplementation:

- Iron supplementation
- Vitamin D and calcium (prevent osteoporosis)
- Multivitamin
- Folate

Monitoring:

- **Serial tTG-IgA levels:** Should decline on gluten-free diet (may take 6-12 months to normalize)
- Repeat biopsy in 1-2 years (verify histologic improvement)
- Nutritional labs (iron, vitamin D, calcium)
- Bone density monitoring
- Screen for complications

Follow-Up Testing:

6 Months on Gluten-Free Diet:

- tTG-IgA: 45 U/mL (decreased but still elevated - improving)
- Symptoms: Diarrhea resolved, weight gain 8 lbs
- Hemoglobin: 12.1 g/dL (improved)
- Dermatitis herpetiformis: Resolved

12 Months:

- tTG-IgA: 18 U/mL (normalized)
- Repeat biopsy: Marsh 1 (near-normal histology, residual increased IEL)
- Nutritional deficiencies corrected

Complications of Untreated Celiac Disease:

- Osteoporosis/osteomalacia
- Infertility, miscarriage
- Neurologic complications (ataxia, peripheral neuropathy)
- **Enteropathy-associated T-cell lymphoma (EATL)** - rare but serious
- Non-Hodgkin lymphoma
- Refractory celiac disease (persistent symptoms despite gluten-free diet)
- Small bowel adenocarcinoma

Teaching Points:

1. **tTG-IgA:** Most sensitive and specific single test; first-line screening test; may be falsely negative in IgA deficiency
2. **Total IgA:** Must be checked with celiac panel; 2-3% of celiac patients are IgA-deficient; if deficient, use IgG-based tests (tTG-IgG, DGP-IgG)
3. **Gluten Challenge:** Patients must be on gluten-containing diet during testing (at least 1-2 slices bread daily for ≥6 weeks); gluten-free diet causes false-negative serology and biopsy
4. **HLA-DQ2/DQ8:** Negative result essentially excludes celiac (99% NPV); positive result does NOT confirm (40% of population positive); useful to rule out in uncertain cases

5. **Biopsy Gold Standard:** Required for definitive diagnosis in adults; children with very high tTG-IgA (>10x ULN) and positive EMA may not need biopsy
6. **Dermatitis Herpetiformis:** Pathognomonic skin manifestation of celiac; intensely pruritic grouped vesicles on extensor surfaces; granular IgA deposits in dermal papillae on skin biopsy
7. **Refractory Celiac:** Persistent symptoms despite strict gluten-free diet for >12 months; Type I (polyclonal IEL) has better prognosis; Type II (clonal IEL) at risk for EATL
8. **Screening Indications:** First-degree relatives, type 1 diabetes, unexplained iron deficiency, chronic diarrhea, elevated transaminases

Related Cases: Selective IgA deficiency with celiac, dermatitis herpetiformis, refractory celiac disease, tropical sprue

---

Case 9.7: Chronic Hepatitis B Serology

Clinical Presentation: A 42-year-old man from China presents for routine physical examination. He is asymptomatic. Laboratory screening reveals elevated liver enzymes. He immigrated to the US 10 years ago. No history of jaundice, blood transfusions, or IV drug use. Family history: Mother died of liver cancer at age 58.

Physical Examination:

- Appears well
- No jaundice, spider angiomas, or palmar erythema
- Liver span 12 cm (normal), non-tender
- No splenomegaly or ascites

Initial Laboratory Findings:

- **AST: 68 U/L** (elevated)
- **ALT: 95 U/L** (elevated)
- Alkaline phosphatase: 88 U/L (normal)
- Total bilirubin: 0.9 mg/dL (normal)
- Albumin: 4.2 g/dL (normal)
- Platelets: 185,000/μL (normal)
- PT-INR: 1.1 (normal)

Diagnostic Reasoning Questions:

1. How do you interpret hepatitis B serologic markers?
2. What is the difference between acute, chronic, and resolved hepatitis B?
3. How do you assess hepatitis B replication and infectivity?
4. When is antiviral treatment indicated?

Sequential Test Results:

Hepatitis B Serology Panel:

Hepatitis B Surface Antigen (HBsAg):

- **HBsAg: POSITIVE**
- Indicates current hepatitis B infection (acute or chronic)
- If positive >6 months = chronic hepatitis B

Hepatitis B Surface Antibody (anti-HBs):

- **Anti-HBs: NEGATIVE**
- Would be positive in: resolved infection OR post-vaccination
- **Cannot have both HBsAg and anti-HBs positive** (mutually exclusive)

Hepatitis B Core Antibody (anti-HBc):

- **Anti-HBc total (IgG + IgM): POSITIVE**
- **Anti-HBc IgM: NEGATIVE**
- Total anti-HBc positive = past or current infection
- IgM anti-HBc positive = acute infection (<6 months)
- IgM negative = chronic or resolved infection

Hepatitis B e Antigen (HBeAg):

- **HBeAg: POSITIVE**
- Indicates active viral replication
- High infectivity
- Marker of immune-tolerant or immune-active phase

Hepatitis B e Antibody (anti-HBe):

- **Anti-HBe: NEGATIVE**
- Would be positive in: inactive carrier OR HBeAg-negative chronic hepatitis
- Seroconversion from HBeAg to anti-HBe indicates decreased replication

Interpretation of Initial Serology: Chronic Hepatitis B Infection, HBeAg-Positive (Immune-Active Phase)

Hepatitis B Serologic Patterns:

Pattern	HBsAg	Anti-HBs	Anti-HBc IgM	Anti-HBc total	HBeAg	Anti-HBe	Interpretation
Acute HBV	+	-	+	+	+/-	-	Acute infection
Chronic HBV	+	-	-	+	+	-	**Chronic, replicating ← PATIENT**
Chronic, inactive	+	-	-	+	-	+	Low replication
Resolved HBV	-	+	-	+	-	+/-	Past infection, immune

357

Pattern	HBsAg	Anti-HBs	Anti-HBc IgM	Anti-HBc total	HBeAg	Anti-HBe	Interpretation
Vaccinated	-	+	-	-	-	-	Immune from vaccine
Window period	-	-	+	+	-	-	Acute infection window

Viral Load and Activity Assessment:

Hepatitis B DNA (Quantitative PCR):

- **HBV DNA: 8.5 x 10^7 IU/mL (7.93 log10) VERY HIGH**
- Indicates active viral replication
- High infectivity
- Levels:
  - Low: <2,000 IU/mL
  - Moderate: 2,000-20,000 IU/mL
  - High: >20,000 IU/mL
  - Very high: >2 million IU/mL

Hepatitis B Genotype:

- **Genotype B** (common in Asia)
- Relevant for treatment decisions and prognosis

Additional Testing:

Hepatitis D (Delta) Serology:

- Anti-HDV: Negative (excludes hepatitis D co-infection)
- HDV is defective virus requiring HBV for replication

Hepatitis C Serology:

- Anti-HCV: Negative (excludes co-infection)

HIV Testing:

- HIV antibody: Negative

Liver Fibrosis Assessment:

FibroScan (Transient Elastography):

- **Liver stiffness: 9.2 kPa**
- Interpretation: F2 fibrosis (moderate) on METAVIR scale
- F0-F1: <7 kPa; F2: 7-9.5 kPa; F3: 9.5-12.5 kPa; F4 (cirrhosis): >12.5 kPa

Non-Invasive Fibrosis Markers:

- FIB-4 score: 1.8 (suggests moderate fibrosis)
- APRI score: 0.9 (moderate)

Hepatocellular Carcinoma (HCC) Screening:

- **Alpha-fetoprotein (AFP): 12 ng/mL** (normal <20)
- **Liver ultrasound:** No focal lesions, normal liver echotexture

Final Diagnosis: Chronic Hepatitis B Infection, HBeAg-Positive, Immune-Active Phase with Moderate Fibrosis (F2)

Phases of Chronic Hepatitis B:

1. **Immune-Tolerant:** High HBV DNA, normal ALT, minimal liver damage (common in perinatally infected)
2. **Immune-Active (HBeAg-positive):** High HBV DNA, elevated ALT, active liver damage ← **PATIENT HERE**
3. **Inactive Carrier:** Low/undetectable HBV DNA, normal ALT, HBeAg-negative, anti-HBe-positive
4. **Reactivation (HBeAg-negative chronic hepatitis):** Moderate HBV DNA, elevated ALT, HBeAg-negative
5. **Resolved/Occult:** HBsAg-negative, anti-HBc/anti-HBs-positive

Treatment Indications Met:

1. ✓ HBV DNA >20,000 IU/mL
2. ✓ Elevated ALT
3. ✓ Evidence of fibrosis (F2)

Treatment Initiated:

- **Entecavir 0.5 mg daily** (nucleoside analog, potent HBV suppression)
- Alternative: Tenofovir disoproxil fumarate (TDF) or tenofovir alafenamide (TAF)
- Goal: HBV DNA suppression to undetectable, ALT normalization, prevent progression to cirrhosis/HCC

Monitoring on Treatment:

- HBV DNA every 3-6 months (goal: undetectable)
- ALT every 3-6 months
- HBeAg/anti-HBe annually (assess seroconversion)
- AFP and ultrasound every 6 months (HCC surveillance)
- FibroScan annually

Follow-Up (12 Months on Entecavir):

- HBV DNA: Undetectable (<20 IU/mL) - excellent response
- ALT: 32 U/L (normalized)
- HBeAg: Still positive (seroconversion may take years)
- AFP: 8 ng/mL
- Ultrasound: No lesions

Teaching Points:

1. **HBsAg:** Hallmark of current infection; positive >6 months = chronic; indicates infectious
2. **Anti-HBs:** Indicates immunity (resolved infection OR vaccination); mutually exclusive with HBsAg
3. **Anti-HBc Total:** Indicates past or current infection; remains positive for life; present in resolved, chronic, and occult HBV
4. **Anti-HBc IgM:** Acute infection (<6 months); may be present in flares of chronic HBV
5. **HBeAg/Anti-HBe:** HBeAg indicates active replication and high infectivity; seroconversion to anti-HBe indicates lower replication (but HBeAg-negative chronic hepatitis can still have high viral load)
6. **Window Period:** HBsAg negative, anti-HBs not yet positive; only anti-HBc IgM positive; occurs between clearance of HBsAg and appearance of anti-HBs in acute infection
7. **Isolated Anti-HBc:** HBsAg negative, anti-HBs negative, anti-HBc positive; may indicate: resolved infection with waning anti-HBs, occult HBV, or false positive
8. **Treatment Indications:** HBV DNA >2000-20,000 IU/mL (depending on HBeAg status) + elevated ALT + evidence of liver disease OR cirrhosis regardless of ALT/HBV DNA
9. **HCC Risk:** Increased in chronic HBV, especially with cirrhosis, family history, Asian males >40, African descent >20; requires surveillance (AFP + ultrasound q6mo)

Related Cases: Acute hepatitis B, occult hepatitis B, hepatitis B/D co-infection, hepatitis B reactivation

Chapter 10: Point-of-Care and Critical Care Testing

Case 10.1: Arterial Blood Gas Interpretation in Respiratory Failure

Clinical Presentation: A 68-year-old man with COPD (FEV1 45% predicted) presents to ED with 3 days of worsening dyspnea, productive cough with yellow sputum, and fever. He appears in moderate respiratory distress, using accessory muscles. He ran out of his inhalers 1 week ago. Smoking history: 45 pack-years, quit 2 years ago.

Physical Examination:

- BP 148/88, HR 112, **RR 32** (tachypneic), Temp 101.4°F, **SpO2 86% on room air**
- Appears dyspneic, diaphoretic
- **Pursed-lip breathing, using accessory muscles**
- Lungs: Decreased breath sounds bilaterally, diffuse wheezes, prolonged expiration
- No cyanosis initially

Diagnostic Reasoning Questions:

1. How do you interpret arterial blood gas results systematically?
2. What is the difference between acute and chronic respiratory acidosis?
3. How do you calculate A-a gradient and what does it indicate?
4. When is non-invasive vs. invasive ventilation indicated?

Sequential Test Results:

Arterial Blood Gas (ABG) - Room Air:

Initial ABG:

- **pH: 7.28 ACIDEMIC** (normal 7.35-7.45)
- **PaCO2: 68 mmHg ELEVATED** (normal 35-45)
- **PaO2: 52 mmHg SEVERELY LOW** (normal 80-100)
- **HCO3-: 31 mEq/L ELEVATED** (normal 22-26)
- **SaO2: 84%** (saturation correlates with PaO2)
- Lactate: 1.8 mmol/L (mildly elevated)

Systematic ABG Interpretation:

Step 1: Assess pH

- pH 7.28 = **ACIDEMIA**

Step 2: Determine Primary Disorder

- PaCO2 68 mmHg (elevated) → **RESPIRATORY ACIDOSIS**
- HCO3- 31 mEq/L (elevated) → metabolic alkalosis or compensation

Step 3: Assess Compensation

- Expected HCO3- for acute respiratory acidosis: HCO3- increases 1 mEq/L for every 10 mmHg rise in PaCO2
  - PaCO2 rose from 40 to 68 = 28 mmHg increase
  - Expected HCO3- = 24 + (28/10) = 24 + 2.8 ≈ 27 mEq/L
- Actual HCO3- = 31 mEq/L (HIGHER than expected for acute)
- Expected HCO3- for chronic respiratory acidosis: HCO3- increases 4 mEq/L for every 10 mmHg rise in PaCO2
  - Expected HCO3- = 24 + (28/10 x 4) = 24 + 11.2 ≈ 35 mEq/L
- Actual HCO3- = 31 mEq/L (close to expected)

Interpretation: CHRONIC RESPIRATORY ACIDOSIS WITH ACUTE EXACERBATION

- Patient has baseline elevated CO2 (COPD) with partial renal compensation (elevated HCO3-)
- Current acute illness causing further CO2 retention

Step 4: Assess Oxygenation

- **PaO2 52 mmHg = SEVERE HYPOXEMIA** (respiratory failure)
- **A-a Gradient Calculation:**
  - PAO2 (alveolar) = (FiO2 x [Patm - PH2O]) - (PaCO2/0.8)
  - PAO2 = (0.21 x [760 - 47]) - (68/0.8)
  - PAO2 = 150 - 85 = 65 mmHg
  - **A-a gradient = PAO2 - PaO2 = 65 - 52 = 13 mmHg**
  - Normal A-a gradient = 10-15 mmHg (age-adjusted: [Age/4] + 4)
  - **NORMAL A-a gradient** → hypoxemia due to **HYPOVENTILATION** (elevated CO2 displacing O2)

Final ABG Interpretation: Acute-on-Chronic Respiratory Acidosis with Severe Hypoxemic Respiratory Failure (Type II Respiratory Failure) due to COPD Exacerbation

Chest X-Ray:

- Hyperinflation, flattened diaphragms (chronic COPD changes)
- Right lower lobe infiltrate (pneumonia trigger)

Additional Labs:

- WBC: 16,500/µL (elevated)
- Procalcitonin: 1.8 ng/mL (suggests bacterial infection)
- BNP: 185 pg/mL (mildly elevated, ? right heart strain)

Treatment Initiated:

Immediate Interventions:

- **Controlled oxygen therapy:** Nasal cannula 2 L/min → SpO2 target 88-92% (avoid hyperoxia in COPD)
- **Bronchodilators:** Albuterol and ipratropium nebulizers
- **Corticosteroids:** Methylprednisolone 125 mg IV
- **Antibiotics:** Ceftriaxone + azithromycin (community-acquired pneumonia)
- **Non-invasive positive pressure ventilation (NIPPV/BiPAP) initiated**

ABG on BiPAP (2 Hours Later):

- pH: 7.34 (improved)
- PaCO2: 58 mmHg (improved)
- PaO2: 68 mmHg (improved)
- HCO3-: 31 mEq/L
- FiO2: 0.30

Interpretation: Improving acute-on-chronic respiratory acidosis; still hypoxemic but better

ABG 24 Hours Later (Still on BiPAP):

- pH: 7.38 (normalized)
- PaCO2: 52 mmHg (closer to baseline for this patient)
- PaO2: 72 mmHg (improved)
- HCO3-: 30 mEq/L
- SpO2: 92%

Patient gradually weaned from BiPAP over 48 hours; transitioned to nasal cannula 2 L/min

Final Diagnosis:

1. Acute Exacerbation of COPD with Acute-on-Chronic Hypercapnic Respiratory Failure (Type II)
2. Community-Acquired Pneumonia (trigger)
3. Baseline Chronic Respiratory Acidosis with Metabolic Compensation

ABG Patterns:

Disorder	pH	PaCO2	HCO3-	Common Causes
Resp Acidosis (Acute)	↓	↑	**Normal/↑1-2**	**Hypoventilation, COPD, drugs**
Resp Acidosis (Chronic)	Normal/↓	↑	↑↑ (compensated)	COPD, neuromuscular
Resp Alkalosis	↑	↓	↓	Hyperventilation, anxiety, PE
Metabolic Acidosis	↓	↓ (comp)	↓	DKA, lactic acidosis, renal failure
Metabolic Alkalosis	↑	↑ (comp)	↑	Vomiting, diuretics, Cushing's

Teaching Points:

1. **Type I vs II Respiratory Failure:** Type I = hypoxemic (PaO2 <60) with normal/low CO2 (pneumonia, ARDS); Type II = hypercapnic (PaCO2 >50) with hypoxemia (COPD, neuromuscular)
2. **A-a Gradient:** Normal (10-15) suggests hypoventilation or low FiO2; elevated (>15) suggests V/Q mismatch, shunt, or diffusion impairment
3. **Compensation:** Acute respiratory acidosis → minimal HCO3- rise (1 mEq/L per 10 mmHg CO2); Chronic → significant rise (4 mEq/L per 10 mmHg)
4. **COPD Oxygen Goals:** Target SpO2 88-92% (not 95-100%); high oxygen can worsen hypercapnia (Haldane effect, V/Q mismatch)
5. **BiPAP Indications:** Acute hypercapnic respiratory failure; pH 7.25-7.35; alert, cooperative patient; reduces intubation rate by 50%
6. **Intubation Indications:** pH <7.25 despite BiPAP; worsening mental status; inability to protect airway; hemodynamic instability; BiPAP failure
7. **Winter's Formula:** Expected PaCO2 in metabolic acidosis = (1.5 x HCO3-) + 8 ± 2; helps identify mixed disorders
8. **Base Excess:** Metabolic component; negative = metabolic acidosis; positive = metabolic alkalosis

Related Cases: ARDS with hypoxemic respiratory failure, metabolic acidosis in DKA, mixed acid-base disorder, permissive hypercapnia

---

Case 10.2: Lactate Elevation in Septic Shock

Clinical Presentation: A 72-year-old woman with history of diabetes and recurrent UTIs presents to ED with 1 day of fever, chills, confusion, and decreased urine output. Family reports she has been lethargic and "not herself" for 2 days. She had dysuria 3 days ago but didn't seek care.

Physical Examination:

- **BP 78/45** (hypotensive), **HR 128** (tachycardic), RR 28, **Temp 102.8°F**, SpO2 94% on room air
- **Altered mental status, confused to time and place**
- Skin: **Warm, flushed** (early septic shock - vasodilatory)
- **Delayed capillary refill >4 seconds**
- Lungs: Clear
- Abdomen: Mild suprapubic tenderness, no peritoneal signs
- **Urine output: 15 mL in past 4 hours** (oliguria)

SIRS Criteria (≥2 = SIRS):

1. √ Temp >38°C (102.8°F)
2. √ HR >90 (128)
3. √ RR >20 (28)
4. WBC >12,000 or <4,000 or >10% bands

Diagnostic Reasoning Questions:

1. What is the significance of lactate in sepsis and septic shock?
2. What are the mechanisms of lactate elevation?

3. How does lactate guide resuscitation and prognosis?
4. What is the role of point-of-care testing in critical illness?

Sequential Test Results:

Point-of-Care Testing (Immediate Results):

Lactate (Venous Blood Gas with Co-Oximetry):

- **Initial lactate: 6.8 mmol/L MARKEDLY ELEVATED** (normal <2.0 mmol/L)
- **Sepsis definition:** Infection + lactate >2 mmol/L indicates organ dysfunction
- **Septic shock definition:** Sepsis + hypotension requiring vasopressors + lactate >2 mmol/L

Blood Glucose (Point-of-Care):

- **Glucose: 245 mg/dL** (hyperglycemia - stress response in diabetic)

Initial Labs (Rapid Turnaround):

- **WBC: 22,400/µL** with 18% bands (leukocytosis with left shift)
- Hemoglobin: 11.2 g/dL
- Platelets: 95,000/µL (thrombocytopenia - early DIC)
- **Creatinine: 2.8 mg/dL** (elevated from baseline 1.1 - acute kidney injury)
- **BUN: 52 mg/dL**
- Potassium: 5.2 mEq/L (hyperkalemia)
- Bicarbonate: 16 mEq/L (metabolic acidosis)

Arterial Blood Gas:

- pH: 7.28 (acidemic)
- $PaCO_2$: 28 mmHg (respiratory compensation)
- PaO_2: 88 mmHg
- **HCO_3^-: 13 mEq/L** (metabolic acidosis)
- **Lactate: 7.2 mmol/L** (confirms elevation)
- Base excess: -12

Interpretation: Lactic Acidosis with Appropriate Respiratory Compensation

Anion Gap Calculation:

- **Anion Gap = Na - (Cl + HCO_3^-)**
- AG = 138 - (102 + 13) = **23** (elevated; normal 10-12)
- **High anion gap metabolic acidosis** (MUDPILES: Methanol, Uremia, DKA, Propylene glycol/Paraldehyde, Iron/Isoniazid, Lactic acidosis, Ethylene glycol, Salicylates)

Urinalysis (Point-of-Care Dipstick):

- **Leukocyte esterase: 3+ (positive)**

- **Nitrites: Positive**
- **WBCs: >100/hpf**
- **Bacteria: Many**
- Confirms urinary tract infection (source of sepsis)

Mechanism of Lactate Elevation:

Type A Lactic Acidosis (Tissue Hypoperfusion/Hypoxia): ← PATIENT

- Septic shock with hypotension
- Inadequate oxygen delivery to tissues
- Anaerobic metabolism → lactate production
- Decreased lactate clearance (liver, kidneys)

Type B Lactic Acidosis (Not from Hypoxia):

- Medications (metformin, linezolid, propofol)
- Malignancy
- Liver failure
- Thiamine deficiency

Septic Shock Diagnosis Confirmed:

1. √ Infection (UTI)
2. √ Hypotension (MAP <65 mmHg)
3. √ Lactate >2 mmol/L (6.8 mmol/L)
4. √ Requiring vasopressors to maintain MAP ≥65

Surviving Sepsis Campaign Bundle Initiated (Within 1 Hour):

Hour 0 (ED Arrival):

- **Measure lactate:** 6.8 mmol/L √
- **Obtain blood cultures before antibiotics** √
- **Administer broad-spectrum antibiotics:** Piperacillin-tazobactam + vancomycin IV √
- **Fluid resuscitation:** 30 mL/kg crystalloid (2 liters) over 30 minutes √
- Vasopressors if hypotensive after fluids √

Hour 1:

- **Repeat lactate:** 5.2 mmol/L (decreased but still elevated - continue resuscitation)
- BP: 88/52 (still hypotensive despite 2 L fluids)
- **Norepinephrine infusion started** (vasopressor)
- Central line placed
- Foley catheter for strict urine output monitoring

Hour 3:

- **Lactate: 3.8 mmol/L** (continued improvement)
- BP: 102/68 on norepinephrine 8 mcg/min
- Urine output: 40 mL/hr (improving)
- Mental status: More alert

Hour 6:

- **Lactate: 2.1 mmol/L** (near-normal)
- **Lactate clearance >50% from initial** (good prognostic sign)
- BP: 112/72 (stable, weaning norepinephrine)
- Transferred to ICU

Blood Culture Results (24 Hours):

- **2/2 bottles positive:** *Escherichia coli*
- Susceptibility: Sensitive to piperacillin-tazobactam, ceftriaxone; resistant to ampicillin

Lactate Clearance Calculation:

- **Lactate clearance = [(Initial lactate - Repeat lactate) / Initial lactate] x 100%**
- Clearance at 6h = [(6.8 - 2.1) / 6.8] x 100% = **69% clearance**
- **Lactate clearance >10% at 6 hours associated with improved survival**

Day 2:

- Lactate: 1.4 mmol/L (normalized)
- Norepinephrine weaned off
- Creatinine: 1.8 mg/dL (improving)
- Mental status: Baseline

Day 5:

- Discharged from ICU
- Antibiotics narrowed to ceftriaxone based on sensitivities
- Completed 10-day course

Final Diagnosis:

1. Septic Shock secondary to *E. coli* Urosepsis
2. Type A Lactic Acidosis (Tissue Hypoperfusion)
3. Acute Kidney Injury (Sepsis-Induced)
4. Sepsis-Associated Encephalopathy

Lactate Levels and Prognosis:

Lactate Level	Interpretation	Mortality Risk
<2.0 mmol/L	Normal	Baseline

Lactate Level	Interpretation	Mortality Risk
2.0-4.0 mmol/L	Elevated, tissue hypoperfusion	10-15%
4.0-8.0 mmol/L	**Severe**	**20-30% ← PATIENT**
>8.0 mmol/L	Critical	>50%

Teaching Points:

1. **Lactate as Biomarker:** Elevated lactate (>2 mmol/L) in sepsis indicates tissue hypoperfusion and organ dysfunction; correlates with mortality
2. **Lactate Clearance:** Serial measurements guide resuscitation; >10-20% clearance in first 6 hours associated with improved survival
3. **Point-of-Care Lactate:** Rapid turnaround (minutes) enables early recognition and treatment; venous lactate acceptable (correlates with arterial)
4. **Sepsis-3 Definitions:** Sepsis = infection + SOFA score ≥2; Septic shock = sepsis + vasopressors to maintain MAP ≥65 + lactate >2 mmol/L despite adequate fluid resuscitation
5. **Surviving Sepsis Bundle:** Within 1 hour: measure lactate, obtain cultures, give antibiotics, administer 30 mL/kg crystalloid; reassess if lactate >2 or hypotension persists
6. **Fluid Resuscitation:** Initial 30 mL/kg crystalloid bolus; reassess after fluids; avoid fluid overload (monitor for pulmonary edema)
7. **Vasopressor Choice:** Norepinephrine first-line; vasopressin or epinephrine second-line; dopamine not recommended
8. **Type A vs B Lactic Acidosis:** Type A from tissue hypoxia (sepsis, shock, severe anemia); Type B from impaired lactate clearance or increased production without hypoxia
9. **Anion Gap:** Lactic acidosis causes high anion gap metabolic acidosis; lactate donates

Teaching Points (continued): 9. **Anion Gap:** Lactic acidosis causes high anion gap metabolic acidosis; lactate donates H+ ions; evaluate with MUDPILES mnemonic 10. **qSOFA Score:** Quick sepsis screening (≥2 of: altered mental status, SBP ≤100, RR ≥22); identifies high-risk patients outside ICU

Related Cases: Cardiogenic shock with elevated lactate, lactic acidosis from metformin, DKA with lactic acidosis, mesenteric ischemia

---

Case 10.3: Cardiac Troponin in Acute Coronary Syndrome

Clinical Presentation: A 58-year-old man with history of hypertension, hyperlipidemia, and smoking presents to ED with 2 hours of severe substernal chest pressure radiating to left arm and jaw. Pain began while shoveling snow. Associated with diaphoresis, nausea, and dyspnea. Denies prior episodes. Takes aspirin, atorvastatin, and lisinopril.

Physical Examination:

- BP 168/95, HR 98, RR 20, SpO2 96% on room air
- Diaphoretic, anxious, in moderate distress
- Cardiac: Regular rhythm, S4 gallop present, no murmurs

- Lungs: Clear bilaterally
- No peripheral edema

Initial ECG (10 Minutes After Arrival):

- **ST-segment elevation 3-4 mm in leads II, III, aVF (Inferior STEMI)**
- Reciprocal ST depression in leads I, aVL
- No prior ECG for comparison

Diagnostic Reasoning Questions:

1. What is the difference between troponin I and troponin T?
2. How are troponin levels interpreted in ACS?
3. What is the role of high-sensitivity troponin?
4. When should serial troponins be obtained?

Sequential Test Results:

Point-of-Care Troponin I (Bedside, Results in 15 Minutes):

- **Time 0 (ED arrival, 2h after symptom onset):**
  - **Troponin I: 0.18 ng/mL** (Elevated; 99th percentile URL = 0.04 ng/mL)
  - Above upper reference limit confirms myocardial injury

Laboratory Troponin I (Central Lab, High-Sensitivity Assay):

- **Time 0 (same sample):**
  - **hs-Troponin I: 285 ng/L** (Markedly elevated; 99th percentile = 26 ng/L for males)

Universal Definition of Myocardial Infarction (4th Definition):

1. √ **Rise and/or fall of troponin** with at least one value above 99th percentile
2. √ **Plus ≥1 of:**
   - Symptoms of myocardial ischemia √
   - New ischemic ECG changes √
   - Development of pathological Q waves
   - Imaging evidence of new loss of viable myocardium
   - Intracoronary thrombus on angiography

Type 1 MI (Spontaneous): Atherosclerotic plaque rupture, ulceration, fissuring, erosion, dissection → thrombus ← **PATIENT**

Additional Labs:

- **CK-MB: 48 ng/mL** (elevated; normal <5)
- CK-MB ratio: (CK-MB/total CK) x 100 = 8% (>5% suggests cardiac origin)
- Total CK: 600 U/L (elevated)
- Myoglobin: 285 ng/mL (elevated - early marker)

369

- BNP: 145 pg/mL (mildly elevated)

Treatment Initiated (STEMI Protocol):

Immediate (Within 10 Minutes of STEMI Diagnosis):

- **Aspirin 325 mg chewed** ✓
- **Clopidogrel 600 mg loading dose** (or ticagrelor 180 mg)
- **Heparin bolus + infusion**
- **Nitroglycerin sublingual** (3 doses)
- Morphine 4 mg IV for pain
- **Activate cardiac catheterization lab** (door-to-balloon goal <90 minutes)

Serial Troponin Monitoring:

3 Hours After Symptom Onset (1h after ED arrival):

- **hs-Troponin I: 2,450 ng/L** (**Rising rapidly** - confirms acute MI)

6 Hours After Symptom Onset:

- **hs-Troponin I: 8,200 ng/L** (Peak elevation)

Coronary Angiography (Performed 65 Minutes After ED Arrival):

- **100% occlusion of proximal right coronary artery (RCA)** with thrombus
- Successful PCI with drug-eluting stent placement
- TIMI 3 flow restored
- LAD: 40% stenosis (non-obstructive)
- LCx: 30% stenosis (non-obstructive)

Post-PCI Troponin:

12 Hours After Symptom Onset (Post-PCI):

- **hs-Troponin I: 12,500 ng/L** (Continued rise despite reperfusion - common in first 12-24h)

24 Hours:

- **hs-Troponin I: 9,800 ng/L** (Beginning to decline)

48 Hours:

- **hs-Troponin I: 4,200 ng/L** (Declining)

72 Hours:

- **hs-Troponin I: 1,850 ng/L** (Continued decline)

370

Day 5:

- **hs-Troponin I: 485 ng/L** (Near baseline, still elevated due to recent MI)

Troponin Kinetics:

- **Rise:** Detectable 2-4 hours after symptom onset
- **Peak:** 12-24 hours (earlier with reperfusion)
- **Return to baseline:** 5-14 days (troponin I); 7-14 days (troponin T)

Echocardiography (Day 2):

- **LVEF: 45%** (mild-moderate systolic dysfunction)
- **Inferior wall hypokinesis** (corresponds to RCA territory)
- No valvular abnormalities
- No pericardial effusion

Final Diagnosis:

1. **ST-Elevation Myocardial Infarction (STEMI) - Inferior Wall**
2. **Type 1 MI** (Spontaneous plaque rupture with thrombosis)
3. 100% RCA Occlusion (Successfully Revascularized)
4. Mild LV Systolic Dysfunction

Troponin Interpretation Scenarios:

Clinical Scenario	Troponin Pattern	Diagnosis
ACS (Type 1 MI)	**Rise & fall, >99th percentile**	**Acute MI ← PATIENT**
Type 2 MI	Rise & fall, demand ischemia	Supply-demand mismatch
Unstable angina	Normal or minimally elevated	ACS without MI
Myocarditis	Elevated, may fluctuate	Inflammatory
Chronic elevation	Stable elevation	CKD, CHF, chronic
Pulmonary embolism	Mild elevation	RV strain

High-Sensitivity Troponin (hs-Tn) Advantages:

1. **Earlier detection:** Positive 1-3 hours after symptom onset (vs 4-6 hours conventional)
2. **Improved sensitivity:** Detects smaller MIs
3. **Rule-out protocols:** 0h/1h or 0h/3h algorithms for rapid MI exclusion
4. **Risk stratification:** Predicts adverse outcomes even below 99th percentile

0-Hour/1-Hour hs-Troponin Algorithm (ESC):

Rule-OUT (Low Risk):

- hs-Tn at 0h <5 ng/L (very low) AND

371

- Δ change <5 ng/L at 1h
- NPV >99%; safe for discharge

Rule-IN (High Risk):

- hs-Tn at 0h ≥52 ng/L OR
- Δ change ≥5 ng/L at 1h (if baseline ≥52)
- Proceed to angiography

Discharge Medications:

- Dual antiplatelet therapy (aspirin + P2Y12 inhibitor) for 12 months
- High-intensity statin (atorvastatin 80 mg)
- Beta-blocker (metoprolol)
- ACE inhibitor (lisinopril)
- Cardiac rehabilitation referral

Teaching Points:

1. **Troponin Specificity:** Cardiac-specific; troponin I and T are regulatory proteins in cardiac muscle; released with myocyte necrosis
2. **99th Percentile URL:** Diagnostic threshold; values above indicate myocardial injury (not necessarily infarction without clinical context)
3. **Rise and Fall Pattern:** Essential for diagnosing acute MI; >20% change between serial measurements suggests acute event vs chronic elevation
4. **Type 1 vs Type 2 MI:** Type 1 = primary coronary event (plaque rupture); Type 2 = supply-demand mismatch (tachycardia, hypotension, anemia, vasospasm)
5. **Troponin Elevation Without ACS:** CKD (most common), CHF, myocarditis, PE, sepsis, stroke, cardiac trauma, post-cardioversion
6. **CK-MB Obsolete:** Troponin more sensitive and specific; CK-MB may help detect reinfarction (normalizes faster)
7. **Serial Testing:** Required for diagnosis; initial troponin may be normal if presenting early (<2-4h); repeat at 3-6 hours
8. **High-Sensitivity Assays:** Detect troponin at 10-100x lower concentrations; enable earlier diagnosis and rapid rule-out protocols
9. **Chronic Troponin Elevation:** Seen in CKD, CHF; stable levels without dynamic changes argue against acute MI
10. **Door-to-Balloon Time:** STEMI goal <90 minutes; immediate cath lab activation; every 30-minute delay increases mortality

Related Cases: Non-STEMI (NSTEMI), unstable angina, type 2 MI from sepsis, troponin elevation in pulmonary embolism, myocarditis

Case 10.4: Glucose Management in ICU - Critical Illness Hyperglycemia

Clinical Presentation: A 45-year-old man with no history of diabetes is admitted to surgical ICU following emergent exploratory laparotomy for perforated diverticulitis with fecal peritonitis. Surgery was complicated by significant blood loss requiring transfusion. Post-operatively, he is intubated, sedated, and hemodynamically unstable on norepinephrine.

Physical Examination (Post-Op Day 1):

- BP 98/62 on norepinephrine 12 mcg/min
- HR 118, Temp 101.8°F
- Intubated, sedated (propofol, fentanyl)
- Abdomen: Surgical wound, drains in place

Initial Laboratory Findings:

- WBC: 18,500/μL
- Lactate: 3.2 mmol/L (elevated)
- Creatinine: 1.8 mg/dL (AKI)

Diagnostic Reasoning Questions:

1. What causes stress hyperglycemia in critical illness?
2. What are the target glucose ranges in different ICU populations?
3. How is insulin therapy managed in the ICU?
4. What are the risks of tight glycemic control?

Sequential Test Results:

Point-of-Care Glucose Monitoring:

Post-Op Hour 6:

- **Glucose: 285 mg/dL** (marked hyperglycemia)
- Patient NPO, on TPN (total parenteral nutrition)
- No personal or family history of diabetes

Diagnosis: Stress-Induced Hyperglycemia (Critical Illness Hyperglycemia)

Mechanisms of Stress Hyperglycemia:

1. **Increased counter-regulatory hormones:** Cortisol, catecholamines, glucagon, growth hormone
2. **Insulin resistance:** Inflammatory cytokines (TNF-α, IL-6)
3. **Increased hepatic glucose production:** Gluconeogenesis
4. **Decreased peripheral glucose uptake**
5. **Iatrogenic:** Vasopressors, corticosteroids, TPN/enteral feeding

ICU Glycemic Control Protocol Initiated:

Target Range for General ICU Patients: 140-180 mg/dL

- Less stringent than prior recommendations (tight control 80-110 mg/dL associated with increased hypoglycemia and mortality)

Insulin Infusion Protocol Started:

- Regular insulin IV infusion
- Initial rate: 2 units/hour
- **Glucose monitoring: q1h until stable, then q2h**

Serial Glucose Measurements:

Hour 0 (Baseline):

- **Glucose: 285 mg/dL**
- Insulin infusion: 2 units/hr started

Hour 1:

- **Glucose: 262 mg/dL** (decreasing)
- Insulin infusion: Increased to 3 units/hr

Hour 2:

- **Glucose: 228 mg/dL**
- Insulin infusion: 4 units/hr

Hour 4:

- **Glucose: 175 mg/dL** (within target range)
- Insulin infusion: Maintained at 4 units/hr

Hour 6:

- **Glucose: 156 mg/dL** (stable)
- Insulin infusion: 4 units/hr
- **Monitoring interval: Extended to q2h** (stable glucose)

Hour 10:

- **Glucose: 68 mg/dL HYPOGLYCEMIA!** (Critical value)
- **IMMEDIATE INTERVENTION:**
  - Insulin infusion STOPPED
  - **D50W 25 mL (12.5g dextrose) IV push**
  - Repeat glucose in 15 minutes

Hour 10 + 15 minutes:

- **Glucose: 92 mg/dL** (corrected)

374

- Insulin infusion: Restarted at 2 units/hr (50% of previous rate)

Hour 12:

- Glucose: 148 mg/dL (stable)
- Insulin: 2 units/hr

Post-Op Day 2:

- Patient more stable, weaning vasopressors
- TPN rate reduced (starting enteral feeds)
- Glucose: 140-165 mg/dL range (well-controlled)
- Insulin: 1.5-2.5 units/hr

Post-Op Day 3:

- Extubated, alert
- Transitioned to **subcutaneous insulin regimen:**
  - **Basal insulin:** Glargine 10 units daily
  - **Nutritional insulin:** Regular insulin with enteral feeds
  - **Correction insulin:** Sliding scale for glucose >180 mg/dL

Post-Op Day 5:

- Tolerating oral diet
- Glucose: 110-140 mg/dL (excellent control)
- Insulin requirements decreasing as acute illness resolves

Post-Op Day 7:

- Glucose: 95-115 mg/dL on minimal insulin
- Insulin discontinued
- **HbA1c: 5.2%** (confirms no underlying diabetes)

Discharge (Day 10):

- No insulin needed
- Glucose normalized (90-110 mg/dL)
- Endocrinology follow-up in 3 months (recheck HbA1c)

Final Diagnosis:

1. Stress-Induced Hyperglycemia (Critical Illness Hyperglycemia)
2. Status Post Perforated Diverticulitis with Peritonitis
3. Iatrogenic Hypoglycemia (ICU-acquired)

Glycemic Targets in Different ICU Settings:

Population	Target Range	Rationale
General ICU	**140-180 mg/dL**	**Balanced safety/efficacy**
Cardiac surgery ICU	140-180 mg/dL	Prior tight control harmful
Diabetic patients	140-180 mg/dL	Same as non-diabetic
Neurocritical care	140-180 mg/dL	Avoid hypoglycemia (brain injury)
Burn ICU	130-150 mg/dL	May tolerate tighter control

Insulin Infusion Management:

Starting Rate Calculation:

- Weight-based: 0.02-0.05 units/kg/hr
- Glucose-based:
    - 150-200 mg/dL: 1-2 units/hr
    - 200-300 mg/dL: 2-4 units/hr
        - 300 mg/dL: 4-6 units/hr

Rate Adjustments:

- **If glucose falling rapidly (>100 mg/dL/hr):** Reduce insulin by 50%
- **If glucose not decreasing:** Increase insulin by 1-2 units/hr
- **If glucose <70 mg/dL:** STOP insulin, give D50W, recheck in 15 min

Monitoring Frequency:

- Hourly until glucose stable in target range
- Every 2 hours once stable
- Every 4 hours if very stable and feeding/medication regimen unchanged

Critical Value Protocols:

Hypoglycemia (<70 mg/dL):

- **Mild (50-69 mg/dL):** D50W 12.5-25g IV, stop insulin temporarily
- **Severe (<50 mg/dL):** D50W 25-50g IV, stop insulin, notify physician, repeat glucose q15min

Severe Hyperglycemia (>400 mg/dL):

- Check for DKA (if known diabetic): ABG, ketones, anion gap
- Aggressive insulin therapy
- Fluid resuscitation

Teaching Points:

1. **Stress Hyperglycemia:** Common in critical illness; caused by counter-regulatory hormones, insulin resistance, and inflammation; transient

2. **Target 140-180 mg/dL:** Landmark studies (NICE-SUGAR) showed tight control (80-110) increased mortality vs moderate control (140-180)
3. **Hypoglycemia Risk:** Most dangerous complication of insulin therapy; associated with increased mortality, arrhythmias, neurologic injury
4. **Continuous IV Insulin:** Preferred in ICU for rapid titration; regular insulin (short-acting) used; infusion allows minute-to-minute adjustment
5. **Glucose Variability:** Wide fluctuations independently predict mortality; stable glucose within target better than mean alone
6. **Nutritional Considerations:** TPN/enteral feeds significantly impact glucose; adjust insulin when nutrition changes
7. **Vasopressor Effect:** Catecholamines (norepinephrine, epinephrine) increase glucose; insulin requirements may decrease as vasopressors wean
8. **Corticosteroids:** Cause significant hyperglycemia; anticipate increased insulin needs; methylprednisolone > hydrocortisone
9. **Transition to Subcutaneous:** Calculate total daily IV insulin requirement; give 50-80% as basal + nutritional + correction insulin
10. **No Underlying Diabetes:** Most stress hyperglycemia resolves; confirm with HbA1c; if HbA1c normal, no long-term diabetes treatment needed

Related Cases: DKA in ICU, hyperosmolar hyperglycemic state, hypoglycemia from insulin overdose, steroid-induced hyperglycemia

---

Case 10.5: Coagulation Monitoring During Anticoagulation - Heparin-Induced Thrombocytopenia

Clinical Presentation: A 62-year-old woman undergoes total knee replacement surgery. Post-operatively, she receives subcutaneous heparin 5,000 units TID for DVT prophylaxis. On post-op day 6, she develops acute right leg swelling and pain. Ultrasound confirms DVT in right popliteal vein. She is started on therapeutic IV unfractionated heparin with plan to bridge to warfarin.

Physical Examination (Day 6):

- Vital signs stable
- Right leg: Swollen, tender, warm
- Surgical site: Healing well, no infection

Initial Laboratory Findings:

- **Platelet count (pre-op baseline): 285,000/µL**
- Hemoglobin: 11.2 g/dL (post-surgical anemia)
- INR: 1.1

Diagnostic Reasoning Questions:

1. How is heparin therapy monitored?
2. What are the characteristics and types of HIT?
3. How is HIT diagnosed and managed?

4. What alternative anticoagulants are used in HIT?

Sequential Test Results:

Heparin Therapy Initiated (Day 6, 4 PM):

- **Unfractionated heparin (UFH) IV:**
    - Bolus: 80 units/kg
    - Infusion: 18 units/kg/hr
- **Monitoring:** aPTT every 6 hours until therapeutic

aPTT Monitoring:

Baseline (Pre-Heparin):

- **aPTT: 32 seconds** (normal 25-35 seconds)

6 Hours After Starting Heparin:

- **aPTT: 48 seconds** (therapeutic goal 60-80 seconds)
- **Subtherapeutic** → Increase heparin by 4 units/kg/hr

12 Hours:

- **aPTT: 72 seconds** (therapeutic range ✓)
- Maintain current heparin rate

18 Hours:

- **aPTT: 68 seconds** (therapeutic ✓)

Platelet Monitoring:

Day 6 (Heparin started):

- Platelets: 285,000/μL

Day 7:

- Platelets: 260,000/μL (normal)

Day 8:

- Platelets: 245,000/μL

Day 9:

- **Platelets: 115,000/μL SUDDEN DROP** (>50% from baseline)

- **CRITICAL ALERT: Possible Heparin-Induced Thrombocytopenia (HIT)**

Clinical Assessment Day 9:

- Patient reports new left chest pain
- CT angiography: **Pulmonary embolism in left lower lobe**
- **Paradoxical thrombosis on anticoagulation!**

4T Score for HIT Probability:

Category	Score	Patient
Thrombocytopenia	2 (>50% fall, nadir 20-100K)	2
Timing	2 (Day 5-10, or <1 day if recent heparin)	2
Thrombosis	2 (New thrombosis, skin necrosis)	2
oTher causes	0 (Other cause likely: 0; Possible: 1; None: 2)	2

Total 4T Score: 8 (High Probability of HIT)

- Score 0-3: Low probability (≤5% HIT)
- Score 4-5: Intermediate (14% HIT)
- **Score 6-8: High probability (64% HIT) ← PATIENT**

Immediate Management:

- **STOP all heparin immediately** (IV heparin, SC heparin, heparin flushes)
- **Start alternative anticoagulation** (cannot wait for confirmatory testing)
- **NO platelet transfusions** (contraindicated in HIT - increases thrombosis risk)

Alternative Anticoagulant Started:

- **Argatroban (direct thrombin inhibitor) IV infusion**
- Initial dose: 2 mcg/kg/min
- Monitor aPTT (target 1.5-3x baseline)

Confirmatory HIT Testing:

Immunoassay (ELISA) for Anti-PF4/Heparin Antibodies:

- **Anti-PF4/Heparin IgG antibodies: STRONGLY POSITIVE**
- Optical density (OD): 2.8 (OD >2.0 highly specific for HIT)

Functional Assay (Serotonin Release Assay - SRA):

- **Positive at low heparin concentration (0.1-0.3 U/mL)**
- **Negative at high heparin concentration (100 U/mL)** (confirmatory pattern for HIT)
- Gold standard test: 95% specificity

Final Diagnosis: Heparin-Induced Thrombocytopenia (HIT) Type II with Thrombosis (HITT)

HIT Type I vs Type II:

Feature	HIT Type I	HIT Type II
Mechanism	Non-immune, direct platelet activation	**Immune-mediated (anti-PF4/heparin Ab)**
Onset	1-2 days	**5-10 days (or <1 day if recent exposure)**
Platelet nadir	>100,000/µL	**<100K or >50% drop**
Thrombosis	No	**YES (30-50%)**
Clinical significance	Benign, self-limited	**Life-threatening**
Management	Continue heparin	**STOP heparin, alternative anticoagulation**

Argatroban Monitoring:

Day 9 (Started Argatroban):

- aPTT: 85 seconds (therapeutic for argatroban 1.5-3x baseline)
- Platelets: 110,000/µL

Day 11:

- **Platelets: 145,000/µL** (recovering)
- aPTT: 78 seconds

Day 13:

- **Platelets: 195,000/µL** (near-normal)
- Begin warfarin overlap (cannot start until platelets >150K)

Transition to Warfarin:

- Warfarin 5 mg daily started (day 13)
- **Overlap argatroban and warfarin for ≥5 days AND INR >2**
- Argatroban affects INR (falsely elevates)

Day 18:

- INR: 2.8 (on argatroban + warfarin)
- Calculate "true INR" (argatroban-free):
  - Reduce argatroban to 2 mcg/kg/min
  - Recheck INR 4 hours later: INR 2.3 (therapeutic)
- **Discontinue argatroban**
- Continue warfarin

Long-Term Management:

- Warfarin for 3-6 months (treat DVT/PE)
- **Lifelong avoidance of all heparin products**
- Medical alert bracelet
- Document HIT in medical record
- Future anticoagulation: Use DOACs (apixaban, rivaroxaban) or fondaparinux

Imaging Follow-Up (3 Months):

- Repeat lower extremity ultrasound: DVT resolved
- Repeat CT chest: PE resolved
- Platelet count: 275,000/μL (normal)

Teaching Points:

1. **HIT Pathophysiology:** IgG antibodies against PF4-heparin complexes activate platelets → thrombocytopenia + paradoxical thrombosis
2. **Timing:** Typically days 5-10 of heparin; can occur <24 hours if heparin exposure within past 100 days (anamnestic response)
3. **Thrombocytopenia:** >50% drop from baseline OR platelet count <150K; often nadir 20-100K (not severe thrombocytopenia)
4. **Thrombosis:** 30-50% of HIT patients develop thrombosis (venous > arterial); can occur before platelet drop
5. **4T Score:** Pre-test probability tool; high score (6-8) warrants stopping heparin and starting alternative anticoagulation immediately
6. **Immunoassay (ELISA):** High sensitivity (>95%), moderate specificity; OD >2.0 highly predictive; negative result essentially rules out HIT
7. **Functional Assay (SRA, HIPA):** Gold standard; high specificity (>95%); slow turnaround (days); positive at low heparin, negative at high heparin = confirmatory
8. **Alternative Anticoagulation:** Argatroban (direct thrombin inhibitor), fondaparinux, DOACs; NEVER platelet transfusions (increases thrombosis)
9. **Warfarin Caution:** Do NOT start until platelets >150K (risk of venous limb gangrene); must overlap with alternative anticoagulant ≥5 days
10. **LMWH Cross-Reactivity:** 80-100% cross-reactivity with anti-PF4/heparin antibodies; AVOID in HIT

Related Cases: Warfarin-induced skin necrosis, over-anticoagulation with bleeding, direct oral anticoagulant monitoring

---

Case 10.6: Electrolyte Management in Critical Illness - Severe Hypokalemia

Clinical Presentation: A 55-year-old woman with history of alcoholism presents to ED with 1 week of intractable nausea, vomiting, and diarrhea. She appears severely dehydrated and weak. Unable to keep down any food or liquids. Takes furosemide 40 mg daily for peripheral edema. EMS reports she was found confused at home.

Physical Examination:

- BP 88/52 (hypotensive), HR 118, RR 22, Temp 98.2°F
- Appears cachectic, dry mucous membranes
- Skin: Tenting, delayed capillary refill
- Neurologic: Confused, generalized weakness
- Decreased bowel sounds

Initial ECG:

- Sinus tachycardia
- **Flattened T waves**
- **Prominent U waves** (characteristic of hypokalemia)
- **Prolonged QT interval**
- Occasional PVCs

Diagnostic Reasoning Questions:

1. What are the causes and clinical manifestations of severe hypokalemia?
2. How should potassium be repleted in critical illness?
3. What are the ECG changes associated with electrolyte abnormalities?
4. What other electrolytes must be monitored and repleted?

Sequential Test Results:

Point-of-Care Chemistry Panel (iStat):

Initial Results (ED Arrival):

- **Potassium: 1.9 mEq/L CRITICAL** (normal 3.5-5.0)
- Sodium: 132 mEq/L (low)
- Chloride: 88 mEq/L (low)
- **Bicarbonate: 38 mEq/L ELEVATED** (metabolic alkalosis)
- **Magnesium: 1.1 mg/dL LOW** (normal 1.7-2.2)
- Calcium: 8.0 mg/dL (low)
- Phosphorus: 2.1 mg/dL (low)
- Glucose: 92 mg/dL
- Creatinine: 1.4 mg/dL (elevated - prerenal azotemia)

Arterial Blood Gas:

- pH: 7.52 (alkalemia)
- $PaCO_2$: 48 mmHg (respiratory compensation for metabolic alkalosis)
- HCO_3^-: 38 mEq/L (elevated)
- **Metabolic alkalosis with appropriate respiratory compensation**

Critical Value Alert: Severe Hypokalemia (K+ 1.9 mEq/L)

Causes of Hypokalemia in This Patient:

1. **GI losses:** Vomiting and diarrhea (major contributor)
2. **Renal losses:** Furosemide (loop diuretic)
3. **Poor oral intake:** Malnutrition, alcoholism
4. **Hypomagnesemia:** Impairs potassium retention (renal K+ wasting)
5. **Metabolic alkalosis:** Shifts K+ intracellularly

Clinical Manifestations of Severe Hypokalemia:

- **Cardiovascular:** Arrhythmias (PVCs, VT, VF), ECG changes, cardiac arrest
- **Neuromuscular:** Weakness, paralysis, rhabdomyolysis, respiratory failure
- **GI:** Ileus, constipation
- **Renal:** Polyuria, impaired concentrating ability
- **Metabolic:** Worsens hyperglycemia

Immediate Management:

Cardiac Monitoring:

- Continuous telemetry (risk of life-threatening arrhythmias)

Aggressive Potassium Repletion:

Peripheral IV (Two Large-Bore):

- **Initial bolus: 40 mEq KCl in 100 mL NS over 1 hour** (via peripheral IV)
- Concentration: 40 mEq/100 mL = 0.4 mEq/mL (safe for peripheral; <0.5 mEq/mL)

Central Line Placed:

- For higher concentration infusion (peripheral max 10-20 mEq/hr)
- **Central line allows 40 mEq/hr** (for severe hypokalemia <2.5 mEq/L)

Magnesium Repletion (Essential):

- **Magnesium sulfate 4 g (32 mEq) IV over 4 hours**
- Hypomagnesemia prevents potassium retention
- **Must correct magnesium to successfully replete potassium**

Serial Potassium Monitoring:

Hour 0:

- **K+: 1.9 mEq/L**
- Started: 40 mEq KCl peripheral IV over 1h + magnesium

Hour 1:

- **K+: 2.3 mEq/L** (rising)
- Central line placed
- **Infusion: 40 mEq/hr KCl via central line**

Hour 2:

- **K+: 2.6 mEq/L**
- Continue 40 mEq/hr
- Magnesium infusion ongoing

Hour 4:

- **K+: 3.1 mEq/L** (improved but still low)
- **Magnesium: 1.7 mg/dL** (repleted to normal)
- Reduce KCl to 20 mEq/hr

Hour 6:

- **K+: 3.6 mEq/L** (normal range ✓)
- ECG: T waves normalizing, U waves resolving
- Continue 10-20 mEq/hr maintenance

Hour 12:

- **K+: 4.2 mEq/L** (therapeutic)
- Transition to oral potassium supplementation
- **KCl 40 mEq PO BID**

ECG Changes with Potassium Levels:

Potassium Level	ECG Findings
<2.5 mEq/L (Severe hypokalemia)	**Flattened T waves, prominent U waves, ST depression, prolonged QT** ← PATIENT
<3.0 mEq/L	T wave flattening, U waves
3.0-3.5 mEq/L	Minimal changes
5.5-6.5 mEq/L	Tall peaked T waves
6.5-8.0 mEq/L	Prolonged PR, wide QRS, flat P waves
>8.0 mEq/L	**Sine wave, VF, asystole (life-threatening)**

Additional Electrolyte Management:

Phosphorus Repletion:

- Phosphorus: 2.1 mg/dL (low)
- Sodium phosphate 15 mmol IV over 6 hours

Calcium Monitoring:

- Calcium: 8.0 mg/dL (ionized calcium ordered)
- Ionized calcium: 1.08 mmol/L (mildly low; normal 1.12-1.32)
- Calcium gluconate 2g IV (given cautiously - alkalosis increases protein binding)

Fluid Resuscitation:

- 2 liters 0.9% normal saline (correct hypovolemia, prerenal azotemia)
- Careful monitoring (risk of fluid overload)

Day 2 Results:

- K+: 3.9 mEq/L (stable)
- Mg: 1.9 mg/dL (normal)
- Phosphorus: 2.8 mg/dL (improved)
- Creatinine: 1.0 mg/dL (resolved prerenal AKI)
- Bicarbonate: 28 mEq/L (alkalosis improving)
- ECG: Normalized

Underlying Cause Investigation:

Urine Electrolytes (After Initial Resuscitation):

- Urine potassium: 35 mEq/L (inappropriately high - suggests renal losses)
- **Transtubular potassium gradient (TTKG): 8.5** (elevated; >4 suggests renal K+ wasting)
- Consistent with diuretic effect + hypomagnesemia

Additional Testing:

- Renin/aldosterone: Within normal limits (excludes primary hyperaldosteronism)
- Cortisol: Normal (excludes Cushing's)
- Thyroid function: Normal

Final Diagnosis:

1. **Severe Hypokalemia (K+ 1.9 mEq/L)** with Critical ECG Changes
2. Hypomagnesemia (Contributing to Refractory Hypokalemia)
3. Hypochloremic Metabolic Alkalosis (Contraction Alkalosis)
4. Multifactorial Etiology:
   - GI losses (vomiting, diarrhea)
   - Renal losses (furosemide, hypomagnesemia)
   - Poor nutritional intake (alcoholism)

Discharge Plan (Day 4):

- K+ stable 4.0-4.5 mEq/L
- **KCl 20 mEq PO BID** (oral supplementation)

- **Magnesium oxide 400 mg PO daily**
- **Discontinue furosemide** (manage edema with compression, leg elevation)
- Nutrition consultation
- Alcohol cessation counseling
- Follow-up electrolytes in 1 week

Potassium Repletion Guidelines:

Mild Hypokalemia (3.0-3.5 mEq/L):

- Oral replacement: KCl 40-80 mEq/day divided doses
- Dietary sources (bananas, oranges, potatoes)

Moderate (2.5-3.0 mEq/L):

- IV replacement: 10-20 mEq/hr peripheral IV
- OR oral if tolerated

Severe (<2.5 mEq/L): ← PATIENT

- **Aggressive IV replacement: 40 mEq/hr via central line**
- Continuous cardiac monitoring
- Recheck K+ every 1-2 hours
- **MUST correct magnesium**

Maximum Infusion Rates:

- Peripheral IV: 10-20 mEq/hr (max concentration 40 mEq/L to prevent phlebitis)
- Central IV: Up to 40 mEq/hr (for life-threatening hypokalemia)
- **NEVER IV push** (causes cardiac arrest)

Teaching Points:

1. **Hypomagnesemia:** Prevents renal potassium retention; MUST correct magnesium to successfully replete potassium; 40% of hypokalemic patients are also hypomagnesemic
2. **ECG Changes:** Reliable indicator of severity; U waves and T wave flattening indicate significant hypokalemia; prolonged QT increases risk of torsades de pointes
3. **Repletion Rate:** Severe hypokalemia (<2.5) requires aggressive replacement (40 mEq/hr central line); every 10 mEq raises serum K+ by ~0.1 mEq/L
4. **Total Body Deficit:** Serum K+ doesn't reflect total body stores; K+ 3.0 = deficit ~100-200 mEq; K+ 2.0 = deficit 200-400 mEq
5. **Metabolic Alkalosis:** Shifts K+ intracellularly (for every 0.1 pH increase, K+ decreases 0.4-0.6 mEq/L); treating alkalosis helps normalize K+
6. **GI vs Renal Losses:** Urine K+ <15 mEq/L = GI/transcellular shift; >15 mEq/L = renal losses (diuretics, RTA, hyperaldosteronism)
7. **Arrhythmia Risk:** Severe hypokalemia (<2.5) + digoxin = very high VT/VF risk; hypokalemia + prolonged QT = torsades de pointes
8. **Peripheral Phlebitis:** Concentrations >40 mEq/L cause severe pain and phlebitis; use central line for higher concentrations

9. **Potassium Sources:** KCl preferred (corrects concurrent hypochloremia); K-phosphate if also hypophosphatemic; avoid K-acetate/bicarbonate if alkalotic
10. **Chronic Diuretic Use:** Requires potassium-sparing diuretics (spironolactone, amiloride) or routine K+ supplementation and monitoring

Related Cases: Hyperkalemia in renal failure, refeeding syndrome with hypophosphatemia, diabetic ketoacidosis with total body potassium depletion, hypocalcemia with QT prolongation

Chapter 11: Pediatric Laboratory Medicine

Case 11.1: Newborn Screening Abnormalities - Phenylketonuria (PKU)

Clinical Presentation: A 10-day-old full-term male infant is referred to pediatric genetics clinic following an abnormal newborn screen. The initial screen (collected at 24 hours of life) showed elevated phenylalanine. Baby is exclusively breastfed, feeding well, and appears healthy. No family history of metabolic disorders. Parents are non-consanguineous. Pregnancy and delivery were uncomplicated.

Physical Examination:

- Weight: 3.4 kg (appropriate for age)
- Vital signs: Normal for age
- Alert, active, normal tone
- No dysmorphic features
- Normal neurologic examination
- No musty/mousy odor (develops later if untreated)

Initial Newborn Screening Results (24 Hours of Life):

- **Phenylalanine: 8.5 mg/dL ELEVATED** (normal <2 mg/dL in newborns)
- Phenylalanine/Tyrosine ratio: 4.2 (elevated; normal <3)
- Other newborn screen analytes: Normal

Diagnostic Reasoning Questions:

1. What disorders are included in newborn screening panels?
2. Why is timing of specimen collection critical for PKU screening?
3. How is PKU diagnosed and what are the different forms?
4. What is the role of phenylalanine hydroxylase (PAH) in metabolism?

Sequential Test Results:

Confirmatory Testing (Day 10):

Quantitative Plasma Amino Acids:

- **Phenylalanine: 22 mg/dL (1,330 µmol/L) MARKEDLY ELEVATED**
  - Normal: <2 mg/dL (120 µmol/L)
  - Hyperphenylalaninemia: 2-6 mg/dL
  - **Classic PKU: >20 mg/dL ← PATIENT**
- **Tyrosine: 0.8 mg/dL (44 µmol/L)** (low-normal)
- **Phenylalanine/Tyrosine ratio: 27.5 VERY ELEVATED** (normal <3)
- Other amino acids: Normal

Urine Organic Acids:

- Phenylpyruvic acid: Present (ketone derivative of phenylalanine)
- Phenyllactic acid: Present
- Phenylacetic acid: Present
- Pattern consistent with PKU

Pterins Analysis (Urine and Blood):

- Biopterin: Normal
- Neopterin: Normal
- Dihydropteridine reductase (DHPR): Normal
- **Excludes BH4 deficiency** (tetrahydrobiopterin cofactor defect)

Molecular Genetic Testing:

PAH Gene Sequencing:

- **Mutation 1: c.1222C>T (p.Arg408Trp)** - Pathogenic, common mutation
- **Mutation 2: c.1066-11G>A (IVS10-11G>A)** - Pathogenic, splicing mutation
- **Genotype: Compound heterozygous**
- Inheritance: Autosomal recessive (one mutation from each parent)

Newborn Screening Panel Components (Varies by State):

Amino Acid Disorders:

- PKU, Maple syrup urine disease, Homocystinuria, Citrullinemia, Argininosuccinic acidemia, Tyrosinemia

Organic Acid Disorders:

- Methylmalonic acidemia, Propionic acidemia, Isovaleric acidemia, Glutaric acidemia type I

Fatty Acid Oxidation Disorders:

- MCAD deficiency, VLCAD deficiency, LCHAD deficiency, Carnitine uptake defect

Hemoglobinopathies:

- Sickle cell disease, Beta-thalassemia

Endocrine Disorders:

- Congenital hypothyroidism, Congenital adrenal hyperplasia

Other:

- Biotinidase deficiency, Galactosemia, Cystic fibrosis, Severe combined immunodeficiency (SCID)

Timing of Newborn Screening:

- **Optimal: 24-48 hours of life** (after protein feeding initiated)
- **Too early (<24h):** False negatives for PKU (insufficient protein intake)
- **Preterm/NICU infants:** Screen at discharge or 7 days, whichever comes first
- **Repeat screen:** Recommended at 1-2 weeks for early discharge or NICU babies

Phenylalanine Metabolism:

1. **Normal pathway:** Phenylalanine → (PAH enzyme + BH4 cofactor) → Tyrosine
2. **PKU defect:** PAH deficiency → phenylalanine accumulates
3. **Alternative pathways:** Excess phenylalanine → phenylpyruvic acid, phenyllactic acid, phenylacetic acid (detected in urine)

Classification of Hyperphenylalaninemia:

Type	Phenylalanine Level	Enzyme Activity	Treatment
Classic PKU	**>20 mg/dL**	**<1% PAH**	**Strict low-phe diet ← PATIENT**
Moderate PKU	10-20 mg/dL	1-5% PAH	Low-phe diet
Mild PKU	6-10 mg/dL	5-10% PAH	Relaxed restriction
Mild HPA	2-6 mg/dL	>10% PAH	Often no treatment
BH4 deficiency	Variable	Normal PAH, cofactor defect	BH4 supplementation

Final Diagnosis: Classic Phenylketonuria (PKU) - Compound Heterozygous PAH Mutations (c.1222C>T / c.1066-11G>A)

Treatment Initiated (Day 10):

Dietary Management:

- **Low-phenylalanine diet** (phenylalanine-restricted medical formula)
- **Target phenylalanine: 2-6 mg/dL** (120-360 μmol/L)
- Breastfeeding combined with phenylalanine-free formula
- Measured phenylalanine intake based on tolerance
- Tyrosine supplementation (becomes essential amino acid in PKU)

Monitoring:

- **Phenylalanine levels twice weekly** (infancy)
- Adjust diet based on levels
- Growth and development assessment
- Neurologic evaluation

Serial Phenylalanine Monitoring:

Week 2 (on diet 1 week):

- Phenylalanine: 5.2 mg/dL (therapeutic range ✓)

Week 4:

- Phenylalanine: 4.8 mg/dL (excellent control)

Month 3:

- Phenylalanine: 3.6 mg/dL (optimal)
- Growth: 50th percentile (normal)
- Development: Appropriate for age

Month 12:

- Phenylalanine: 4.2 mg/dL (well-controlled)
- Developmental milestones: All achieved on time
- IQ testing (later): Normal range

Untreated PKU Consequences (Prevented by Early Treatment):

- **Intellectual disability** (IQ 50-70 if untreated)
- Seizures (25-50%)
- Behavioral problems (hyperactivity, autism-like features)
- Eczema, musty odor
- Hypopigmentation (phenylalanine competes with tyrosine for melanin synthesis)
- Microcephaly

Maternal PKU Considerations:

- Female patients must maintain strict diet during reproductive years
- **Maternal PKU syndrome:** High maternal phenylalanine causes fetal microcephaly, intellectual disability, congenital heart disease, growth restriction
- Pre-conception counseling essential

Parental Testing:

Mother:

- Heterozygous carrier for c.1222C>T
- Phenylalanine: 1.2 mg/dL (normal)

Father:

- Heterozygous carrier for c.1066-11G>A
- Phenylalanine: 1.0 mg/dL (normal)

Genetic Counseling:

- 25% recurrence risk with each pregnancy
- Prenatal diagnosis available
- Carrier screening for extended family

Teaching Points:

1. **Newborn Screening Rationale:** PKU is asymptomatic at birth; early detection (before 2 weeks) and treatment prevent intellectual disability
2. **Phenylalanine/Tyrosine Ratio:** More specific than phenylalanine alone; ratio >3 suggestive of PKU; helps distinguish from transient tyrosinemia of newborn
3. **Timing Critical:** Screen at 24-48 hours (protein feeding established); too early = false negative; repeat screen if <24h or NICU
4. **BH4 Deficiency:** Rare cause of hyperphenylalaninemia (2-3%); requires BH4, neurotransmitter supplementation; screened with pterins analysis
5. **Dietary Treatment:** Lifelong low-phenylalanine diet; phenylalanine is essential amino acid (cannot eliminate completely); target 2-6 mg/dL
6. **Age-Specific Targets:** Stricter control in infancy/childhood (2-6 mg/dL); may relax in adolescence (2-10 mg/dL); strict again for pregnancy
7. **Sapropterin (Kuvan):** BH4 supplement; 20-50% of PKU patients responsive (PAH activity increases); allows more dietary flexibility
8. **False Positives:** Prematurity, parenteral nutrition (amino acid solutions), liver disease; confirm with quantitative amino acids
9. **Tandem Mass Spectrometry:** Modern screening uses MS/MS; measures phenylalanine and multiple metabolites simultaneously from dried blood spot

Related Cases: Maple syrup urine disease, homocystinuria, tyrosinemia, BH4 deficiency, maternal PKU syndrome

---

Case 11.2: Failure to Thrive with Metabolic Evaluation

Clinical Presentation: A 6-month-old female infant is brought to pediatrician for poor weight gain and developmental concerns. Born at term with normal birth weight (3.2 kg), she initially fed well but has had progressive feeding difficulties over the past 3 months. Mother reports poor appetite, frequent vomiting after feeds, and lethargy. Recent upper respiratory infection seemed to worsen symptoms. No seizures. First child to healthy non-consanguineous parents.

Physical Examination:

- **Weight: 5.8 kg** (well below 3rd percentile; expected ~7.5 kg)
- **Length: 63 cm** (10th percentile; expected ~65 cm)
- **Head circumference: 41 cm** (5th percentile; expected ~43 cm)
- **Failure to thrive** (weight <3rd percentile)
- Appears lethargic, poor muscle tone (hypotonia)
- Hepatomegaly (liver 3 cm below costal margin)
- Developmental delay (not sitting independently; should at 6 months)

- No dysmorphic features

Initial Laboratory Findings:

- Glucose: 48 mg/dL (hypoglycemia)
- Hemoglobin: 9.2 g/dL (anemia)
- Albumin: 3.0 g/dL (low)

Diagnostic Reasoning Questions:

1. What is the differential diagnosis for failure to thrive with hypoglycemia and hepatomegaly?
2. How are inborn errors of metabolism evaluated?
3. What is the significance of metabolic decompensation during illness?
4. How do storage diseases present in infancy?

Sequential Test Results:

Comprehensive Metabolic Workup:

Basic Metabolic Panel:

- Glucose: 45 mg/dL (persistent hypoglycemia)
- **Bicarbonate: 18 mEq/L** (metabolic acidosis)
- Creatinine: 0.3 mg/dL (normal for age)
- **Anion gap: 16** (elevated; normal 8-12)

Liver Function Tests:

- **AST: 285 U/L** (elevated)
- **ALT: 320 U/L** (elevated)
- Alkaline phosphatase: 250 U/L (normal for age)
- **Total bilirubin: 2.8 mg/dL** (elevated)
- Direct bilirubin: 0.4 mg/dL
- **PT-INR: 1.6** (prolonged - coagulopathy)

Lactate and Ammonia:

- **Lactate: 6.8 mmol/L** (elevated; normal <2.0)
- **Ammonia: 125 µmol/L** (elevated; normal <100)

Lipid Panel:

- Total cholesterol: 285 mg/dL (elevated)
- **Triglycerides: 420 mg/dL MARKEDLY ELEVATED**
- HDL: 28 mg/dL (low)

Uric Acid:

- **Uric acid: 8.5 mg/dL** (elevated for age; normal <5.5)

Pattern Recognition: Hypoglycemia + hepatomegaly + elevated lactate + hypertriglyceridemia + hyperuricemia → **Glycogen Storage Disease (GSD)**

Targeted Metabolic Testing:

Plasma Acylcarnitine Profile (MS/MS):

- Free carnitine: Low
- C2 (acetylcarnitine): Elevated
- Long-chain acylcarnitines: Normal
- Pattern: Non-specific but suggests impaired fatty acid oxidation

Urine Organic Acids (GC-MS):

- **Lactic acid: Markedly elevated**
- 3-hydroxybutyric acid: Decreased (ketone production impaired)
- **Uric acid: Elevated**
- No abnormal organic acids (excludes organic acidemias)

Fasting Study (Supervised, Critical Diagnostic Test):

Baseline (Fed State):

- Glucose: 68 mg/dL

After 4 Hours Fasting:

- **Glucose: 38 mg/dL** (hypoglycemia)
- Insulin: <2 µU/mL (appropriately suppressed)
- Cortisol: 18 µg/dL (appropriate stress response)
- Growth hormone: 12 ng/mL (appropriate)
- **Free fatty acids: 0.3 mmol/L** (LOW - should be elevated during fasting)
- **Beta-hydroxybutyrate: 0.2 mmol/L** (LOW - impaired ketogenesis)
- Lactate: 5.2 mmol/L (elevated)

Fasting study terminated at 4 hours due to hypoglycemia (normal infants can fast 12-18 hours)

Interpretation: Hypoketotic hypoglycemia - impaired fatty acid oxidation and/or gluconeogenesis

Glucagon Stimulation Test:

- **Baseline glucose: 52 mg/dL**
- Glucagon 0.03 mg/kg IV given
- **30 minutes post-glucagon: Glucose 125 mg/dL (Robust response - rise of 73 mg/dL)**
- Normal response: >40 mg/dL rise

Interpretation: Excellent glucagon response suggests **adequate glycogen stores that can be mobilized** → Excludes GSD Type I (glucose-6-phosphatase deficiency would have minimal response)

Enzyme Analysis:

Liver Biopsy (Performed for Definitive Diagnosis):

Histopathology:

- **Marked glycogen accumulation in hepatocytes** (PAS-positive)
- Hepatocyte ballooning
- Minimal fibrosis
- No cirrhosis

Biochemical Enzyme Assay on Liver Tissue:

- Glucose-6-phosphatase: Normal (excludes GSD I)
- **Debranching enzyme (AGL): <5% of normal activity SEVERELY DEFICIENT**
- Phosphorylase: Normal
- Phosphorylase kinase: Normal

Molecular Genetic Testing:

AGL Gene Sequencing (Debranching Enzyme Gene):

- *Mutation 1: c.3964G>T (p.Glu1322)** - Nonsense mutation (truncating)
- **Mutation 2: c.4455delT** - Frameshift mutation
- **Compound heterozygous mutations**
- Inheritance: Autosomal recessive

Final Diagnosis: Glycogen Storage Disease Type III (GSD III, Cori Disease, Forbes Disease) - Debranching Enzyme Deficiency (AGL Mutations)

GSD Type III Characteristics:

Subtype IIIa (75%): Liver + muscle involvement **Subtype IIIb (25%):** Liver only

Clinical Features (This Patient):

- Hepatomegaly (prominent)
- Fasting hypoglycemia (moderate)
- Growth retardation
- Hyperlipidemia
- Elevated transaminases
- **GOOD glucagon response** (distinguishes from GSD I)

Comparison of Glycogen Storage Diseases:

Type	Enzyme Deficiency	Glucagon Response	Lactate	Key Features
I (Von Gierke)	Glucose-6-phosphatase	**POOR**	**Very high**	Severe hypoglycemia, lactic acidosis
III (Cori)	Debranching enzyme	**GOOD**	**Mild elevation**	Milder, improves with age ← PATIENT
IV (Andersen)	Branching enzyme	Variable	Normal	Cirrhosis, early death
V (McArdle)	Muscle phosphorylase	N/A	Normal	Exercise intolerance, myoglobinuria
VI (Hers)	Liver phosphorylase	Good	Normal	Mild hepatomegaly

Treatment Initiated:

Nutritional Management:

- **Frequent feeding every 3-4 hours** (prevent hypoglycemia)
- **Nighttime continuous gastric feeding** (via NG tube)
- **Uncooked cornstarch** (slow-release glucose source): 1.6 g/kg every 4-6 hours
- High-protein diet (25% of calories from protein)
- Complex carbohydrates

Monitoring:

- Avoid fasting >4 hours
- Glucose monitoring
- Growth parameters
- Liver enzymes, lipids
- Echocardiogram (screen for cardiomyopathy - can occur in GSD III)

Prevent Metabolic Decompensation During Illness:

- Maintain glucose intake during infections
- Emergency protocol for illness (frequent feeds, cornstarch)

Follow-Up (6 Months Later, Age 12 Months):

- Weight: 8.2 kg (25th percentile - improved!)
- Glucose: 70-90 mg/dL (stable)
- Liver size: Decreased to 2 cm below costal margin
- Transaminases: AST 85, ALT 95 (improved)
- Development: Sitting, crawling (catching up)
- Hepatomegaly typically improves with age

Long-Term Prognosis:

- GSD III generally milder than GSD I
- Hepatomegaly and hypoglycemia often improve after puberty

- Monitor for myopathy, cardiomyopathy (develop in adulthood)
- Normal lifespan with good management
- Risk of hepatic adenomas, cirrhosis (less than GSD I)

Teaching Points:

1. **Failure to Thrive Workup:** Weight <3rd percentile or crossing percentiles; evaluate for: inadequate intake, malabsorption, increased losses, increased metabolic demand, or metabolic disorders
2. **Hepatomegaly + Hypoglycemia:** Classic for glycogen storage diseases; also consider: fatty acid oxidation defects, gluconeogenesis defects
3. **Hypoketotic Hypoglycemia:** Low ketones during hypoglycemia abnormal; suggests hyperinsulinism, fatty acid oxidation defect, or GSD
4. **Glucagon Response:** Distinguishes GSD types; GSD I minimal response (no glucose-6-phosphatase); GSD III robust response (can mobilize glycogen, but only outer branches)
5. **Debranching Enzyme:** Required to release glucose from branch points in glycogen; deficiency causes abnormal glycogen accumulation (limit dextrin)
6. **Metabolic Decompensation:** Illness triggers catabolism; GSD patients cannot maintain glucose → severe hypoglycemia, acidosis
7. **Cornstarch Therapy:** Slowly digested complex carbohydrate; provides sustained glucose release; revolutionized GSD management
8. **Age-Specific Reference Ranges:** Critical in pediatrics; glucose <50 mg/dL concerning in infant; ammonia, uric acid, transaminases have different normals
9. **GSD vs Fatty Acid Oxidation Defects:** Both cause hypoketotic hypoglycemia + hepatomegaly; GSD has elevated lactate, good glucagon response; FAO defects have elevated acylcarnitines

Related Cases: GSD Type I (Von Gierke), MCAD deficiency, hyperinsulinism, propionic acidemia, galactosemia

---

Case 11.3: Pediatric Acute Lymphoblastic Leukemia (ALL)

Clinical Presentation: A 4-year-old boy presents to pediatrician with 3 weeks of fatigue, pallor, and easy bruising. Mother reports he has been less active, complaining of leg pain at night, and had several nosebleeds this week. Low-grade fevers for 5 days. No significant past medical history. Denies recent infections, travel, or toxic exposures.

Physical Examination:

- Appears pale, lethargic
- Temp 100.8°F, HR 118, RR 24
- **Petechiae on lower extremities**
- **Ecchymoses on arms and legs** (bruising)
- **Cervical and axillary lymphadenopathy** (1-2 cm, non-tender)
- **Hepatomegaly:** Liver 3 cm below costal margin
- **Splenomegaly:** Spleen palpable 2 cm below costal margin
- No bone tenderness on examination (though history of leg pain)

Diagnostic Reasoning Questions:

1. What is the differential diagnosis for pancytopenia with organomegaly in a child?
2. How is ALL diagnosed and classified?
3. What laboratory findings predict prognosis in pediatric ALL?
4. How does pediatric ALL differ from adult ALL?

Sequential Test Results:

Complete Blood Count (CBC) with Differential:

Initial CBC:

- **WBC: 42,000/µL ELEVATED** (normal 5,000-15,000 for age)
- **Hemoglobin: 6.8 g/dL SEVERELY LOW** (normal 11-13 for age)
- **Hematocrit: 20%**
- **Platelets: 18,000/µL SEVERELY LOW** (normal 150,000-450,000)
- **MCV: 88 fL** (normocytic)

Differential Count:

- Neutrophils: 8% (absolute count: 3,360/µL - neutropenia)
- **Lymphocytes: 82%** (absolute count: 34,440/µL)
- Monocytes: 6%
- Eosinophils: 2%
- Basophils: 2%
- **Blasts: 68% MARKEDLY ELEVATED** (normal 0%)

Peripheral Blood Smear:

- **Numerous lymphoblasts** (large cells, high nuclear:cytoplasmic ratio, nucleoli visible)
- Blasts comprise majority of WBCs
- Normocytic, normochromic RBCs (appropriate for anemia of malignancy)
- Marked thrombocytopenia
- No schistocytes (excludes hemolytic process)

Chemistry and Coagulation:

- **LDH: 1,850 U/L MARKEDLY ELEVATED** (normal <500; tumor burden marker)
- **Uric acid: 8.2 mg/dL** (elevated; tumor lysis)
- Creatinine: 0.4 mg/dL (normal for age)
- Potassium: 4.8 mEq/L (monitor for tumor lysis)
- Phosphorus: 5.2 mg/dL (high-normal)
- Calcium: 9.0 mg/dL (normal)
- PT-INR: 1.2 (mildly prolonged)
- aPTT: 35 seconds (normal)
- Fibrinogen: 285 mg/dL (normal)

Bone Marrow Aspiration and Biopsy:

Bone Marrow Aspirate:

- **Hypercellular marrow (>95% cellularity)**
- **Lymphoblasts: 92%** (normal <5%) **DIAGNOSTIC OF ACUTE LEUKEMIA**
- Erythroid precursors: Markedly decreased
- Myeloid precursors: Markedly decreased
- Megakaryocytes: Absent

Morphology:

- **Small to medium-sized lymphoblasts**
- Scant cytoplasm
- Fine chromatin, small nucleoli
- **L1 morphology (FAB classification):** Small uniform blasts

Bone Marrow Biopsy:

- **>90% replacement by lymphoblasts**
- Normal hematopoiesis suppressed

Immunophenotyping (Flow Cytometry):

Surface Markers:

- **CD19: Positive** (B-cell marker)
- **CD10 (CALLA): Positive** (common ALL antigen)
- **CD20: Positive** (weak)
- **TdT (terminal deoxynucleotidyl transferase): Positive** (immature lymphoid marker)
- **CD34: Positive** (stem cell marker)
- **HLA-DR: Positive**
- CD3: Negative (excludes T-cell lineage)
- CD13, CD33: Negative (excludes myeloid lineage)
- MPO (myeloperoxidase): Negative

Diagnosis: B-cell Precursor Acute Lymphoblastic Leukemia (B-ALL) - Common/Pre-B Immunophenotype

Cytogenetics and Molecular Studies:

Conventional Karyotype:

- **Hyperdiploidy (>50 chromosomes):** 54 chromosomes
- Trisomies of chromosomes 4, 10, 17
- No t(9;22) BCR-ABL (Philadelphia chromosome - negative)
- No t(4;11) MLL rearrangement
- No hypodiploidy (<44 chromosomes)

FISH (Fluorescence In Situ Hybridization):

- **BCR-ABL1 fusion: NEGATIVE** (good; Philadelphia chromosome associated with poor prognosis)
- **MLL (KMT2A) rearrangement: NEGATIVE** (good; MLL associated with poor prognosis in infants)
- **ETV6-RUNX1 fusion: POSITIVE** (favorable prognosis)

Minimal Residual Disease (MRD) Testing:

- Will be assessed after induction chemotherapy (day 29)
- MRD negative (<0.01% blasts) = excellent prognosis

CNS Evaluation (CNS Involvement Assessment):

Lumbar Puncture with CSF Analysis:

- **WBC: 2 cells/µL** (normal <5)
- **No blasts identified** (CNS1 status - CNS negative)
- Protein: Normal
- Glucose: Normal

CSF Status Classification:

- **CNS1:** No blasts (this patient)
- CNS2: <5 WBC with blasts, or ≥5 WBC with <50% blasts
- CNS3: ≥5 WBC with blasts, or cranial nerve involvement

Imaging:

Chest X-ray:

- **No mediastinal mass** (thymic enlargement more common in T-ALL)
- No pleural effusions

Abdominal Ultrasound:

- Confirms hepatosplenomegaly
- No renal involvement
- No abdominal lymphadenopathy beyond what's palpable

Risk Stratification (COG/NCI Criteria):

Age and WBC Count (NCI Criteria):

- **Age: 4 years** (standard risk 1-9.99 years)
- **WBC: 42,000/µL** (standard risk <50,000)
- **NCI Standard Risk** ✓

Additional Favorable Prognostic Features:

- Hyperdiploidy (54 chromosomes) - **FAVORABLE**
- ETV6-RUNX1 fusion - **FAVORABLE**
- No BCR-ABL (Philadelphia chromosome) - **FAVORABLE**
- No MLL rearrangement - **FAVORABLE**
- CNS1 status (no CNS involvement) - **FAVORABLE**
- B-cell precursor (vs T-cell) - **FAVORABLE**

Risk Category: Standard Risk B-ALL (85-90% cure rate)

Final Diagnosis: B-Cell Precursor Acute Lymphoblastic Leukemia (B-ALL)

- Common/Pre-B Immunophenotype (CD10+, CD19+, CD34+, TdT+)
- Favorable Cytogenetics (Hyperdiploidy, ETV6-RUNX1 fusion)
- NCI Standard Risk
- CNS1 (No CNS involvement)

Treatment Protocol (COG AALL0331 or Similar):

Phase 1: Induction (4 weeks):

- Vincristine (weekly x 4)
- Daunorubicin or doxorubicin (anthracycline)
- PEG-asparaginase
- Prednisone (daily x 28 days)
- IT chemotherapy (intrathecal methotrexate - CNS prophylaxis)

Tumor Lysis Syndrome Prophylaxis:

- **Allopurinol** or **rasburicase** (reduce uric acid)
- IV hydration (3 L/m²/day)
- Monitor: Potassium, phosphorus, calcium, uric acid, creatinine

Day 8 Response Assessment:

- Peripheral blood blast count (early response predictor)

Day 29 End-Induction Assessment:

- **Bone marrow aspirate: <5% blasts = Morphologic remission √**
- **MRD testing (flow cytometry): <0.01% = MRD negative √** (excellent prognosis)

Phase 2: Consolidation (8 weeks):

- High-dose methotrexate
- 6-mercaptopurine
- Vincristine, asparaginase

Phase 3: Interim Maintenance (8 weeks):

- Vincristine, methotrexate, asparaginase

Phase 4: Delayed Intensification (8 weeks):

- Repeat induction-like therapy

Phase 5: Maintenance (Until 2-3 years from diagnosis):

- Daily 6-mercaptopurine
- Weekly methotrexate
- Monthly vincristine + prednisone pulses
- Periodic IT chemotherapy

Monitoring During Treatment:

- **CBC:** Weekly (monitor for cytopenias)
- **Metabolic panel:** Regular (monitor for tumor lysis, organ toxicity)
- **MRD:** End-induction, end-consolidation (risk-stratify)
- **Growth and development**
- **Late effects screening:** Cardiac (anthracycline), endocrine, neurocognitive

Follow-Up (3 Months Post-Diagnosis):

- **Complete remission maintained**
- MRD: <0.01% (negative - excellent)
- Tolerating chemotherapy
- Attending school with precautions

Follow-Up (2 Years Post-Diagnosis):

- Continuous complete remission
- On maintenance chemotherapy
- Normal growth and development
- **5-year event-free survival expected: 85-90%** (standard risk B-ALL)

Teaching Points:

1. **ALL Diagnosis:** Requires ≥20% blasts in bone marrow (WHO criteria); <20% = lymphoblastic lymphoma
2. **Immunophenotyping:** Essential for lineage determination; B-ALL (80-85%): CD19+, CD10+ most common; T-ALL (15-20%): CD3+, often mediastinal mass
3. **Cytogenetic Risk Factors:** Hyperdiploidy (>50 chr) and ETV6-RUNX1 = favorable; t(9;22) BCR-ABL, t(4;11) MLL, hypodiploidy (<44) = poor prognosis
4. **Age and WBC:** NCI criteria - standard risk: age 1-9.99 years + WBC <50,000; high risk: age <1 or ≥10 years or WBC ≥50,000
5. **MRD (Minimal Residual Disease):** Most important prognostic factor; <0.01% at end-induction = excellent outcome; ≥0.01% = high risk, intensified therapy
6. **Pediatric vs Adult ALL:** Pediatric cure rate 85-90%; adult 40%; children tolerate intensive therapy better; different biology (more favorable cytogenetics in children)

7. **Tumor Lysis Syndrome:** Life-threatening complication; hyperuricemia, hyperkalemia, hyperphosphatemia, hypocalcemia; prevent with hydration, allopurinol/rasburicase
8. **CNS Prophylaxis:** ALL has CNS tropism; intrathecal chemotherapy prevents CNS relapse (historically 50-75% without prophylaxis, now <5%)
9. **Late Effects:** Monitor for anthracycline cardiomyopathy, asparaginase pancreatitis, methotrexate hepatotoxicity, secondary malignancies, neurocognitive effects
10. **TdT (Terminal Deoxynucleotidyl Transferase):** Nuclear enzyme in immature lymphoid cells; positive in ALL (95%), negative in mature lymphomas; helps distinguish ALL from Burkitt lymphoma

Related Cases: T-cell ALL, infant ALL with MLL rearrangement, Philadelphia chromosome-positive ALL, AML in children, aplastic anemia

---

Case 11.4: Hemolytic Disease of the Fetus and Newborn (HDFN) - ABO Incompatibility

Clinical Presentation: A term newborn male (39 weeks gestation) is noted to be jaundiced at 18 hours of life. Mother is blood type O-positive, first pregnancy, uncomplicated prenatal course. Baby was born via normal vaginal delivery, Apgar scores 8 and 9. Breastfeeding well. Nursing staff reports increasing jaundice.

Physical Examination (18 Hours of Life):

- Weight: 3.4 kg (appropriate for gestational age)
- Vital signs: Normal for age
- **Jaundice:** Visible on face, chest, and abdomen (zone 3)
- **Mild hepatosplenomegaly**
- No petechiae or bruising
- Otherwise well-appearing, active

Maternal Information:

- Blood type: **O-positive**
- Prenatal labs: Antibody screen negative (no alloantibodies detected)
- No prior pregnancies, no history of transfusions

Initial Laboratory Findings (18 Hours of Life):

Newborn Blood Type:

- **Blood type: A-positive** (ABO incompatibility with mother)

Total Serum Bilirubin:

- **Total bilirubin: 14.2 mg/dL** at 18 hours of life
- **Direct bilirubin: 0.6 mg/dL** (indirect/unconjugated: 13.6 mg/dL)
- Plotted on Bhutani nomogram: **High-risk zone** (approaching exchange transfusion threshold)

Diagnostic Reasoning Questions:

1. What causes ABO hemolytic disease of the newborn?
2. How does ABO HDFN differ from Rh HDFN?
3. How is severity of hemolysis assessed?
4. When is phototherapy vs. exchange transfusion indicated?

Sequential Test Results:

Complete Blood Count:

- Hemoglobin: 13.2 g/dL (normal 14-20 for term newborn)
- Hematocrit: 40% (slightly low)
- **Reticulocyte count: 8.5% ELEVATED** (normal 3-7% in newborn; indicates hemolysis)
- Platelets: 245,000/µL (normal)
- **WBC: 18,500/µL** (normal for newborn)

Peripheral Blood Smear:

- **Spherocytes: Present** (classic for ABO HDFN)
- **Polychromasia** (young RBCs)
- Nucleated RBCs: 12 per 100 WBC (elevated; stress erythropoiesis)
- No fragmented cells

Direct Antiglobulin Test (DAT, Direct Coombs):

- **DAT (IgG): Weakly positive (1+)** - detects maternal anti-A IgG on baby's RBCs
- **DAT (C3d): Positive (2+)** - complement activation
- Pattern: **Mixed field agglutination** (characteristic of ABO HDFN)

Indirect Antiglobulin Test (IAT, Indirect Coombs):

- **Maternal serum tested against A cells: Strongly positive**
- Anti-A titer (IgG): 1:512 (elevated; normal anti-A is IgM which doesn't cross placenta)
- **Maternal IgG anti-A antibodies detected**

Blood Smear Comparison:

ABO HDFN: Spherocytes, weakly positive DAT **Rh HDFN:** No spherocytes, strongly positive DAT, more severe anemia

Bilirubin Trends (Critical for Management):

Hour 18 (Initial):

- Total bilirubin: 14.2 mg/dL (high-risk zone)
- **Phototherapy started immediately** (double phototherapy - lights above and below)

Hour 24:

- Total bilirubin: 16.8 mg/dL (rising despite phototherapy)
- Rate of rise: 2.6 mg/dL over 6 hours (0.43 mg/dL/hr - rapid)

Hour 30:

- **Total bilirubin: 18.5 mg/dL APPROACHING EXCHANGE THRESHOLD**
- Hemoglobin: 11.8 g/dL (declining - ongoing hemolysis)

Management Decision Point:

- Exchange transfusion threshold for term infant: ~20 mg/dL (varies by risk factors)
- Rising bilirubin despite intensive phototherapy
- **Decision: Prepare for exchange transfusion if continues to rise**

IVIG (Intravenous Immunoglobulin) Administration:

- **IVIG 0.5 g/kg over 2 hours** (blocks Fc receptors, reduces hemolysis)
- Given when bilirubin rising rapidly despite phototherapy

Hour 36 (Post-IVIG):

- Total bilirubin: 18.2 mg/dL (plateaued!)
- Hemoglobin: 11.5 g/dL (stable)

Hour 48:

- Total bilirubin: 16.4 mg/dL (declining ✓)
- Hemoglobin: 11.8 g/dL (stable)

Hour 72 (Day 3):

- Total bilirubin: 12.8 mg/dL (continued decline)
- **Exchange transfusion avoided ✓**

Day 5:

- Total bilirubin: 8.2 mg/dL (safe range)
- Phototherapy discontinued
- Hemoglobin: 10.2 g/dL (mild anemia persists)
- Reticulocyte count: 6% (ongoing compensation)

Follow-Up (2 Weeks):

- Total bilirubin: 1.2 mg/dL (normal)
- **Hemoglobin: 8.9 g/dL** (anemia of hemolysis - nadir typically 2-6 weeks)
- Reticulocyte count: 4% (compensating)

- Plan: Monitor, may need iron supplementation or transfusion if Hgb <7 g/dL

Follow-Up (8 Weeks):

- Hemoglobin: 10.8 g/dL (recovering)
- Development: Normal

Final Diagnosis: ABO Hemolytic Disease of the Fetus and Newborn (ABO HDFN)

- Mother: O-positive with IgG anti-A antibodies
- Baby: A-positive
- Severe hyperbilirubinemia requiring intensive phototherapy and IVIG
- Exchange transfusion avoided

ABO HDFN Pathophysiology:

Setup:

1. Mother: Blood type O (has naturally occurring anti-A and anti-B antibodies)
2. Fetus/baby: Blood type A or B
3. Maternal anti-A or anti-B antibodies are usually **IgM** (don't cross placenta)
4. **Some mothers produce IgG anti-A or anti-B** (these cross placenta)
5. Maternal IgG coats fetal RBCs → hemolysis

ABO vs Rh HDFN:

Feature	ABO HDFN	Rh HDFN
First pregnancy	**YES (common)**	**NO (requires sensitization)**
Severity	Usually mild-moderate	Can be severe (hydrops)
DAT	Weakly positive	Strongly positive
Spherocytes	Present	Absent
Anemia at birth	Mild	Can be severe
Hyperbilirubinemia	Common	Common
Prevention	None	RhoGAM

Bhutani Nomogram (Hour-Specific Bilirubin):

- Plots total bilirubin vs. age in hours
- Risk zones: Low, low-intermediate, high-intermediate, high
- Guides phototherapy and exchange transfusion decisions
- Patient at 18h with 14.2 mg/dL = **high-risk zone**

Phototherapy:

- **Mechanism:** Blue light (460-490 nm) converts unconjugated bilirubin to water-soluble isomers
- **Intensive phototherapy:** Multiple lights, high irradiance

- **Indications:** Based on hour-specific nomogram and risk factors

Exchange Transfusion:

- **Indications:**
  - ○ Bilirubin exceeds exchange threshold (~20 mg/dL term, lower if risk factors)
  - ○ Rising rapidly despite intensive phototherapy + IVIG
  - ○ Signs of bilirubin encephalopathy
- **Procedure:** Remove baby's blood, replace with donor blood (double volume exchange)
- **Risks:** Electrolyte abnormalities, infections, NEC, death (1%)

IVIG in ABO HDFN:

- **Mechanism:** Blocks Fc receptors on macrophages → decreases hemolysis
- **Indications:** Rapidly rising bilirubin despite phototherapy, approaching exchange levels
- **Dose:** 0.5-1 g/kg over 2-4 hours
- **Efficacy:** Reduces need for exchange transfusion by 50-75%

Kernicterus (Bilirubin Encephalopathy):

- **Acute:** Lethargy, hypotonia, poor feeding, high-pitched cry, opisthotonus
- **Chronic:** Choreoathetoid cerebral palsy, auditory neuropathy, dental enamel dysplasia, upward gaze paralysis
- **Prevention:** Early detection and aggressive treatment of hyperbilirubinemia

Teaching Points:

1. **ABO HDFN Can Occur in First Pregnancy:** Unlike Rh disease (requires prior sensitization); ~15% of pregnancies have ABO incompatibility, but only 1-3% develop significant hemolysis
2. **IgG vs IgM:** Only IgG crosses placenta; some type O mothers produce IgG anti-A/B (most have only IgM)
3. **Spherocytes:** Characteristic of ABO HDFN; partial antibody coating causes membrane loss → spherocyte formation
4. **Weakly Positive DAT:** ABO HDFN typically 0-1+ DAT (fewer antigen sites on baby RBCs); Rh HDFN typically 3-4+ DAT
5. **Mixed Field Agglutination:** In ABO HDFN, not all RBCs agglutinate (Type A baby has both A and O donor RBCs from mother); characteristic pattern
6. **Bhutani Nomogram:** Must use hour-specific bilirubin; cannot use "rule of thumb" (e.g., 5x age in days); nomogram accounts for age in hours
7. **Late Anemia:** Nadir hemoglobin at 2-6 weeks; ongoing hemolysis + decreased erythropoietin; monitor and may need transfusion
8. **No Prevention for ABO HDFN:** Unlike Rh (RhoGAM), no prevention available; cannot predict which type O mothers will produce IgG antibodies
9. **Reticulocyte Count:** Elevated in hemolysis (normal newborn 3-7%; hemolysis >7%); indicates bone marrow response
10. **G6PD Deficiency:** Consider if severe jaundice in at-risk populations (Mediterranean, African, Asian); exacerbated by hemolysis

Related Cases: Rh hemolytic disease, G6PD deficiency with neonatal jaundice, hereditary spherocytosis in newborn, breast milk jaundice

Case 11.5: Congenital Hypothyroidism

Clinical Presentation: A 14-day-old female term infant is referred to pediatric endocrinology clinic for abnormal newborn screen showing low T4 and elevated TSH. Baby was born at 39 weeks via normal vaginal delivery, birth weight 3.3 kg. Mother had uncomplicated pregnancy, no thyroid disease, no medications. Baby is currently breastfeeding well, having normal stools, and appears healthy to parents.

Physical Examination:

- Weight: 3.5 kg (appropriate weight gain)
- Vital signs: Temp 36.8°C (slightly low), HR 120, RR 38
- **Appears "well" but subtle signs on careful examination:**
- Large anterior and posterior fontanelles (>2.5 cm anterior)
- **Umbilical hernia** (small, reducible)
- **Hypotonia** (decreased muscle tone, frog-leg posture)
- **Prolonged jaundice** (mild, day 14 - should be resolving)
- Dry skin
- **Coarse facial features** (subtle - thick lips, macroglossia)
- **Hoarse cry**
- No goiter palpable

Newborn Screening Results (24-48 Hours of Life):

- **T4: 3.2 µg/dL LOW** (normal 6-12 µg/dL for newborn)
- **TSH: 88 mIU/L MARKEDLY ELEVATED** (normal <20 mIU/L)

Diagnostic Reasoning Questions:

1. What are the causes of congenital hypothyroidism?
2. Why is early detection and treatment critical?
3. How do thyroid function tests differ in newborns vs. adults?
4. What imaging studies help determine etiology?

Sequential Test Results:

Confirmatory Serum Thyroid Function Tests (Day 14):

Thyroid Panel:

- **Free T4: 0.4 ng/dL SEVERELY LOW** (normal 0.8-2.0 for newborn)
- **Total T4: 2.8 µg/dL LOW** (normal 6-12)
- **TSH: 145 mIU/L MARKEDLY ELEVATED** (normal 0.5-5.0 after first week)
- **T3: Low-normal** (less reliable in newborns)

Interpretation: Primary Congenital Hypothyroidism (low T4, elevated TSH indicates thyroid gland failure)

Thyroid Antibodies (Maternal and Infant):

- Infant anti-TPO antibodies: Negative
- Infant anti-thyroglobulin antibodies: Negative
- Maternal thyroid antibodies: Negative (excludes transplacental maternal antibodies)

Additional Labs:

- **Thyroglobulin: Undetectable** (suggests thyroid dysgenesis)
- Cholesterol: 185 mg/dL (elevated for age - hypothyroidism increases cholesterol)
- Newborn screen amino acids: Normal (excludes other metabolic disorders)

Imaging Studies:

Thyroid Ultrasound:

- **No thyroid tissue visualized in normal location (neck)**
- Thyroid bed empty
- No ectopic thyroid tissue identified on ultrasound

Thyroid Scintigraphy (Technetium-99m or I-123 Scan):

- **No uptake in normal thyroid location**
- **Uptake visualized at base of tongue** (lingual thyroid - ectopic thyroid tissue)
- Confirms: **Thyroid dysgenesis with ectopic gland**

Bone Age (Left Hand X-ray):

- **No distal femoral epiphysis visible** (should be present at term)
- **Delayed bone maturation** (suggests hypothyroidism was present in utero)

Final Diagnosis: Primary Congenital Hypothyroidism due to Thyroid Dysgenesis (Ectopic Lingual Thyroid)

Etiology of Congenital Hypothyroidism:

1. Thyroid Dysgenesis (85%): ← THIS PATIENT

- **Agenesis:** Complete absence of thyroid
- **Ectopia:** Ectopic thyroid tissue (lingual, sublingual) ← **PATIENT**
- **Hypoplasia:** Small, underdeveloped gland
- Usually sporadic, not inherited

2. Dyshormonogenesis (10-15%):

- Inherited defects in thyroid hormone synthesis
- Genes: TPO, DUOX2, SLC5A5, etc.
- Autosomal recessive
- Goiter often present

3. Transient Hypothyroidism (5-10%):

- Maternal antibodies (blocking TSH receptor)
- Iodine deficiency or excess
- Maternal antithyroid drugs
- Resolves within weeks to months

4. Central (Secondary/Tertiary) Hypothyroidism (Rare):

- Pituitary (TSH deficiency) or hypothalamic (TRH deficiency)
- Low/normal TSH with low T4
- Associated with hypopituitarism

Treatment Initiated Immediately (Day 14):

Levothyroxine (L-thyroxine):

- **Starting dose: 10-15 μg/kg/day** (37.5 μg daily for 3.5 kg infant)
- **IMMEDIATE TREATMENT CRITICAL** (every day of delay risks neurodevelopmental damage)
- Liquid formulation or crushed tablet mixed with breast milk
- Administer in morning, avoid soy formula (decreases absorption)

Monitoring Plan:

- Repeat thyroid function tests in **2 weeks** (ensure adequate dosing)
- Then every 1-2 months in first year (rapid growth, dose adjustments needed)
- **Goal: Normalize T4 within 2 weeks, TSH within 4 weeks**

Target Thyroid Levels on Treatment:

First 3 Years (Critical for Brain Development):

- Free T4: Upper half of normal range (1.2-2.0 ng/dL)
- TSH: 0.5-2.0 mIU/L (maintain slightly suppressed)

After Age 3:

- Free T4: Mid-normal range
- TSH: 0.5-4.0 mIU/L

Follow-Up Thyroid Testing:

2 Weeks (on 37.5 µg levothyroxine):

- Free T4: 1.6 ng/dL (excellent - upper normal)
- TSH: 8.2 mIU/L (decreasing but still elevated)
- Continue current dose

4 Weeks:

- Free T4: 1.8 ng/dL (excellent)
- TSH: 2.1 mIU/L (normalized ✓)
- Dose appropriate

3 Months:

- Free T4: 1.4 ng/dL (therapeutic)
- TSH: 1.8 mIU/L (excellent)
- Weight: 5.2 kg
- **Dose increased to 50 µg daily** (growth-based adjustment)

6 Months:

- Free T4: 1.5 ng/dL
- TSH: 1.2 mIU/L (well-controlled)
- Developmentally appropriate
- Sitting independently

12 Months:

- Free T4: 1.6 ng/dL
- TSH: 1.5 mIU/L
- Dose: 62.5 µg daily
- **Developmental milestones: All achieved on time ✓**
- Walking independently

Age 3 Years:

- **Developmental assessment: NORMAL cognition, language, motor skills ✓**
- IQ testing: Normal range
- **Treatment lifelong, excellent prognosis if treated early**

Neurodevelopmental Outcomes Based on Treatment Timing:

Treatment Started	IQ Outcome
<2 weeks	**Normal (85-115)** ← PATIENT
2-4 weeks	Mildly reduced (80-100)
1-3 months	Moderately reduced (70-85)
>3 months	Severely reduced (<70)

Treatment Started	IQ Outcome
Untreated	Severe intellectual disability (cretinism)

Clinical Features of Untreated Congenital Hypothyroidism:

- Severe intellectual disability (cretinism)
- Growth failure (short stature)
- Delayed bone age
- Coarse facial features, large tongue
- Umbilical hernia
- Constipation
- Prolonged jaundice
- Hypotonia, lethargy
- Bradycardia, hypothermia

Newborn Screening for Congenital Hypothyroidism:

Screening Strategies:

1. **Primary T4 + backup TSH** (used in some states)
2. **Primary TSH + backup T4** (more common)
3. **Simultaneous T4 and TSH** (most comprehensive)

Timing:

- Screen at 24-48 hours of life (after TSH surge)
- **TSH surge:** Physiologic TSH rise to 60-80 mIU/L at birth, then declines to <20 by 24-48h
- Screening too early (<24h): False positives from physiologic surge
- Preterm/sick infants: Repeat screen at discharge or 2 weeks

Recall/Confirmatory Testing:

- Abnormal screen → immediate serum T4 and TSH
- **DO NOT WAIT** for confirmatory results to start treatment if highly suspicious

Teaching Points:

1. **Early Treatment Critical:** Every day of delay risks permanent neurodevelopmental damage; start treatment immediately if screen abnormal, even before confirmation
2. **Thyroid Dysgenesis:** Most common cause (85%); ectopic thyroid (lingual most common), agenesis, or hypoplasia; usually sporadic, not inherited
3. **Normal-Appearing Newborn:** Most infants with congenital hypothyroidism appear normal at birth; subtle signs (prolonged jaundice, umbilical hernia, hypotonia, large fontanelles); newborn screening is essential
4. **TSH Surge:** Physiologic TSH peak (60-80 mIU/L) at birth, falls by 24-48h; screen after 24h to avoid false positives
5. **Age-Specific Reference Ranges:** Newborn T4 and TSH levels much higher than adults; first week TSH can be 5-20 mIU/L (normal); use age-appropriate ranges

6. **Treatment Goals:** Normalize T4 within 2 weeks, TSH within 4 weeks; maintain T4 in upper-normal range first 3 years (critical brain development)
7. **Dose Adjustments:** Frequent monitoring in infancy (rapid growth); dose based on weight, adjusted every 1-2 months first year
8. **Ectopic Thyroid:** Lingual thyroid most common ectopic location; functional but insufficient hormone production; scintigraphy confirms location
9. **Bone Age:** Delayed bone maturation in hypothyroidism; useful to assess duration and severity; distal femoral epiphysis absent = in utero hypothyroidism
10. **Lifelong Treatment:** Congenital hypothyroidism is permanent (except transient forms); annual monitoring once stable; excellent outcomes if treated early

Related Cases: Transient hypothyroidism from maternal antibodies, dyshormonogenesis with goiter, central hypothyroidism, iodine deficiency

---

Case 11.6: Inborn Error of Metabolism - Maple Syrup Urine Disease (MSUD)

Clinical Presentation: A 5-day-old term male infant is brought to ED by parents reporting poor feeding, lethargy, and unusual sweet odor to his urine for the past day. He was born at home and has not had newborn screening yet. Initially breastfed well but over the past 24 hours has become increasingly sleepy, refusing feeds, and developed vomiting. Parents are Mennonite (increased carrier frequency for MSUD in this population).

Physical Examination:

- **Lethargic, poor responsiveness**
- Temp 36.2°C (hypothermia), HR 160 (tachycardia), RR 44 (tachypnea)
- Weight: 3.1 kg (birth weight 3.4 kg - **10% weight loss**)
- **Abnormal movements:** Dystonia, intermittent opisthotonus (extensor posturing)
- **"Fencing" posture** (tonic neck reflex exaggerated)
- **Sweet, maple syrup/burnt sugar odor** in urine and cerumen (ear wax)
- Fontanelle full, not bulging
- Tone: Increased (hypertonia)

Initial Laboratory Findings (ED):

- **Glucose: 65 mg/dL** (low-normal, concerning in sick neonate)
- **Sodium: 128 mEq/L** (hyponatremia)
- **Bicarbonate: 12 mEq/L** (metabolic acidosis)
- **Anion gap: 22** (elevated)
- Ammonia: 45 μmol/L (normal; <100)
- Lactate: 2.8 mmol/L (mildly elevated)

Diagnostic Reasoning Questions:

1. What inborn errors of metabolism present in the neonatal period?
2. What is the significance of the "maple syrup" odor?
3. How are branched-chain amino acids metabolized?

413

4. What is the acute management of metabolic crisis?

Sequential Test Results:

Arterial Blood Gas:

- pH: 7.22 (acidemia)
- PaCO2: 32 mmHg (respiratory compensation)
- HCO3-: 12 mEq/L (metabolic acidosis)
- **Severe metabolic acidosis with appropriate respiratory compensation**

Urine Ketones:

- **Strongly positive (3+)** (ketonuria with minimal fasting concerning for metabolic disorder)

Plasma Amino Acid Analysis (STAT - Results in 4 Hours):

Branched-Chain Amino Acids (BCAAs):

- **Leucine: 3,850 μmol/L MARKEDLY ELEVATED** (normal 48-160)
- **Isoleucine: 980 μmol/L MARKEDLY ELEVATED** (normal 26-91)
- **Valine: 1,240 μmol/L MARKEDLY ELEVATED** (normal 74-321)
- **Alloisoleucine: Present** (pathognomonic for MSUD; not normally present)

Other Amino Acids:

- Alanine: Decreased
- Glutamine: Decreased
- All other amino acids: Relatively decreased (BCAAs dominate)

Urine Organic Acids (GC-MS):

- **Branched-chain ketoacids:**
    - **Ketoisocaproic acid** (from leucine)
    - **Ketoisovaleric acid** (from valine)
    - **Keto-β-methylvaleric acid** (from isoleucine)
- **Branched-chain hydroxy acids** also present
- **"Maple syrup" odor from sotolone** (compound in branched-chain ketoacids)

CRITICAL DIAGNOSIS: Classic Maple Syrup Urine Disease (MSUD) - Acute Neonatal Metabolic Crisis

MSUD Biochemistry:

Normal BCAA Metabolism:

1. Leucine, isoleucine, valine (branched-chain amino acids from protein)
2. Transamination → branched-chain ketoacids

414

3. **Branched-chain α-ketoacid dehydrogenase (BCKD) complex** → CoA derivatives
4. Further metabolism to acetyl-CoA, succinyl-CoA

MSUD Defect:

- **BCKD complex deficiency** (E1α, E1β, E2, or E3 subunit mutations)
- BCAAs and branched-chain ketoacids accumulate
- **Leucine is neurotoxic** (inhibits neurotransmitter transport, causes cerebral edema)

Immediate Management (Life-Saving):

Stop Protein Intake:

- **NPO (nothing by mouth)** - stop all protein/breast milk
- **Prevent further BCAA accumulation**

High-Calorie IV Fluids:

- **D10W with electrolytes** (10% dextrose promotes anabolism, reduces catabolism)
- Goal: 150-200 kcal/kg/day
- **Reverse catabolic state** (stops protein breakdown)

Correct Metabolic Acidosis:

- Sodium bicarbonate IV (target pH >7.30, HCO3 >18)

Hemodialysis (Gold Standard for Severe MSUD Crisis):

- **Urgent hemodialysis** for leucine >1,000 μmol/L or neurologic symptoms
- Rapidly removes BCAAs and ketoacids
- **CANNOT use peritoneal dialysis** (inadequate clearance)

Supportive Care:

- Treat cerebral edema: Elevate head, osmotherapy if needed
- Anticonvulsants if seizures
- Close neurologic monitoring

Serial BCAA Monitoring:

Hour 0 (Diagnosis):

- Leucine: 3,850 μmol/L (severe)
- Patient: Lethargic, dystonic

Hour 6 (On D10W, awaiting dialysis):

- Leucine: 3,920 μmol/L (stable/rising)

- Neurologic status: Worsening, decreased responsiveness

Hour 12 (After 6 hours of hemodialysis):

- **Leucine: 980 µmol/L** (significant improvement)
- Neurologic status: Improved alertness

Hour 24:

- Leucine: 450 µmol/L (near target)
- **Target leucine: 80-200 µmol/L**
- Patient: Alert, feeding BCAA-free formula

Day 3:

- Leucine: 180 µmol/L (therapeutic range)
- Isoleucine: 85 µmol/L
- Valine: 220 µmol/L
- **Reintroduce small amount of protein** (BCAA-restricted diet)

Day 7:

- Leucine: 145 µmol/L (excellent control)
- Neurologic exam: Normal tone, no dystonia
- Feeding: BCAA-free medical formula + measured amounts of breastmilk

Molecular Genetic Testing:

BCKDHA Gene Sequencing (E1α Subunit):

- **Mutation 1: c.1036C>T (p.Arg346Trp)** - Pathogenic
- **Mutation 2: c.632C>T (p.Thr211Met)** - Pathogenic, Mennonite founder mutation
- **Compound heterozygous**
- Inheritance: Autosomal recessive

Enzyme Activity:

- Lymphocyte BCKD activity: <2% of normal (classic MSUD)

MSUD Subtypes:

Type	BCKD Activity	Phenotype
Classic	**<2%**	**Neonatal crisis, severe ← PATIENT**
Intermediate	3-30%	Later onset, less severe
Intermittent	5-20%	Normal until stress, episodic crises
Thiamine-responsive	Variable	Responds to vitamin B1

416

Type	BCKD Activity	Phenotype
E3-deficient	<2%	MSUD + lactic acidosis

Long-Term Management:

Dietary Therapy:

- **BCAA-restricted diet** (lifelong)
- BCAA-free medical formula (Ketonex®)
- Measured amounts of natural protein (breast milk/foods)
- **Target plasma leucine: 80-200 µmol/L** (isoleucine, valine also monitored)
- Avoid fasting >4 hours (infancy)

Monitoring:

- **Plasma amino acids:** 2-3x/week (infancy), weekly (childhood), then as needed
- Adjust diet based on leucine levels
- Growth and development assessment

Sick Day Protocol:

- **At first sign of illness:** Stop natural protein, increase calories (simple sugars)
- Frequent BCAA monitoring
- May need hospitalization for IV fluids
- **Prevent catabolism** (protein breakdown releases BCAAs)

Liver Transplantation:

- Curative (liver produces majority of BCKD)
- Considered for severe cases, poor metabolic control
- Normalizes BCAA metabolism

Follow-Up (3 Months):

- Leucine: 120-180 µmol/L (excellent control)
- Weight: 5.8 kg (50th percentile)
- Development: Meeting milestones

Follow-Up (12 Months):

- Leucine: 100-160 µmol/L (well-controlled)
- Development: Normal cognition, language, motor
- Walking independently

Follow-Up (3 Years):

- IQ testing: Normal range (early treatment prevented brain damage)
- Continues BCAA-restricted diet

- Tolerates illness with sick day protocol

Newborn Screening for MSUD:

- **Tandem mass spectrometry (MS/MS)** detects elevated leucine/isoleucine
- Leucine/phenylalanine ratio, leucine/alanine ratio used
- Screen at 24-48 hours
- **This patient born at home, missed screening** - highlights importance

Untreated MSUD Outcomes:

- Neonatal death (without treatment)
- Severe intellectual disability
- Recurrent metabolic crises
- Cerebral edema, seizures
- Permanent neurologic damage

Teaching Points:

1. **MSUD Presentation:** Classic form presents 4-7 days of life with poor feeding, vomiting, lethargy, sweet odor, dystonia; untreated → coma, cerebral edema, death
2. **Maple Syrup Odor:** Pathognomonic; from sotolone in branched-chain ketoacids; detected in urine, sweat, cerumen; not all clinicians can detect
3. **Leucine Neurotoxicity:** Leucine >1,000 μmol/L causes cerebral edema, inhibits large neutral amino acid transport across blood-brain barrier, impairs neurotransmitter synthesis
4. **Alloisoleucine:** Stereoisomer of isoleucine; **pathognomonic for MSUD**; not normally present; formed when ketoacids accumulate
5. **Hemodialysis:** Acute treatment of choice for severe crisis; removes BCAAs rapidly; peritoneal dialysis inadequate; may need 12-24 hours
6. **Anabolic Therapy:** High-calorie IV fluids (D10W or higher) reverse catabolism, stop protein breakdown, prevent further BCAA release
7. **Sick Day Protocol:** Any illness = catabolic stress → protein breakdown → BCAA rise → crisis; aggressive early intervention essential
8. **BCAA Balance:** Must provide minimal amounts of leucine, isoleucine, valine (essential amino acids); cannot eliminate completely; balance is critical
9. **Thiamine-Responsive MSUD:** 25-40% of patients responsive to vitamin B1 (thiamine pyrophosphate is BCKD cofactor); trial of thiamine 10-1,000 mg/day
10. **Mennonite Population:** Founder mutation (c.632C>T) in BCKDHA gene; carrier frequency 1:71 (vs 1:150 general population); genetic screening available

Related Cases: Isovaleric acidemia, propionic acidemia, methylmalonic acidemia, urea cycle disorders, other organic acidemias

Chapter 12: Geriatric and Special Population Cases

Case 12.1: Anemia of Chronic Disease in Elderly Patient

Clinical Presentation: An 82-year-old woman presents to her primary care physician for routine follow-up. She has chronic complaints of fatigue, weakness, and decreased exercise tolerance over the past year. Medical history significant for rheumatoid arthritis (RA) for 15 years (moderately controlled), chronic kidney disease stage 3, and heart failure with preserved ejection fraction. She takes multiple medications and lives independently.

Physical Examination:

- BP 142/78, HR 78, RR 16, BMI 24
- Appears chronically ill, pale conjunctivae
- Cardiac: Regular rhythm, 2/6 systolic murmur
- Lungs: Clear
- Abdomen: Soft, no organomegaly
- Extremities: Bilateral hand deformities (RA), trace edema
- No lymphadenopathy

Current Medications:

- Methotrexate 15 mg weekly (RA)
- Prednisone 5 mg daily (RA)
- Furosemide 20 mg daily (CHF)
- Lisinopril 10 mg daily
- Atorvastatin 20 mg daily
- Omeprazole 20 mg daily (chronic use - 8 years)

Initial Laboratory Findings:

- **Hemoglobin: 9.8 g/dL LOW** (normal 12-16 for women)
- **MCV: 84 fL** (normocytic; normal 80-100)
- **MCHC: 32 g/dL** (normal)
- **RDW: 15.2%** (mildly elevated; normal 11.5-14.5)

Diagnostic Reasoning Questions:

1. What is the differential diagnosis for normocytic anemia in an elderly patient?
2. How does anemia of chronic disease differ from iron deficiency?
3. What role does inflammation play in anemia of chronic disease?
4. How do comorbidities and polypharmacy contribute to anemia?

Sequential Test Results:

Complete Blood Count:

- WBC: 7,800/μL (normal)
- Hemoglobin: 9.8 g/dL (anemia)
- Hematocrit: 29%
- **MCV: 84 fL** (normocytic, though borderline microcytic)
- Platelets: 425,000/μL (elevated - inflammation)
- **Reticulocyte count: 1.2%** (absolute 48,000/μL)
- **Reticulocyte production index (RPI): 0.7** (hypoproliferative; normal >2)

Peripheral Blood Smear:

- Normocytic, normochromic RBCs
- Mild anisocytosis (size variation)
- Mild rouleaux formation (stacking of RBCs - seen in inflammation)
- No schistocytes
- WBC morphology: Normal
- Platelets: Adequate

Iron Studies:

- **Serum iron: 28 μg/dL LOW** (normal 50-170)
- **TIBC: 210 μg/dL LOW** (normal 250-400)
- **Transferrin saturation: 13% LOW** (normal 20-50%)
- **Ferritin: 245 ng/mL NORMAL-HIGH** (normal 12-150 for women; often elevated in elderly)

Pattern: Low iron, **low TIBC**, normal/elevated ferritin → **Anemia of Chronic Disease (ACD)**

Comparison: ACD vs Iron Deficiency Anemia (IDA):

Parameter	ACD	IDA	Combined (ACD + IDA)
Serum iron	↓	↓	↓↓
TIBC	**↓ or normal**	↑	Normal or ↓
Transferrin sat	↓	↓↓	↓↓
Ferritin	**Normal or ↑**	↓↓ (<15)	Low-normal or ↓
Soluble transferrin receptor (sTfR)	Normal	↑	↑
sTfR/log ferritin ratio	<1	>2	1-2

Soluble Transferrin Receptor (sTfR):

- **sTfR: 18 nmol/L** (normal 10-28)
- **sTfR/log ferritin ratio: 0.8** (<1 suggests ACD alone, not IDA)
- Interpretation: **Pure ACD** (no evidence of true iron deficiency)

Hepcidin Level (Research/Specialty Lab):

- **Hepcidin: Elevated** (key mediator of ACD)
- Mechanism: Inflammation → IL-6 → hepatic hepcidin production → blocks ferroportin → iron sequestered in macrophages → functional iron deficiency

Inflammatory Markers:

- **ESR: 68 mm/hr ELEVATED** (normal <30 for age; RA activity)
- **CRP: 4.8 mg/dL ELEVATED** (normal <0.3; chronic inflammation)
- IL-6: Elevated (if measured; drives hepcidin)

Additional Workup:

Renal Function:

- Creatinine: 1.6 mg/dL (baseline 1.4-1.7)
- **eGFR: 32 mL/min/1.73m²** (CKD stage 3b)
- **Erythropoietin (EPO) level: 18 mIU/mL** (inappropriately low for degree of anemia)
- Expected EPO for Hgb 9.8 g/dL: >50-100 mIU/mL
- **Relative EPO deficiency** (CKD contributes to anemia)

Vitamin Levels:

- **Vitamin B12: 285 pg/mL** (low-normal; normal 200-900)
- **Folate: 6.2 ng/mL** (low-normal; normal >5.4)
- **Consider subclinical deficiency** (chronic PPI use impairs B12 absorption)

Methylmalonic Acid (MMA) and Homocysteine (Sensitive B12 Markers):

- **MMA: 485 nmol/L** (elevated; normal <270; suggests functional B12 deficiency)
- **Homocysteine: 22 µmol/L** (elevated; normal <15; suggests B12 and/or folate deficiency)
- **Interpretation:** Subclinical B12 deficiency contributing to anemia

Stool Occult Blood:

- **Negative x3** (no GI bleeding)

Additional Causes Considered:

Hemolysis Workup:

- LDH: 185 U/L (normal; no hemolysis)
- Haptoglobin: Normal
- Indirect bilirubin: Normal
- **No evidence of hemolysis**

Bone Marrow Evaluation (Not Initially Done - Reserved for Unclear Cases):

- Would show: Adequate iron stores (Prussian blue stain), but iron trapped in macrophages, decreased sideroblasts (RBC precursors with iron)

Final Diagnosis: Multifactorial Anemia in Elderly Patient:

1. **Anemia of Chronic Disease (Primary)** - Due to Rheumatoid Arthritis
2. **Anemia of Chronic Kidney Disease** - Relative EPO Deficiency
3. **Subclinical Vitamin B12 Deficiency** - Chronic PPI Use
4. **Medication-Related** - Methotrexate (folate antagonist)

Pathophysiology of Anemia of Chronic Disease:

1. **Hepcidin-mediated iron sequestration:** Inflammation → IL-6 → hepcidin → blocks iron release from macrophages
2. **Blunted EPO response:** Inflammatory cytokines suppress EPO production
3. **Shortened RBC lifespan:** Inflammatory cytokines, macrophage activation
4. **Bone marrow suppression:** TNF-α, IL-1, IFN-γ suppress erythropoiesis

Management:

Treat Underlying Inflammatory Condition:

- Optimize RA treatment (consider biologic DMARD if needed)
- Goal: Reduce CRP, ESR

Address Contributory Factors:

1. Vitamin B12 Supplementation:

- **Cyanocobalamin 1,000 µg IM monthly** OR
- **Oral B12 1,000-2,000 µg daily** (high-dose overcomes absorption issues)
- Discontinue or reduce PPI if possible (8 years is excessive)

2. Folate Supplementation:

- **Folic acid 1 mg daily** (especially important with methotrexate)

3. Consider EPO-Stimulating Agent (ESA):

- **Indications:** CKD + Hgb <10 g/dL, symptoms
- **Epoetin alfa or darbepoetin**
- Target Hgb: 10-11.5 g/dL (higher targets increase cardiovascular risk in elderly)
- **Must ensure adequate iron** (functional iron deficiency may require IV iron)

4. Iron Supplementation (Controversial in ACD):

- **Oral iron usually ineffective** (hepcidin blocks absorption)
- **IV iron (e.g., iron sucrose, ferric carboxymaltose):** May be beneficial in select cases

- Consider if ferritin <100 ng/mL and transferrin sat <20%
- This patient: Ferritin 245, likely will not respond to oral iron

5. Medication Review:

- Methotrexate: Continue (RA control priority), ensure folate supplementation
- Omeprazole: **Reduce or discontinue** (contributes to B12 malabsorption)

Follow-Up (3 Months):

- Hemoglobin: 10.8 g/dL (improved)
- B12: 485 pg/mL (repleted)
- MMA: 220 nmol/L (normalized)
- Homocysteine: 14 μmol/L (improved)
- ESR: 48 mm/hr (improved RA control)
- Patient reports improved energy

Follow-Up (6 Months with EPO + IV Iron):

- Hemoglobin: 11.2 g/dL (target achieved)
- Ferritin: 180 ng/mL
- Transferrin saturation: 22%
- ESR: 38 mm/hr
- Patient: Significantly improved functional status

Considerations in Elderly Anemia:

"Unexplained" Anemia of Aging:

- 30% of elderly anemia has no clear cause (myelodysplasia, clonal hematopoiesis, inflammaging)

Age-Specific Hemoglobin Thresholds:

- WHO anemia definition: <12 g/dL (women), <13 g/dL (men)
- Elderly often tolerate lower Hgb (cardiovascular adaptation)
- Symptomatic threshold varies (assess functional status)

Polypharmacy Effects:

- PPIs → B12 malabsorption
- NSAIDs → GI bleeding, renal impairment
- Anticoagulants → bleeding risk
- Chemotherapy (methotrexate) → bone marrow suppression

Teaching Points:

1. **ACD Diagnostic Criteria:** Normocytic anemia + chronic disease + low/normal TIBC + normal/elevated ferritin; may be microcytic if prolonged

2. **Iron Studies Interpretation:** ACD has low iron AND low TIBC (vs IDA: low iron, HIGH TIBC); ferritin elevated in ACD (acute phase reactant)
3. **Hepcidin Pathophysiology:** Master iron regulator; inflammation → hepcidin → blocks ferroportin → iron trapped in macrophages → functional iron deficiency
4. **Soluble Transferrin Receptor:** Distinguishes ACD from IDA; sTfR elevated in IDA (increased erythropoiesis demand), normal in pure ACD; sTfR/log ferritin ratio >2 = IDA
5. **Reticulocyte Production Index (RPI):** Corrects reticulocyte count for anemia and maturation time; RPI <2 = hypoproliferative (ACD, CKD, nutritional); RPI >2 = hyperproliferative (hemolysis, bleeding)
6. **CKD Anemia:** EPO deficiency primary mechanism; consider ESA if Hgb <10 g/dL; target 10-11.5 g/dL (higher targets increase CV risk)
7. **Multifactorial Anemia in Elderly:** Often multiple contributors (inflammation, CKD, nutritional deficiency, medication, GI loss); systematic workup essential
8. **PPI and B12:** Long-term PPI use (>12 months) increases B12 deficiency risk (requires gastric acid for B12-protein dissociation); measure MMA/homocysteine if B12 borderline
9. **IV Iron in ACD:** Oral iron ineffective (hepcidin blocks absorption); IV iron may overcome hepcidin, especially with ESA therapy
10. **Functional Status Priority:** In elderly, focus on symptoms, quality of life, functional capacity; transfusion thresholds lower (Hgb 7-8 g/dL unless symptomatic/cardiovascular disease)

Related Cases: Pure iron deficiency anemia, myelodysplastic syndrome in elderly, B12 deficiency with neurologic manifestations, anemia in heart failure

Case 12.2: Polypharmacy and Drug Interactions

Clinical Presentation: An 78-year-old man presents to ED with confusion, generalized weakness, and a fall at home. His wife reports he has been "not himself" for 3 days, with increased confusion and unsteady gait. She found him on the bathroom floor this morning. No witnessed loss of consciousness. He sees multiple specialists and takes "a lot of medications."

Medical History:

- Atrial fibrillation (on warfarin)
- Heart failure with reduced EF (30%)
- Chronic kidney disease stage 3
- Type 2 diabetes
- Hypertension
- Depression
- Benign prostatic hyperplasia
- Chronic pain (osteoarthritis)
- GERD

Physical Examination:

- BP 98/62 (hypotensive), HR 52 (bradycardic), RR 18, Temp 98.4°F
- **Confused, disoriented to time and place**
- **Dry mucous membranes** (dehydration)
- Cardiac: Irregularly irregular rhythm (AF), no murmurs
- **Delayed capillary refill**
- Neuro: **Generalized weakness, tremor**
- **Ecchymoses on arms** (bruising)

Medication List (Brought by Wife - 14 Medications):

1. Warfarin 5 mg daily
2. Metoprolol 100 mg BID
3. Furosemide 40 mg BID
4. Lisinopril 20 mg daily
5. Digoxin 0.25 mg daily
6. Metformin 1,000 mg BID
7. Insulin glargine 30 units qHS
8. Sertraline 100 mg daily
9. Tamsulosin 0.4 mg daily
10. Omeprazole 40 mg daily
11. **Ibuprofen 600 mg TID** (recently added for back pain - over-the-counter)
12. **Ciprofloxacin 500 mg BID** (started 5 days ago for UTI by urgent care)
13. Acetaminophen 650 mg PRN
14. Docusate 100 mg daily

Diagnostic Reasoning Questions:

1. What drug-drug interactions may be contributing to this presentation?
2. How do age-related physiologic changes affect drug metabolism?
3. What laboratory abnormalities suggest drug toxicity?
4. How should polypharmacy be deprescribed safely?

Sequential Test Results:

Initial Laboratory Findings:

Basic Metabolic Panel:

- **Sodium: 128 mEq/L LOW** (hyponatremia)
- **Potassium: 5.8 mEq/L ELEVATED** (hyperkalemia)
- Chloride: 96 mEq/L
- **Bicarbonate: 18 mEq/L** (metabolic acidosis)
- **BUN: 58 mg/dL ELEVATED**
- **Creatinine: 2.8 mg/dL ELEVATED** (baseline 1.4 mg/dL - **acute kidney injury**)
- **eGFR: 22 mL/min/1.73m²** (acute decline from baseline 45)
- Glucose: 68 mg/dL (hypoglycemia)

Coagulation:

- **PT: 38 seconds MARKEDLY PROLONGED** (normal 11-13.5)
- **INR: 6.8 CRITICAL** (target 2-3 for AF)
- aPTT: 48 seconds (prolonged)

Complete Blood Count:

- Hemoglobin: 10.2 g/dL (baseline 11.5 - decreased)
- **Platelets: 95,000/µL** (thrombocytopenia)
- WBC: 12,500/µL

Liver Function:

- AST: 45 U/L (mildly elevated)
- ALT: 52 U/L (mildly elevated)
- Alkaline phosphatase: 85 U/L (normal)

Cardiac Biomarkers:

- **Digoxin level: 2.8 ng/mL TOXIC** (therapeutic 0.5-2.0 ng/mL)
- Troponin: Mildly elevated (demand ischemia)
- BNP: 850 pg/mL (elevated)

ECG:

- **Heart rate: 48 bpm** (bradycardia)
- Atrial fibrillation with slow ventricular response

- **ST depression, T wave changes** ("scooped" ST segments - digitalis effect)
- **Occasional PVCs**

Urinalysis:

- WBC: 15-20/hpf
- Bacteria: Many
- Nitrites: Positive
- Confirms UTI (reason for ciprofloxacin)

CRITICAL FINDINGS:

1. **Digoxin toxicity** (level 2.8 ng/mL, bradycardia, ECG changes)
2. **Over-anticoagulation** (INR 6.8, bleeding risk)
3. **Acute kidney injury** (Cr 2.8 from 1.4)
4. **Hyperkalemia** (5.8 mEq/L)
5. **Hyponatremia** (128 mEq/L)
6. **Hypoglycemia** (68 mg/dL)

Drug Interaction Analysis:

Interaction #1: Ciprofloxacin + Warfarin

- **Mechanism:** Ciprofloxacin inhibits CYP2C9 (warfarin metabolism) → increased warfarin levels → over-anticoagulation
- **Result:** INR 6.8 (critical)
- **Clinical impact:** Bruising, bleeding risk

Interaction #2: Ciprofloxacin + Digoxin

- **Mechanism:** Ciprofloxacin inhibits P-glycoprotein (digoxin transport) → decreased renal clearance → digoxin accumulation
- **Result:** Digoxin 2.8 ng/mL (toxic)
- **Clinical impact:** Bradycardia, confusion, weakness, nausea

Interaction #3: NSAIDs (Ibuprofen) + ACE Inhibitor (Lisinopril) + Diuretic (Furosemide) = "Triple Whammy"

- **Mechanism:** NSAIDs → renal vasoconstriction, ACE-I → efferent arteriole dilation, diuretic → volume depletion → **acute kidney injury**
- **Result:** Cr 2.8 (from 1.4), eGFR 22
- **Clinical impact:** AKI, hyperkalemia, hypotension

Interaction #4: AKI → Accumulation of Renally Cleared Drugs

- **Digoxin** (70% renal excretion): Levels increase with reduced GFR
- **Metformin** (renal excretion): Risk of lactic acidosis (contraindicated if eGFR <30)

Interaction #5: ACE Inhibitor + ARB/K+-Sparing Diuretic + AKI

- **Mechanism:** Lisinopril + AKI → hyperkalemia
- **Result:** K+ 5.8 mEq/L

Interaction #6: SSRI (Sertraline) + Warfarin

- **Mechanism:** SSRIs inhibit platelet function, sertraline may inhibit CYP2C9 → increased bleeding risk
- **Result:** Contributes to elevated INR

Interaction #7: Metformin + AKI

- **Lactic acidosis risk:** Metformin accumulates with eGFR <30
- Bicarbonate 18 mEq/L (metabolic acidosis - early lactic acidosis?)

Age-Related Pharmacokinetic Changes:

Absorption:

- Decreased gastric acid (↓ B12, iron absorption)
- Decreased GI motility

Distribution:

- ↓ Lean body mass, ↑ body fat → lipophilic drugs (digoxin, benzodiazepines) have increased half-life
- ↓ Albumin → more free drug (warfarin, phenytoin)
- ↓ Total body water → higher drug concentrations (digoxin)

Metabolism:

- ↓ Hepatic mass (30% by age 80)
- ↓ CYP enzyme activity → slower phase I metabolism
- Phase II metabolism (conjugation) preserved

Excretion:

- ↓ Renal mass (30-50% by age 80)
- ↓ GFR (eGFR declines ~1 mL/min/year after age 40)
- Renally cleared drugs accumulate (digoxin, metformin, antibiotics)

Immediate Management:

1. Digoxin Toxicity:

- **STOP digoxin**

- **Digoxin-specific antibody fragments (DigiFab):** Consider if life-threatening (severe bradycardia, VT, K+ >5.5)
- Cardiac monitoring
- Avoid calcium (precipitates arrhythmias in digoxin toxicity)
- Correct electrolytes cautiously

2. Over-Anticoagulation (INR 6.8):

- **HOLD warfarin**
- **Vitamin K 2.5-5 mg PO** (lowers INR in 12-24 hours)
- Monitor for bleeding
- Recheck INR in 24 hours

3. Acute Kidney Injury:

- **STOP nephrotoxic drugs:** Ibuprofen, lisinopril (temporarily)
- **IV fluids:** NS 100 mL/hr (cautious in heart failure)
- Monitor urine output, electrolytes

4. Hyperkalemia (K+ 5.8):

- **Calcium gluconate 1g IV** (cardiac membrane stabilization)
- **Insulin 10 units + D50W 25g IV** (shift K+ intracellularly)
- **Sodium polystyrene sulfonate (Kayexalate)** (bind K+ in GI tract)
- **Stop ACE inhibitor** temporarily

5. Hyponatremia (Na 128):

- **Free water restrict**
- Evaluate for SIADH (sertraline can cause)
- Monitor carefully (correct slowly, <8 mEq/L/24h to avoid osmotic demyelination)

6. Hypoglycemia:

- **D50W 25g IV** (immediate)
- Reduce insulin dose (AKI decreases insulin clearance)
- **STOP metformin** (eGFR <30 contraindication)

7. Ciprofloxacin:

- Complete UTI treatment but **no further drug interactions**
- Consider alternative antibiotic if longer course needed

Drug Reconciliation and Deprescribing:

Medications to STOP:

1. **Digoxin** - Toxic, questionable benefit in this patient

2. **Ibuprofen** - Caused AKI, bleeding risk with warfarin
3. **Metformin** - Contraindicated with eGFR <30
4. **Lisinopril** - Hold temporarily (AKI, hyperkalemia); reassess after recovery

Medications to ADJUST: 5. **Warfarin** - Hold until INR therapeutic, then restart at lower dose (monitor with ciprofloxacin) 6. **Furosemide** - Reduce to 20 mg daily (volume depleted) 7. **Metoprolol** - Reduce to 50 mg BID (bradycardia) 8. **Insulin glargine** - Reduce to 20 units (AKI, hypoglycemia)

Medications to CONTINUE: 9. Sertraline (but monitor for SIADH/hyponatremia) 10. Tamsulosin (BPH symptoms) 11. Omeprazole (though consider reducing dose or PPI holiday) 12. Acetaminophen PRN 13. Docusate

Follow-Up Labs (24 Hours):

- Digoxin: 1.8 ng/mL (decreasing)
- INR: 3.2 (improving)
- Creatinine: 2.1 mg/dL (improving with fluids, stopping NSAIDs)
- Potassium: 4.8 mEq/L (corrected)
- Sodium: 131 mEq/L (improving)
- Glucose: 105 mg/dL (stable)

Follow-Up (48 Hours):

- **Clinically improved:** Alert, oriented, no bradycardia (HR 68)
- Digoxin: 1.2 ng/mL
- INR: 2.4
- Creatinine: 1.6 mg/dL (near baseline)
- K+: 4.4 mEq/L

Discharge (Day 4):

- **Medication list reduced from 14 to 10**
- Patient and wife educated on drug interactions
- Medication reconciliation with primary care
- Avoid OTC NSAIDs
- Alert bracelet for warfarin

Follow-Up (2 Weeks, Outpatient):

- Creatinine: 1.5 mg/dL (baseline)
- INR: 2.6 (therapeutic on lower warfarin dose)
- Patient doing well, no confusion

Final Diagnosis: Polypharmacy with Multiple Drug-Drug Interactions Leading to:

1. Digoxin Toxicity (ciprofloxacin interaction + AKI)
2. Over-Anticoagulation (ciprofloxacin-warfarin interaction)
3. Acute Kidney Injury ("Triple Whammy" - NSAID + ACE-I + Diuretic)
4. Hyperkalemia (ACE-I + AKI)

5. Hypoglycemia (AKI impairing insulin/metformin clearance)
6. Hyponatremia (SSRI-induced SIADH + diuretics)

Teaching Points:

1. **Polypharmacy Definition:** ≥5 medications (this patient had 14); associated with adverse drug events, falls, cognitive impairment, hospitalization
2. **Drug-Drug Interactions:** Ciprofloxacin is potent CYP and P-gp inhibitor (interacts with warfarin, digoxin, theophylline); always check interactions when adding medications
3. **"Triple Whammy":** NSAID + ACE-I/ARB + Diuretic = high risk for AKI; avoid in elderly, CKD; counsel patients on OTC NSAID dangers
4. **Digoxin in Elderly:** Narrow therapeutic index; highly protein-bound and renally cleared; toxicity common with AKI, drug interactions; consider discontinuation (marginal benefit in AF)
5. **Beers Criteria:** List of potentially inappropriate medications in elderly; includes: digoxin >0.125 mg, NSAIDs, benzodiazepines, anticholinergics, PPIs >8 weeks
6. **Age-Related Pharmacokinetics:** ↓ renal function (most important), ↓ hepatic metabolism, ↑ fat distribution, ↓ albumin → adjust doses, avoid nephrotoxic/hepatotoxic drugs
7. **Deprescribing:** Systematic process of stopping medications when harm outweighs benefit; prioritize: anticholinergics, sedatives, NSAIDs, duplicate therapies
8. **Warfarin Monitoring:** Highly susceptible to interactions (CYP2C9, CYP3A4, vitamin K, protein binding); antibiotics commonly increase INR (ciprofloxacin, metronidazole, TMP-SMX)
9. **Metformin and AKI:** Contraindicated if eGFR <30 (lactic acidosis risk); hold if acute illness, contrast administration, or AKI; restart when eGFR >30 and stable
10. **Medication Reconciliation:** Essential at every encounter; include OTC medications, herbals, supplements; use teach-back method to ensure understanding

Related Cases: Warfarin-drug interactions, NSAID-induced AKI, digoxin toxicity, lactic acidosis from metformin, serotonin syndrome

---

Case 12.3: Vitamin Deficiencies in Malabsorption

Clinical Presentation: A 76-year-old woman presents to her physician with progressive weakness, numbness and tingling in her feet for 6 months, and recent difficulty with balance leading to two falls. She also reports chronic diarrhea (3-4 loose stools daily for years), unintentional 20-pound weight loss over 1 year, and easy bruising. History of celiac disease diagnosed 15 years ago, though admits poor adherence to gluten-free diet. Also has chronic pancreatitis from alcohol use (sober 10 years).

Physical Examination:

- BMI: 18.5 (underweight)
- Appears cachectic, pale
- **Glossitis** (smooth, beefy red tongue)
- **Angular cheilitis** (mouth corner cracks)
- **Petechiae on lower extremities**
- **Ecchymoses on arms**

431

- Abdomen: Soft, mild epigastric tenderness, no organomegaly
- **Neurologic:**
  - **Decreased vibration sense in feet** (posterior column)
  - **Decreased position sense**
  - **Absent ankle reflexes**
  - **Positive Romberg sign** (sensory ataxia)
  - **Gait ataxia**

Current Medications:

- Pancreatic enzyme replacement (often forgets)
- Calcium/Vitamin D supplement (intermittent)

Diagnostic Reasoning Questions:

1. What vitamin deficiencies occur with malabsorption?
2. How do celiac disease and chronic pancreatitis cause malabsorption?
3. What are the neurologic manifestations of vitamin deficiencies?
4. How are fat-soluble vs. water-soluble vitamin deficiencies diagnosed?

Sequential Test Results:

Complete Blood Count:

- **Hemoglobin: 8.2 g/dL SEVERELY LOW** (normal 12-16)
- **MCV: 118 fL MARKEDLY ELEVATED** (macrocytic; normal 80-100)
- **WBC: 3,200/μL** (leukopenia)
- **Platelets: 85,000/μL** (thrombocytopenia)
- **Pancytopenia with macrocytic anemia**

Peripheral Blood Smear:

- **Macro-ovalocytes** (large, oval RBCs - B12/folate deficiency)
- **Hypersegmented neutrophils** (>5% with ≥6 lobes; pathognomonic for megaloblastic anemia)
- Anisocytosis, poikilocytosis
- No schistocytes

Reticulocyte Count:

- **0.5%** (absolute 16,000/μL) **LOW** (hypoproliferative; expected >2% with anemia)

Vitamin B12 and Folate:

- **Vitamin B12: 110 pg/mL SEVERELY LOW** (normal 200-900)
- **Folate: 2.8 ng/mL LOW** (normal >5.4)
- **Combined B12 and folate deficiency**

Metabolites (Confirm Functional Deficiency):

- **Methylmalonic acid (MMA): 1,850 nmol/L MARKEDLY ELEVATED** (normal <270)
  - Elevated in B12 deficiency (B12 cofactor for methylmalonyl-CoA mutase)
- **Homocysteine: 68 μmol/L MARKEDLY ELEVATED** (normal <15)
  - Elevated in both B12 and folate deficiency

Interpretation:

- **MMA elevated + Homocysteine elevated = B12 deficiency**
- **Homocysteine elevated with normal MMA** = Folate deficiency or B6 deficiency
- Both B12 and folate deficient in this patient

Coagulation Studies:

- **PT-INR: 1.8 PROLONGED** (normal 0.9-1.1)
- **aPTT: 42 seconds** (mildly prolonged; normal 25-35)
- **Vitamin K deficiency suspected** (fat-soluble vitamin malabsorption)

Fat-Soluble Vitamins:

Vitamin A:

- **Serum retinol: 18 μg/dL LOW** (normal 30-80)
- Clinical: Night blindness reported on questioning

Vitamin D:

- **25-OH Vitamin D: 8 ng/mL SEVERELY DEFICIENT** (normal >30)
- **Calcium: 7.8 mg/dL LOW** (normal 8.5-10.5)
- **Phosphorus: 2.1 mg/dL** (low-normal)
- **PTH: 125 pg/mL ELEVATED** (normal 10-65; secondary hyperparathyroidism)
- **Alkaline phosphatase: 185 U/L ELEVATED** (bone turnover)

Vitamin E:

- **Alpha-tocopherol: 3.2 mg/L LOW** (normal 5-20)
- Can contribute to neuropathy

Vitamin K:

- Measured indirectly by coagulation studies (PT prolonged)
- **PIVKA-II (Protein Induced by Vitamin K Absence): Elevated** (if measured)

Other Deficiencies:

Iron Studies:

- Serum iron: 28 μg/dL (low)
- TIBC: 420 μg/dL (elevated)

- Ferritin: 12 ng/mL (low)
- **Iron deficiency** (from malabsorption and possible GI blood loss from celiac)

Zinc:

- **Serum zinc: 42 µg/dL LOW** (normal 70-120)
- Clinical: Hair loss, skin changes, impaired wound healing

Malabsorption Workup:

Celiac Serology (Assess Disease Activity):

- **tTG-IgA: 125 U/mL POSITIVE** (normal <20)
- Total IgA: Normal
- **Active celiac disease** (poor diet adherence)

Fecal Elastase:

- **<50 µg/g stool SEVERELY LOW** (normal >200)
- Confirms **pancreatic exocrine insufficiency** (chronic pancreatitis)

Fecal Fat (72-Hour Collection):

- **28 g/day ELEVATED** (normal <7 g/day)
- **Steatorrhea** (fat malabsorption)

Small Bowel Imaging:

- **CT enterography:** Dilated small bowel loops, mucosal edema (active celiac)

Bone Density (DEXA Scan):

- **T-score: -3.2 (spine) OSTEOPOROSIS**
- Multiple vertebral compression fractures
- Result of chronic vitamin D/calcium malabsorption

Neurologic Testing:

Nerve Conduction Studies:

- **Reduced sensory nerve action potentials** (peripheral neuropathy)
- Motor conduction: Mildly reduced

MRI Spine:

- **Posterior column signal changes** (subacute combined degeneration from B12 deficiency)

Final Diagnosis: Multiple Vitamin Deficiencies Secondary to Malabsorption:

1. **Severe Vitamin B12 Deficiency** - Megaloblastic anemia, subacute combined degeneration (neurologic)
2. **Folate Deficiency** - Contributing to megaloblastic anemia
3. **Vitamin D Deficiency** - Secondary hyperparathyroidism, osteoporosis
4. **Vitamin K Deficiency** - Coagulopathy
5. **Vitamin A Deficiency** - Night blindness
6. **Vitamin E Deficiency** - Peripheral neuropathy
7. **Iron Deficiency** - Microcytic component (mixed anemia)
8. **Zinc Deficiency**

Underlying Causes:

- **Active celiac disease** (small bowel villous atrophy → malabsorption)
- **Pancreatic exocrine insufficiency** (fat malabsorption → fat-soluble vitamins)

Pathophysiology of Malabsorption:

Celiac Disease:

- Villous atrophy in duodenum/proximal jejunum
- Impaired absorption: Iron, folate, B12 (if extensive), calcium, fat-soluble vitamins
- Brush border enzyme loss

Chronic Pancreatitis:

- Pancreatic enzyme deficiency (lipase, protease, amylase)
- **Fat malabsorption** (lipase deficiency → steatorrhea)
- **Fat-soluble vitamins** (A, D, E, K) require bile and pancreatic lipase

Treatment:

Immediate Replacement:

1. Vitamin B12:

- **Cyanocobalamin 1,000 μg IM daily x 1 week**
- Then 1,000 μg IM weekly x 4 weeks
- Then 1,000 μg IM monthly lifelong
- **Oral ineffective** (malabsorption)

2. Folate:

- **Folic acid 5 mg PO daily**
- Continue 3-4 months, reassess

3. Vitamin D:

- **Ergocalciferol 50,000 IU weekly x 8-12 weeks** (repletion)

435

- Then 1,000-2,000 IU daily (maintenance)
- **Calcium carbonate 1,200 mg daily**

4. Vitamin K:

- **Phytonadione (Vitamin K1) 10 mg PO daily x 3 days**
- Monitor INR

5. Vitamin A:

- **Retinol 10,000-25,000 IU PO daily x 1-2 weeks**
- Then maintenance 5,000 IU daily

6. Vitamin E:

- **Alpha-tocopherol 400-800 IU PO daily**

7. Iron:

- **Ferrous sulfate 325 mg PO BID**
- Take with vitamin C (enhances absorption)

8. Zinc:

- **Zinc sulfate 220 mg PO daily**

9. Pancreatic Enzyme Replacement:

- **Increase dose and ensure compliance**
- Take with all meals and snacks
- Goal: Reduce steatorrhea, improve fat-soluble vitamin absorption

Address Underlying Causes:

Celiac Disease:

- **Strict gluten-free diet** (essential)
- Dietitian referral
- Repeat tTG in 6-12 months (confirm response)

Neurologic Monitoring:

- **Urgent B12 replacement** (prevent permanent neurologic damage)
- Subacute combined degeneration may partially reverse if caught early

Follow-Up Labs (4 Weeks):

- Hemoglobin: 10.8 g/dL (improving)

436

- MCV: 102 fL (decreasing)
- Reticulocyte count: 8% (brisk response to B12/folate)
- B12: 485 pg/mL (repleted)
- Folate: 12 ng/mL (repleted)
- MMA: 420 nmol/L (improving but still elevated)
- Homocysteine: 22 μmol/L (improving)
- Calcium: 8.9 mg/dL (improving)
- 25-OH Vitamin D: 28 ng/mL (improving)
- INR: 1.1 (normalized with vitamin K)

Follow-Up (3 Months):

- Hemoglobin: 12.2 g/dL (normalized)
- MCV: 92 fL (normalized)
- Neurologic exam: **Improved vibration/position sense** (partial recovery)
- Gait: Improved, still mild ataxia (may be permanent)
- Weight: Gained 8 pounds (on gluten-free diet, compliant with enzymes)

Follow-Up (6 Months):

- tTG-IgA: 18 U/mL (normalized - celiac controlled)
- Repeat fecal fat: 5 g/day (normalized with enzyme replacement)
- All vitamin levels: Therapeutic ranges
- DEXA scan (12 months): T-score -2.6 (osteopenia; improved from -3.2)

Long-Term Management:

- **Lifelong strict gluten-free diet**
- **Lifelong B12 injections** (malabsorption)
- **Pancreatic enzyme replacement** with all meals
- **Fat-soluble vitamin supplementation**
- **Annual vitamin level monitoring**
- **Bone density monitoring** every 1-2 years
- **Neurologic exams** (monitor for progression)

Neurologic Outcomes:

- **Subacute combined degeneration:** Partially reversible if treated within 6 months; permanent if >12 months
- This patient: Mixed outcome (some improvement, residual deficits)

Teaching Points:

1. **Malabsorption Sites:** Duodenum (iron, folate, calcium); Jejunum (fat-soluble vitamins, B12-intrinsic factor complex); Ileum (B12, bile salts)
2. **Megaloblastic Anemia:** Macrocytic anemia (MCV >100) + hypersegmented neutrophils; caused by B12 or folate deficiency; impaired DNA synthesis
3. **MMA vs. Homocysteine:** MMA specific for B12 (elevated in B12 deficiency only); Homocysteine elevated in both B12 and folate deficiency; use to distinguish

4. **Subacute Combined Degeneration:** B12 deficiency → demyelination of posterior columns (vibration/position) and lateral corticospinal tracts (spasticity, weakness); IRREVERSIBLE if untreated >6-12 months
5. **Fat-Soluble Vitamins (ADEK):** Require bile salts and pancreatic lipase for absorption; deficient in cholestasis, pancreatic insufficiency, celiac disease
6. **Celiac Disease:** Prevalence 1%; screen with tTG-IgA + total IgA; confirm with small bowel biopsy; lifelong gluten-free diet; complications include lymphoma, osteoporosis
7. **Pancreatic Exocrine Insufficiency:** Diagnosed with fecal elastase <200 µg/g; treat with pancreatic enzyme replacement (lipase >40,000-90,000 units per meal)
8. **Vitamin K Deficiency:** Prolonged PT (factors II, VII, IX, X depend on vitamin K); aPTT prolonged in severe cases; treat with phytonadione (K1)
9. **Secondary Hyperparathyroidism:** Vitamin D deficiency → low calcium → PTH elevation → bone resorption (elevated alkaline phosphatase)
10. **Osteomalacia/Osteoporosis:** Vitamin D/calcium malabsorption → poor bone mineralization; increased fracture risk; DEXA screening essential in malabsorption

Related Cases: Pernicious anemia (intrinsic factor deficiency), tropical sprue, Whipple disease, short bowel syndrome, bariatric surgery malabsorption

---

Case 12.4: Monoclonal Gammopathy of Undetermined Significance (MGUS) vs. Multiple Myeloma

Clinical Presentation: A 72-year-old man presents to his primary care physician for routine follow-up. He has been generally well but reports mild fatigue and occasional low back pain for several months, which he attributes to "getting older." Incidentally, total protein was noted to be elevated (9.2 g/dL) on recent metabolic panel done for medication monitoring. No weight loss, fevers, night sweats, or infections. No bone pain except mild chronic back pain.

Physical Examination:

- Vital signs: Normal
- Appears well, no acute distress
- No pallor, no lymphadenopathy
- Cardiovascular, respiratory, abdominal exams: Normal
- Musculoskeletal: Mild lumbar tenderness, no bony tenderness elsewhere
- Neurologic: Normal

Past Medical History:

- Hypertension (well-controlled)
- Hyperlipidemia
- Osteoarthritis
- No prior malignancies

Initial Laboratory Findings:

- **Total protein: 9.2 g/dL ELEVATED** (normal 6.0-8.0)

438

- **Albumin: 3.8 g/dL** (normal)
- **Globulin (calculated): 5.4 g/dL ELEVATED** (normal 2.0-3.5)
- **Albumin/Globulin ratio: 0.7 REVERSED** (normal >1.0)

Diagnostic Reasoning Questions:

1. What is the differential diagnosis for elevated globulin fraction?
2. How are monoclonal gammopathies evaluated?
3. What distinguishes MGUS from multiple myeloma?
4. What are the criteria for smoldering vs. active myeloma?

Sequential Test Results:

Serum Protein Electrophoresis (SPEP):

- **M-spike present in gamma region**
- **M-protein concentration: 2.8 g/dL**
- Albumin: Normal
- Alpha-1, Alpha-2, Beta globulins: Normal
- **Gamma region:** Tall, narrow peak (monoclonal protein)

Immunofixation Electrophoresis (IFE):

- **Monoclonal IgG kappa detected**
- Heavy chain: IgG
- Light chain: Kappa
- **Diagnosis: IgG kappa monoclonal gammopathy**

Quantitative Immunoglobulins:

- **IgG: 3,250 mg/dL ELEVATED** (normal 700-1,600)
- IgA: 180 mg/dL (normal)
- IgM: 95 mg/dL (normal)
- **Immunoparesis:** Suppression of uninvolved immunoglobulins (IgA, IgM normal - no suppression)

Serum Free Light Chains (FLC):

- **Kappa FLC: 42 mg/L** (normal 3.3-19.4) **ELEVATED**
- **Lambda FLC: 18 mg/L** (normal 5.7-26.3)
- **Kappa/Lambda ratio: 2.3** (normal 0.26-1.65) **ABNORMAL**
- Involved/uninvolved ratio: 2.3 (involved FLC is kappa)

Urine Studies:

24-Hour Urine Protein Electrophoresis (UPEP):

- **Bence Jones protein (monoclonal kappa light chains): Present**

- **Quantification: 180 mg/24 hours** (small amount)

Complete Blood Count:

- Hemoglobin: 12.8 g/dL (normal 13.5-17.5 for men; borderline low)
- WBC: 6,200/μL (normal)
- Platelets: 245,000/μL (normal)
- **No cytopenias**

Comprehensive Metabolic Panel:

- **Creatinine: 1.3 mg/dL** (baseline; eGFR 55 mL/min - CKD stage 3)
- **Calcium: 10.8 mg/dL ELEVATED** (normal 8.5-10.5)
- Corrected for albumin: 10.9 mg/dL (still elevated)
- Albumin: 3.8 g/dL (normal)

Additional Labs:

Beta-2 Microglobulin:

- **β2M: 2.8 mg/L** (normal <2.5; mildly elevated)
- Prognostic marker in myeloma

LDH:

- 185 U/L (normal)

Bone Marrow Biopsy:

Indication: Evaluate extent of plasma cell infiltration

Bone Marrow Aspirate and Biopsy:

- **Plasma cells: 12%** (normal <5%)
- **Clonality confirmed:** Kappa light chain restriction by flow cytometry
- **Morphology:** Mixture of normal and abnormal plasma cells, no increased blasts
- Megakaryocytes, erythroid, myeloid lineages: Normal

Flow Cytometry:

- **Clonal plasma cells: CD138+, CD38+, cytoplasmic kappa+**
- Aberrant expression: CD56+ (associated with myeloma)
- Lambda light chain: Negative (confirms kappa restriction)

Imaging Studies:

Skeletal Survey (X-rays of skull, spine, ribs, pelvis, long bones):

- **Multiple lytic lesions:**
  - 2 cm lytic lesion in left humeral head
  - 1.5 cm lytic lesion in right pelvic bone
  - Compression fracture of L2 vertebra (pathologic fracture)
- Punched-out lesions in skull (multiple)
- **CRAB criteria: Bone lesions present**

Whole-Body Low-Dose CT (or PET-CT if available):

- Confirms multiple lytic bone lesions
- No extramedullary plasmacytomas

MRI Spine:

- Multiple focal lesions in vertebral bodies
- L2 compression fracture with spinal canal narrowing

Evaluation for CRAB Criteria (End-Organ Damage):

C - Calcium elevation (Hypercalcemia):

- √ **Calcium 10.8 mg/dL** (>11 mg/dL or >1 mg/dL above upper limit = significant)
- **Borderline elevated** (10.8 mg/dL; ULN 10.5)

R - Renal insufficiency:

- √ Creatinine 1.3 mg/dL (eGFR 55)
- **Renal impairment present** (eGFR <60 but >40; not severe)

A - Anemia:

- Hemoglobin 12.8 g/dL (>10 g/dL)
- **No significant anemia** (mild, borderline)

B - Bone lesions:

- √ **Multiple lytic lesions on skeletal survey**
- **CRAB criteria MET**

Myeloma-Defining Events (SLiM Criteria - Alternative to CRAB):

- Sixty percent or more clonal plasma cells on bone marrow: **NO** (12%)
- Light chain ratio (involved/uninvolved) ≥100: **NO** (ratio 2.3)
- More than one focal lesion on MRI: **YES** (multiple lesions)

Diagnosis:

Criteria Assessment:

Criterion	MGUS	Smoldering Myeloma	Active Myeloma	This Patient
M-protein	<3 g/dL	≥3 g/dL	Any	**2.8 g/dL**
BM plasma cells	<10%	10-60%	≥10% or ≥60%	**12%**
CRAB/SLiM	Absent	Absent	**Present**	**Bone lesions present**
Risk of progression	1%/year	10%/year	Active disease	-

Final Diagnosis: Multiple Myeloma (IgG kappa) - Revised International Staging System (R-ISS) Stage II

- M-protein: 2.8 g/dL (IgG kappa)
- Bone marrow plasma cells: 12%
- **CRAB criteria: Bone lesions (lytic lesions, pathologic fracture)**
- **Myeloma-defining event: >1 focal lesion on MRI**

R-ISS Staging:

- **Stage I:** β2M <3.5, albumin ≥3.5, standard-risk cytogenetics, normal LDH
- **Stage II:** Not Stage I or III ← **PATIENT**
- **Stage III:** β2M ≥5.5 OR high-risk cytogenetics OR high LDH

Cytogenetic/FISH Analysis (Prognostic):

- **Standard risk:** No high-risk abnormalities detected
- No del(17p), t(4;14), t(14;16) (high-risk)
- Hyperdiploidy present (favorable)

Why This Is NOT MGUS:

- **MGUS requires:** M-protein <3 g/dL AND BM plasma cells <10% AND **NO end-organ damage (no CRAB)**
- This patient has **bone lesions** → Active myeloma

Why This Is NOT Smoldering Myeloma:

- **Smoldering myeloma:** M-protein ≥3 g/dL OR BM plasma cells 10-60% BUT **NO CRAB/SLiM criteria**
- This patient has **CRAB criteria (bone lesions)** → Active myeloma

Treatment Plan:

Induction Therapy (First-Line for Transplant-Ineligible):

- Age 72, comorbidities (CKD) → **Not a transplant candidate**
- **Regimen: DRd (Daratumumab-Lenalidomide-Dexamethasone)**
  - Daratumumab (anti-CD38 monoclonal antibody) IV weekly x 8, then every 2 weeks
  - Lenalidomide 25 mg PO days 1-21 of 28-day cycle (adjust for renal function)
  - Dexamethasone 40 mg weekly

Supportive Care:

1. Bone Health:

- **Zoledronic acid 4 mg IV monthly** (bisphosphonate - prevent skeletal events)
- Dose adjust for renal function
- Dental evaluation before starting (risk of osteonecrosis of jaw)

2. Infection Prophylaxis:

- **Antibiotic prophylaxis:** TMP-SMX or levofloxacin (immunosuppression)
- **Antiviral:** Acyclovir or valacyclovir (VZV reactivation with daratumumab)
- **IVIG** if recurrent infections

3. Thromboprophylaxis:

- **Aspirin 81 mg daily** (lenalidomide increases VTE risk)

4. Renal Protection:

- Hydration (2-3 L/day)
- Avoid nephrotoxins (NSAIDs, IV contrast)

5. Radiation Therapy:

- **Localized radiation to L2** (pathologic fracture, pain control)
- Analgesics for bone pain

Response Assessment (After 4 Cycles):

Labs:

- **M-protein: 0.8 g/dL** (decreased from 2.8 g/dL) - **Partial response**
- Kappa FLC: 22 mg/L (decreased)
- Kappa/Lambda ratio: 1.2 (near normal)
- Hemoglobin: 13.5 g/dL (improved)
- Calcium: 9.8 mg/dL (normalized)

Imaging:

- **PET-CT:** Decreased metabolic activity in bone lesions
- No new lesions

Bone Marrow:

- Plasma cells: 4% (decreased from 12%)

Response: Partial Response (PR)

- M-protein reduction ≥50%
- Continue treatment, monitor for progression

Long-Term Management:

- **Maintenance therapy:** Lenalidomide indefinitely (until progression)
- **Monthly zoledronic acid** (skeletal protection)
- **Monitor:** M-protein, FLC, CBC, renal function every 1-3 months
- **Annual:** Skeletal survey or PET-CT

Prognosis:

- Median survival with modern therapy: 5-10 years (R-ISS Stage II)
- Response to treatment: Good (partial response achieved)

MGUS Follow-Up Strategy (For Comparison):

- If this were MGUS: Monitor M-protein, CBC, calcium, creatinine every 6-12 months
- Risk of progression to myeloma: 1% per year (lifetime risk ~25%)
- High-risk MGUS (M-protein >1.5 g/dL, non-IgG type, abnormal FLC ratio): Consider closer follow-up

Teaching Points:

1. **MGUS Definition:** M-protein <3 g/dL + BM plasma cells <10% + NO end-organ damage (CRAB); asymptomatic; 1%/year progression to myeloma
2. **Smoldering Myeloma:** M-protein ≥3 g/dL OR BM plasma cells 10-60% + NO CRAB/SLiM; 10%/year progression; observation vs. clinical trials
3. **Active Myeloma:** CRAB criteria (Calcium >11, Renal impairment Cr >2, Anemia Hgb <10, Bone lesions) OR SLiM criteria (≥60% plasma cells, FLC ratio ≥100, >1 focal lesion MRI)
4. **CRAB Criteria:** End-organ damage attributable to myeloma; any CRAB criterion = active myeloma requiring treatment
5. **Free Light Chain Ratio:** Kappa/lambda ratio (normal 0.26-1.65); abnormal ratio indicates clonality; ratio ≥100 (involved/uninvolved) = myeloma-defining event
6. **Skeletal Survey:** Low-dose X-rays (skull, spine, ribs, pelvis, long bones); detects lytic lesions; insensitive (30% bone loss required); PET-CT or whole-body MRI more sensitive
7. **Immunoparesis:** Suppression of uninvolved immunoglobulins; indicates advanced disease; increases infection risk
8. **R-ISS Staging:** Combines β2-microglobulin, albumin, LDH, cytogenetics; Stage I (best, median survival >10 years), Stage III (worst, median survival 3-4 years)
9. **Daratumumab:** Anti-CD38 monoclonal antibody; highly effective; can interfere with blood bank crossmatch (phenotype before starting)
10. **Bisphosphonates:** Zoledronic acid or pamidronate reduce skeletal events (pathologic fractures, hypercalcemia); continue monthly indefinitely; risk of osteonecrosis of jaw (ONJ), renal toxicity

Related Cases: MGUS, smoldering myeloma, Waldenström macroglobulinemia, light chain myeloma, AL amyloidosis

Chapter 13: Integrated Multisystem Complex Cases

Case 13.1: Multi-Organ Failure Requiring Comprehensive Workup

Clinical Presentation: A 45-year-old previously healthy woman presents to ED with 1 week of fever (102-104°F), progressive dyspnea, oliguria, confusion, and diffuse petechiae. She had a mild upper respiratory infection 2 weeks ago that resolved. No recent travel, no sick contacts, no known toxic exposures. Taking no medications. Non-smoker, occasional alcohol.

Physical Examination:

- BP 88/52 (hypotensive), HR 128 (tachycardic), RR 32, Temp 103.2°F, SpO2 88% on room air
- **Altered mental status:** Confused, disoriented
- **Petechiae and purpura:** Diffuse on trunk and extremities
- **Jaundice:** Scleral icterus
- **Tachypneic, labored breathing**
- Cardiac: Tachycardic, no murmurs
- Abdomen: Mild hepatosplenomegaly
- **Urine output: 15 mL in past 4 hours** (oliguria/anuria)

Initial Laboratory Findings:

- **WBC: 18,500/µL** (leukocytosis with left shift)
- **Hemoglobin: 6.8 g/dL SEVERE ANEMIA** (baseline unknown, likely 12-14)
- **Platelets: 12,000/µL SEVERE THROMBOCYTOPENIA**
- **Creatinine: 4.8 mg/dL ACUTE KIDNEY INJURY**
- **Total bilirubin: 6.2 mg/dL ELEVATED** (indirect 5.8 mg/dL)
- **LDH: 2,850 U/L MARKEDLY ELEVATED**

Diagnostic Reasoning Questions:

1. What is the differential diagnosis for the triad of anemia, thrombocytopenia, and acute kidney injury?
2. What features distinguish thrombotic microangiopathies (TTP, HUS, DIC)?
3. How should a critically ill patient with multi-organ failure be systematically evaluated?
4. What urgent therapeutic interventions are required?

Sequential Test Results:

Peripheral Blood Smear (CRITICAL):

- **Schistocytes: 8-10 per high-power field MARKEDLY ELEVATED** (normal <1%)
- **Fragmented RBCs** (helmet cells, microspherocytes)

- **Severe thrombocytopenia** confirmed
- **Polychromasia** (reticulocytosis)
- Nucleated RBCs present
- **NO MALARIA PARASITES** seen

Interpretation: Microangiopathic Hemolytic Anemia (MAHA)

Coagulation Studies:

- PT-INR: 1.2 (normal)
- aPTT: 32 seconds (normal)
- **Fibrinogen: 385 mg/dL NORMAL** (normal 200-400)
- **D-dimer: 1,200 ng/mL** (elevated but not markedly)
- **NORMAL coagulation** (excludes DIC)

Hemolysis Workup:

- **LDH: 2,850 U/L** (markedly elevated - hemolysis)
- **Haptoglobin: <10 mg/dL UNDETECTABLE** (consumed - hemolysis)
- **Indirect bilirubin: 5.8 mg/dL** (elevated - hemolysis)
- **Reticulocyte count: 18% ELEVATED** (compensatory response)
- **Direct Coombs (DAT): Negative** (not autoimmune hemolysis)

Renal Function:

- Creatinine: 4.8 mg/dL (severe AKI)
- BUN: 85 mg/dL
- eGFR: 8 mL/min (near dialysis threshold)
- **Urinalysis:**
    - Blood: 3+ (positive dipstick)
    - **RBC casts: Present** (glomerular injury)
    - **RBCs: Too numerous to count**
    - Protein: 3+ (500 mg/dL)
    - **Granular casts, epithelial casts**

Neurologic Findings:

- **Fluctuating mental status**
- Confusion, disorientation
- **Focal neurologic signs:** Transient right arm weakness (resolved)
- **Headache**

Classic Pentad of TTP (Thrombotic Thrombocytopenic Purpura):

1. √ **Microangiopathic hemolytic anemia** (schistocytes, elevated LDH, low haptoglobin)
2. √ **Thrombocytopenia** (platelets 12,000/μL)
3. √ **Neurologic symptoms** (confusion, focal deficits)
4. √ **Renal impairment** (Cr 4.8 mg/dL)

446

5. √ **Fever** (103.2°F)

Note: Classic pentad seen in only 5-10% of TTP cases; triad of MAHA + thrombocytopenia + any organ dysfunction is sufficient for presumptive diagnosis

ADAMTS13 Testing (Confirmatory for TTP):

- **ADAMTS13 activity: <5% SEVERELY DEFICIENT** (normal >50%)
- **ADAMTS13 inhibitor (antibody): Detected** (autoimmune TTP)
- Confirms: **Acquired (Immune-Mediated) Thrombotic Thrombocytopenic Purpura**

Additional Workup:

Infection Screen:

- Blood cultures: Negative (no sepsis)
- **Shiga toxin (Stx) PCR: Negative** (excludes Shiga toxin-producing E. coli HUS)
- HIV, Hepatitis B/C: Negative

Autoimmune Panel:

- ANA: Negative
- Anti-dsDNA: Negative
- Complement (C3, C4): Normal
- (TTP can be associated with SLE, but not in this case)

Pregnancy Test:

- Negative (TTP can present in pregnancy)

Imaging:

- **CT Head (non-contrast):** No acute hemorrhage, no mass effect
- **Chest X-ray:** Bilateral patchy infiltrates (pulmonary edema, ARDS)
- **Abdominal ultrasound:** Hepatosplenomegaly, normal kidneys (no hydronephrosis)

Differential Diagnosis of Thrombotic Microangiopathies:

Feature	TTP	HUS	DIC	HELLP
Schistocytes	+++	+++	++	++
Platelets	↓↓↓	↓↓	↓	↓
Coagulation	Normal	Normal	↑PT, ↑aPTT, ↓Fibrinogen	Normal/↑PT
Renal failure	Moderate	Severe (>50%)	Variable	Moderate

Feature	TTP	HUS	DIC	HELLP
Neuro symptoms	+++	+	Variable	Seizures, eclampsia
Cause	ADAMTS13 deficiency	Shiga toxin	Sepsis, malignancy	Pregnancy

This patient: Normal coagulation (excludes DIC), severe neuro symptoms, ADAMTS13 <5% → **TTP**

Final Diagnosis: Acquired (Autoimmune) Thrombotic Thrombocytopenic Purpura (TTP) with Multi-Organ Failure:

1. Microangiopathic Hemolytic Anemia
2. Severe Thrombocytopenia
3. Acute Kidney Injury (Stage 3)
4. Neurologic Dysfunction (encephalopathy, focal deficits)
5. Respiratory Failure (ARDS)

Immediate Life-Saving Treatment:

1. Therapeutic Plasma Exchange (TPE/Plasmapheresis) - URGENT:

- **1-1.5 plasma volumes daily** (removes ADAMTS13 antibodies, replaces ADAMTS13)
- Continue until platelets >150,000 x 2 days AND LDH normalizing
- **CANNOT WAIT for ADAMTS13 results** (start empirically if TTP suspected)

2. Immunosuppression:

- **Corticosteroids:** Methylprednisolone 1 g IV daily x 3 days, then prednisone 1 mg/kg
- **Rituximab 375 mg/m² IV weekly x 4** (anti-CD20, depletes B cells producing antibodies)

3. Supportive Care:

- **DO NOT transfuse platelets** (can worsen thrombosis; only if life-threatening bleeding)
- **RBC transfusion PRN** for symptomatic anemia
- **Renal replacement therapy (hemodialysis):** Initiated for severe AKI, oliguria
- **Mechanical ventilation:** For ARDS, hypoxemia
- **Avoid antiplatelet agents initially** (increased bleeding risk)

4. Caplacizumab (If Available):

- **Anti-von Willebrand factor nanobody**
- Prevents platelet adhesion to ultra-large VWF multimers
- Accelerates platelet recovery, reduces TPE duration

Serial Monitoring:

Day 1 (TPE initiated):

- Platelets: 15,000/μL
- LDH: 2,650 U/L
- Creatinine: 5.1 mg/dL (worsening)
- Mental status: Confused
- **Daily TPE started**

Day 3:

- **Platelets: 45,000/μL** (improving!)
- LDH: 1,200 U/L (declining)
- Creatinine: 3.8 mg/dL (improving)
- Mental status: Alert, oriented x3 (resolved!)
- Hemoglobin: 8.2 g/dL (transfused 2 units PRBCs)

Day 7:

- **Platelets: 125,000/μL**
- LDH: 450 U/L (near normal)
- Creatinine: 2.1 mg/dL (improving)
- Schistocytes: <1% (resolved)
- Extubated (off ventilator)

Day 10:

- **Platelets: 180,000/μL** (normalized x2 days)
- LDH: 285 U/L (normal)
- Creatinine: 1.4 mg/dL
- **TPE discontinued** (response achieved)

Day 14:

- Platelets: 220,000/μL (stable)
- Creatinine: 1.2 mg/dL (near baseline)
- Off dialysis
- **Discharged home on prednisone taper + rituximab (completing 4 doses)**

Follow-Up (3 Months):

- ADAMTS13 activity: 45% (improved but not fully normalized)
- ADAMTS13 inhibitor: Negative (antibody cleared)
- Platelets: 245,000/μL (normal)
- Creatinine: 1.0 mg/dL (normal)
- **Complete clinical remission**

Follow-Up (1 Year):

- ADAMTS13 activity: 62% (normalized)
- Remains in remission
- Monitoring every 3-6 months for relapse

Pathophysiology of TTP:

1. **ADAMTS13 deficiency** (acquired autoantibodies or congenital mutation)
2. **Accumulation of ultra-large VWF multimers** (not cleaved)
3. **Platelet adhesion and aggregation** → microthrombi in arterioles/capillaries
4. **Microangiopathic hemolysis** (RBCs sheared by fibrin strands → schistocytes)
5. **Organ ischemia** (brain, kidneys most affected)

Teaching Points:

1. **TTP Diagnosis:** Triad of MAHA (schistocytes) + thrombocytopenia + organ dysfunction; ADAMTS13 <10% confirms; do NOT wait for results to start TPE
2. **ADAMTS13:** Metalloprotease that cleaves ultra-large VWF multimers; deficiency (acquired antibody or congenital mutation) causes TTP
3. **TPE (Plasmapheresis):** Removes antibodies + replaces ADAMTS13; mortality reduced from 90% to 10-20%; continue until platelet/LDH normalized x2 days
4. **Schistocytes:** Fragmented RBCs; >1% suggests microangiopathic process; seen in TTP, HUS, DIC, HELLP, malignant hypertension, mechanical heart valves
5. **TTP vs. HUS:** TTP has neuro symptoms, ADAMTS13 deficiency; HUS has severe renal failure, Shiga toxin (children with bloody diarrhea); significant overlap exists
6. **Normal Coagulation:** Key feature distinguishing TTP/HUS from DIC; PT/aPTT/fibrinogen normal in TTP; prolonged PT/aPTT, low fibrinogen in DIC
7. **Platelet Transfusion Contraindicated:** Can worsen thrombosis in TTP; only give for life-threatening bleeding or procedure
8. **Rituximab:** Anti-CD20 depletes B cells; reduces relapse rate from 50% to 10-20%; now standard adjunct therapy
9. **Relapse Risk:** 30-50% relapse within 10 years; monitor ADAMTS13 activity; relapse treated with repeat TPE + immunosuppression
10. **Multi-Organ Approach:** Systematic evaluation of hemolysis (LDH, haptoglobin, bilirubin), thrombocytopenia (smear, coagulation), renal (Cr, UA), neuro (exam, imaging), infection (cultures)

Related Cases: Atypical HUS (complement-mediated), Shiga toxin HUS, DIC, HELLP syndrome, catastrophic antiphospholipid syndrome

---

Case 13.2: Undiagnosed Disease Requiring Systematic Approach

Clinical Presentation: A 32-year-old woman presents with 6 months of progressive fatigue, arthralgias, weight loss (25 lbs), intermittent fevers, and painful oral ulcers. Recently developed a facial rash that worsens with sun exposure. She has seen multiple physicians without a clear diagnosis. Labs from outside facilities show "anemia and elevated inflammatory markers." No significant past medical history. No family history of autoimmune disease.

Physical Examination:

- BP 158/95 (elevated), HR 92, Temp 100.4°F
- **Malar rash:** Erythematous, sparing nasolabial folds

- **Photosensitive rash on arms**
- **Oral ulcers:** Painless, on hard palate
- **Synovitis:** Bilateral wrists, MCPs, knees (symmetric, non-erosive)
- **Alopecia:** Diffuse, non-scarring
- **2+ pitting edema bilateral lower extremities**
- No lymphadenopathy, hepatosplenomegaly

Systematic Diagnostic Approach:

Step 1: Broad Screening Labs

CBC with Differential:

- **WBC: 2,800/μL LEUKOPENIA**
- **Hemoglobin: 9.2 g/dL ANEMIA**
- **MCV: 88 fL** (normocytic)
- **Platelets: 95,000/μL THROMBOCYTOPENIA**
- **Pancytopenia** (all three cell lines decreased)

Comprehensive Metabolic Panel:

- **Creatinine: 2.1 mg/dL ELEVATED** (AKI)
- BUN: 42 mg/dL
- eGFR: 28 mL/min
- Albumin: 2.8 g/dL (low)
- **Proteinuria suspected**

Inflammatory Markers:

- **ESR: 85 mm/hr MARKEDLY ELEVATED**
- **CRP: 3.2 mg/dL ELEVATED**

Urinalysis:

- **Protein: 4+** (>300 mg/dL)
- **Blood: 3+**
- **RBCs: >100/hpf**
- **RBC casts: Present** (glomerulonephritis)
- **WBCs: 20-30/hpf**

Step 2: Pattern Recognition

- Young woman + malar rash + photosensitivity + oral ulcers + arthritis + cytopenias + renal disease + RBC casts
- **Pattern suggests: Systemic Lupus Erythematosus (SLE)**

Step 3: Targeted Autoimmune Workup

ANA (Antinuclear Antibody):

- **ANA titer: 1:1280 STRONGLY POSITIVE**
- **Pattern: Homogeneous**
- Sensitivity for SLE: 95-98%

Extractable Nuclear Antigens (ENA Panel):

- **Anti-dsDNA: 285 IU/mL STRONGLY POSITIVE** (specific for SLE, correlates with lupus nephritis)
- **Anti-Smith (Sm): POSITIVE** (98% specific for SLE)
- Anti-RNP: Negative
- **Anti-Ro/SSA: POSITIVE**
- Anti-La/SSB: Negative

Complement Levels:

- **C3: 38 mg/dL LOW** (normal 90-180)
- **C4: 6 mg/dL LOW** (normal 10-40)
- **CH50: 12 U/mL LOW** (normal 30-75)
- **Hypocomplementemia** (active SLE with immune complex formation)

Direct Coombs Test (DAT):

- **Positive (IgG)** - autoimmune hemolytic anemia

Antiphospholipid Antibodies:

- **Anticardiolipin IgG: 58 GPL units** (elevated; normal <20)
- **Lupus anticoagulant: POSITIVE**
- Beta-2 glycoprotein I antibodies: Positive
- **Antiphospholipid syndrome (secondary to SLE)**

Step 4: Organ-Specific Evaluation

Renal Biopsy (Nephrology):

- **Indication:** Active urinary sediment, rising creatinine, proteinuria
- **Histology: Class IV lupus nephritis** (diffuse proliferative GN)
- Immunofluorescence: "Full house" pattern (IgG, IgM, IgA, C3, C1q)
- Electron microscopy: Subendothelial deposits
- Activity index: 12/24 (active inflammation)
- Chronicity index: 2/12 (minimal scarring - good prognosis)

24-Hour Urine:

- **Total protein: 4.2 g/24h** (nephrotic range)
- Creatinine clearance: 32 mL/min

Cardiac Evaluation:

- **Echocardiogram:** Small pericardial effusion (serositis)
- No valvular disease

Pulmonary:

- **Chest X-ray:** Small bilateral pleural effusions
- **Pleuritis/serositis**

Neurologic:

- No active CNS involvement
- No seizures, psychosis

Hematologic:

- **Reticulocyte count: 8%** (elevated - compensating for hemolysis)
- **Haptoglobin: <10 mg/dL** (hemolysis)
- **LDH: 850 U/L** (elevated)
- **Coombs-positive hemolytic anemia**

Step 5: Apply Diagnostic Criteria

2019 EULAR/ACR SLE Classification Criteria:

- Requires: ANA ≥1:80 (entry criterion) + Score ≥10 points

Domains and Points:

Constitutional (0-2):

- Fever: 2 points ✓

Hematologic (0-4):

- Leukopenia: 3 points ✓
- Thrombocytopenia: 4 points ✓
- Autoimmune hemolysis: 4 points ✓

Neuropsychiatric (0-5):

- None (0 points)

Mucocutaneous (0-6):

- Acute cutaneous lupus (malar rash): 6 points ✓

- Oral ulcers: 2 points ✓
- Alopecia: 2 points ✓

Serosal (0-5):

- Pleural/pericardial effusion: 5 points ✓

Musculoskeletal (0-6):

- Joint involvement: 6 points ✓

Renal (0-10):

- Class III or IV lupus nephritis: 10 points ✓
- Proteinuria >0.5 g/24h: 4 points

Immunologic (0-6):

- Anti-dsDNA: 6 points ✓
- Anti-Smith: 6 points ✓
- Low complement: 3 points ✓
- Antiphospholipid antibodies: 2 points ✓

Total Score: >50 points (threshold ≥10) → **Definite SLE**

Final Diagnosis: Systemic Lupus Erythematosus (SLE) with:

1. Class IV Lupus Nephritis (WHO classification)
2. Autoimmune Hemolytic Anemia (Coombs-positive)
3. Serositis (pleural and pericardial effusions)
4. Secondary Antiphospholipid Syndrome
5. Cytopenias (pancytopenia)

Treatment Plan:

Induction Therapy (Severe Lupus Nephritis):

- **High-dose corticosteroids:** Methylprednisolone 1 g IV daily x 3 days, then prednisone 1 mg/kg/day
- **Mycophenolate mofetil (MMF) 3 g/day** (divided BID) OR **Cyclophosphamide** IV monthly x 6 months
- Hydroxychloroquine 400 mg daily (all SLE patients)

Supportive:

- **ACE inhibitor:** Lisinopril (proteinuria reduction, BP control)
- **Anticoagulation:** Consider for antiphospholipid syndrome (warfarin if thrombosis)

- **Aspirin 81 mg** (antiphospholipid antibodies present)
- **PCP prophylaxis:** TMP-SMX (immunosuppression)
- **Calcium/Vitamin D:** Bone protection (steroids)
- **Sunscreen, sun avoidance**

Response Assessment (3 Months):

- Creatinine: 1.2 mg/dL (improved)
- Proteinuria: 0.8 g/24h (decreased)
- Anti-dsDNA: 85 IU/mL (decreased)
- C3, C4: Normalized
- Rash, oral ulcers: Resolved
- **Partial renal response**

Maintenance Therapy (After 6 Months Induction):

- **Mycophenolate mofetil** continued (2-3 years)
- **Prednisone taper** to 5-10 mg/day
- **Hydroxychloroquine** lifelong

Teaching Points:

1. **Systematic Approach to Undiagnosed Disease:** (1) Broad screening labs; (2) Pattern recognition; (3) Targeted testing; (4) Organ-specific evaluation; (5) Apply diagnostic criteria
2. **SLE Diagnosis:** Clinical features + ANA positive + specific autoantibodies (anti-dsDNA, anti-Sm); 2019 EULAR/ACR criteria most current
3. **Anti-dsDNA and Anti-Sm:** Most specific SLE antibodies; anti-dsDNA correlates with disease activity and lupus nephritis; anti-Sm does not correlate with activity
4. **Hypocomplementemia:** Low C3/C4 indicates active disease with immune complex formation; monitor for disease activity
5. **Lupus Nephritis:** Biopsy essential for classification (Class I-VI); Class III/IV require aggressive immunosuppression; "full house" IF pattern pathognomonic
6. **Antiphospholipid Syndrome:** Can be primary or secondary (to SLE); requires ≥2 positive tests ≥12 weeks apart; increases thrombosis/pregnancy loss risk
7. **Cytopenias in SLE:** Leukopenia (most common), thrombocytopenia, autoimmune hemolytic anemia (Coombs-positive); part of disease activity
8. **Hydroxychloroquine:** Reduces flares, improves survival, prevents damage accrual; all SLE patients should be on it unless contraindicated
9. **Drug-Induced Lupus:** Hydralazine, procainamide, isoniazid, minocycline; anti-histone antibodies; resolves with drug discontinuation
10. **Monitoring:** Serial anti-dsDNA, complement, CBC, UA, Cr; increasing anti-dsDNA + falling complement often precedes flare

Related Cases: Mixed connective tissue disease, undifferentiated connective tissue disease, drug-induced lupus, rheumatoid arthritis with extra-articular manifestations

Case 13.3: Conflicting Laboratory Results Requiring Resolution

Clinical Presentation: A 52-year-old man with type 2 diabetes presents for routine follow-up. His home glucose monitor shows average readings of 180-220 mg/dL fasting. He reports good medication compliance. HbA1c was ordered to assess glycemic control.

Initial Results:

- **Fingerstick glucose (office): 215 mg/dL**
- **HbA1c: 5.2%** (normal <5.7%) **DISCREPANCY!**
- Expected HbA1c for average glucose 200 mg/dL: ~8.5%

Diagnostic Reasoning:

- HbA1c and glucose measurements are **conflicting**
- HbA1c falsely low OR glucose measurements falsely high?
- **Systematic approach to resolve discrepancy**

Step 1: Verify HbA1c Method and Specimen

- **Repeat HbA1c (same lab): 5.1%** (confirms low HbA1c)
- Method: Immunoassay
- Specimen: Proper EDTA tube, no hemolysis

Step 2: Rule Out HbA1c Interference

Hemoglobin Variant Testing:

- **Hemoglobin electrophoresis:**
    - **HbA: 58%** (decreased; normal ~97%)
    - **HbS: 40%** (sickle hemoglobin trait)
    - **HbA2: 2%** (normal)
- **Diagnosis: Hemoglobin S Trait (Sickle Cell Trait)**

Mechanism of Interference:

- HbA1c assays measure glycated HbA (not HbS)
- Patient has only 58% HbA (rest is HbS)
- **HbA1c underestimates glycemic control** in hemoglobinopathies

Step 3: Alternative Glycemic Marker

Fructosamine:

- **Fructosamine: 385 μmol/L ELEVATED** (normal 200-285)
- Reflects glycemic control over 2-3 weeks
- **Not affected by hemoglobin variants**

Glycated Albumin:

- **Glycated albumin: 22% ELEVATED** (normal <15%)
- Reflects 2-3 week glycemic control
- Alternative when HbA1c unreliable

Continuous Glucose Monitor (CGM) Data:

- **Average glucose: 198 mg/dL** (confirms poor control)
- **Time in range (70-180 mg/dL): 35%** (goal >70%)

Resolution:

- **True glycemic control: POOR** (average glucose ~200 mg/dL)
- **HbA1c 5.2%: FALSELY LOW** due to HbS trait
- **Use fructosamine or glycated albumin for monitoring**

Final Diagnosis: Poorly Controlled Type 2 Diabetes with Falsely Low HbA1c due to Hemoglobin S Trait

Other Causes of HbA1c Discrepancies:

Falsely Low HbA1c:

- **Hemoglobinopathies:** HbS, HbC, HbE traits/disease
- **Hemolytic anemia:** Reduced RBC lifespan (less time to glycate)
- **Recent blood loss/transfusion:** Young RBCs
- **Chronic kidney disease (EPO therapy):** Increased RBC turnover
- **Splenomegaly:** Increased RBC clearance
- **High-dose vitamin C, E:** Antioxidant interference

Falsely Elevated HbA1c:

- **Iron deficiency anemia:** Increased glycation of iron-deficient Hgb
- **Uremia:** Carbamylated hemoglobin (cross-reacts with some assays)
- **High-dose aspirin:** Acetylated Hgb
- **Alcoholism:** Acetaldehyde adducts
- **Hypertriglyceridemia:** Turbidity interference

Alternative Glycemic Markers:

Marker	Timeframe	Advantages	Limitations
HbA1c	2-3 months	Standard, widely available	Hemoglobinopathies, anemia
Fructosamine	2-3 weeks	Not affected by Hgb variants	Affected by albumin levels
Glycated albumin	2-3 weeks	Hgb-independent	Not widely available
CGM	Real-time	Detailed patterns	Expensive, requires training

Teaching Points:

1. **HbA1c Discrepancies:** Always correlate HbA1c with home glucose monitoring; significant discrepancy warrants investigation
2. **Hemoglobin Variants:** HbS, HbC, HbE traits affect HbA1c (most assays measure HbA glycation); order hemoglobin electrophoresis if suspected
3. **Hemolytic Anemia:** Shortened RBC lifespan → less time for glycation → falsely low HbA1c; use fructosamine or glycated albumin
4. **Iron Deficiency:** Falsely elevates HbA1c; iron-deficient Hgb glycates more readily; check ferritin, treat iron deficiency, recheck HbA1c
5. **CKD and HbA1c:** Variable effects; uremia may elevate (carbamylation); EPO therapy may lower (increased RBC turnover); use with caution in dialysis
6. **Fructosamine:** Glycated serum proteins (mainly albumin); reflects 2-3 weeks; falsely low if hypoalbuminemia (nephrotic syndrome, cirrhosis)
7. **Assay-Specific Interference:** Different HbA1c methods (HPLC, immunoassay, enzymatic); some more prone to interference; lab should note method
8. **Clinical Context:** Always interpret lab results in clinical context; discrepancies require investigation, not assumption
9. **Patient Education:** Explain why HbA1c may not be reliable; emphasize importance of alternative monitoring
10. **Documentation:** Note hemoglobin variant in chart; alert lab to use fructosamine or other markers

Related Cases: Iron deficiency causing falsely elevated HbA1c, hemolytic anemia with low HbA1c, uremia causing assay interference

---

Case 13.4: Pre-Analytical Variables Causing Erroneous Results

Clinical Presentation: A 45-year-old woman presents for routine physical exam. She feels well, no complaints. Fasting labs ordered. Results show severe hyperkalemia.

Initial Results:

- **Potassium: 7.2 mEq/L CRITICAL** (normal 3.5-5.0)
- Sodium: 140 mEq/L (normal)
- Other electrolytes: Normal
- **CRITICAL VALUE CALLED TO PHYSICIAN**

Clinical Assessment:

- Patient appears well, no symptoms
- **No EKG changes** (normal, no peaked T waves, no QRS widening)
- No muscle weakness
- Taking no medications that cause hyperkalemia

Diagnostic Reasoning:

- **Asymptomatic severe hyperkalemia** is unusual
- Normal EKG makes true hyperkalemia unlikely (K 7.2 should cause EKG changes)
- **Suspect pseudohyperkalemia (false elevation)**

Step 1: Investigate Pre-Analytical Variables

Specimen Collection Review:

- **Difficult venipuncture:** Required 3 attempts
- **Prolonged tourniquet time:** >2 minutes
- **Fist pumping:** Patient asked to pump fist repeatedly
- **Small vein, slow flow**

Specimen Appearance:

- **Hemolysis index: 3+** (significant hemolysis)
- Serum appears pink-red

Mechanism:

- **Hemolysis releases intracellular K+** (RBC K+ ~140 mEq/L)
- Causes **pseudohyperkalemia** (false elevation)

Step 2: Repeat with Proper Technique

Repeat Potassium (Proper Collection):

- **Proper venipuncture:** Single attempt, minimal tourniquet time
- No fist pumping
- Free-flowing sample
- **Potassium: 4.1 mEq/L NORMAL**
- Hemolysis index: Negative

Resolution: Pseudohyperkalemia due to hemolysis

Other Pre-Analytical Causes of Pseudohyperkalemia:

1. In Vitro Hemolysis:

- Difficult venipuncture, small needle, vigorous mixing, prolonged transport/storage
- **Most common cause**

2. Thrombocytosis (>500,000/µL):

- Platelets release K+ during clotting (serum sample)
- **Use heparinized plasma instead of serum**

3. Leukocytosis (>100,000/µL):

- WBCs release K+ during clotting or if delayed processing
- Process sample quickly, use plasma

4. Hereditary Spherocytosis/Familial Pseudohyperkalemia:

- RBC membrane leak at room temperature
- **Keep sample at 37°C, process immediately**

5. Tourniquet Effect:

- Prolonged tourniquet + fist pumping → K+ leaks from muscle cells

Additional Pre-Analytical Errors:

Case A: Falsely Elevated Glucose

- Glucose measured on whole blood left at room temperature x 4 hours
- RBCs/WBCs consume glucose (glycolysis)
- **Measured glucose: 65 mg/dL** (falsely low)
- **Prevention:** Use fluoride tube (inhibits glycolysis) or process immediately

Case B: Falsely Low Ionized Calcium

- Ionized calcium drawn in heparinized tube
- **Heparin binds calcium** → falsely low ionized Ca
- **Prevention:** Use specific ionized calcium syringe (balanced heparin)

Case C: Contaminated Sample

- Blood drawn from IV line with running fluids
- Sample diluted with IV fluid (D5W)
- **All electrolytes falsely low, glucose falsely high**
- **Prevention:** Draw from different site or discard first 5-10 mL

Case D: Wrong Tube

- CBC drawn in serum separator tube (no anticoagulant)
- Blood clots, platelets consumed
- **Platelet count: 0** (falsely low)
- **Prevention:** Follow order of draw, use correct tubes

Case E: Prolonged Storage

- Blood stored at room temperature overnight
- **pH decrease** (CO_2 production), **K+ increase, glucose decrease**
- **Prevention:** Process within 1-2 hours or refrigerate

Step-by-Step Pre-Analytical Error Investigation:

1. Review Clinical Context:

- Does result match clinical picture?
- Patient symptomatic?

2. Check Delta Check:

- Compare to prior results
- Sudden drastic change without clinical explanation?

3. Examine Specimen:

- Hemolysis? Lipemia? Icterus?
- Tube type correct?
- Adequate volume?

4. Review Collection:

- Venipuncture difficulty?
- Tourniquet time?
- IV line contamination?
- Order of draw correct?

5. Review Processing:

- Time to processing?
- Storage temperature?
- Centrifugation appropriate?

6. Repeat with Optimal Conditions:

- Proper technique
- Correct tube
- Immediate processing

Final Diagnosis: Pseudohyperkalemia due to In Vitro Hemolysis (Pre-Analytical Error)

Teaching Points:

1. **Pseudohyperkalemia:** Falsely elevated K+ due to specimen issue (hemolysis, thrombocytosis, leukocytosis, hereditary disorders); suspect if asymptomatic, normal EKG
2. **Hemolysis Detection:** Visual inspection (pink/red serum), hemolysis index (automated); causes falsely elevated K+, LDH, AST, falsely decreased haptoglobin
3. **Thrombocytosis and K+:** Platelets release K+ during clotting; if platelets >500K, use heparinized plasma (prevents clotting, no K+ release)
4. **Proper Venipuncture:** Minimal tourniquet time (<1 min), no fist pumping, free-flowing sample, proper needle size (21-22G)
5. **Order of Draw:** Blood culture → sodium citrate (blue) → serum (red/gold) → heparin (green) → EDTA (purple) → fluoride (gray); prevents cross-contamination

6. **Critical Value Verification:** Always verify critical values with clinical picture; if discrepant, suspect pre-analytical error and repeat
7. **Delta Check:** Automated comparison to prior results; flags significant changes; helps identify specimen mix-ups, analytical errors
8. **Time-Sensitive Analytes:** Glucose ($\downarrow$ with time), K+ ($\uparrow$ with time), ionized Ca (affected by pH change); process immediately or use stabilizer tubes
9. **Temperature Effects:** Some analytes stable only at specific temperatures (cold agglutinins 37°C, familial pseudohyperkalemia 37°C, cryoglobulins room temp)
10. **Communication:** Lab should note specimen issues (hemolysis, lipemia); physician should provide clinical context; teamwork resolves discrepancies

Related Cases: Falsely low glucose from glycolysis, IV contamination causing abnormal results, wrong tube causing clotting

Case 13.5: Rare Disease Diagnosis - Fabry Disease

Clinical Presentation: A 28-year-old man presents to a general medicine clinic with lifelong burning pain in his hands and feet that he has been told is "just growing pains" or "fibromyalgia." Pain is worse with exercise, heat, and stress. Recently, he developed new proteinuria on routine urinalysis. He also reports decreased sweating (hypohidrosis), recurrent abdominal pain with diarrhea, and early satiety. Family history: maternal uncle died of "kidney failure" at age 42, maternal grandfather had a "stroke" at age 45.

Physical Examination:

BP 145/88, HR 82, Temp 98.6°F

Skin: Clusters of dark red/purple papules (angiokeratomas) in "bathing trunk" distribution (umbilicus to knees, especially scrotum)

Eyes: Slit lamp examination shows **cornea verticillata** (whorl-like corneal deposits)

Cardiovascular: Regular rhythm, no murmurs

Neurologic:

Decreased pain sensation in hands and feet (small fiber neuropathy)

Decreased temperature sensation

Normal strength, reflexes

No hepatosplenomegaly

No lymphadenopathy

Past Medical History:

Chronic pain since childhood (age 7-8)

"Heat intolerance"

Multiple ED visits for severe pain crises

Previously diagnosed with "fibromyalgia," "Raynaud's," "neuropathy of unknown cause"

Diagnostic Reasoning Questions:

What is the differential diagnosis for acral pain, angiokeratomas, and corneal changes?

How are lysosomal storage disorders diagnosed?

What is the pathophysiology of Fabry disease?

What are the systemic manifestations of this disorder?

Sequential Test Results:

Initial Laboratory Findings:

Urinalysis:

Protein: 3+ (300 mg/dL)

Blood: Trace

Lipid-laden cells in urine sediment

No casts initially

Basic Metabolic Panel:

Creatinine: 1.6 mg/dL ELEVATED (normal 0.7-1.3)

eGFR: 52 mL/min/1.73m² (CKD stage 3)

BUN: 32 mg/dL

24-Hour Urine:

Total protein: 2.8 g/24h (nephrotic range)

Echocardiography (Due to Family History of Early Death):

Left ventricular hypertrophy (LVH): Septal thickness 14 mm (normal <12 mm)

Preserved ejection fraction (55%)

Mild mitral regurgitation

No regional wall motion abnormalities

ECG:

Short PR interval (110 ms) (normal 120-200 ms)

Left ventricular hypertrophy by voltage criteria

No pre-excitation (Wolff-Parkinson-White excluded)

Pattern Recognition:

Young man + acral pain + angiokeratomas + cornea verticillata + proteinuria + LVH + family history of early renal/cardiac death

Consider: Fabry Disease (X-linked lysosomal storage disorder)

Targeted Diagnostic Testing:

Enzyme Assay (Plasma or Leukocytes):

Alpha-galactosidase A (α-Gal A) activity: 0.8 nmol/hr/mg protein SEVERELY DEFICIENT

Normal: 40-100 nmol/hr/mg protein

<1% of normal activity → Classic Fabry disease

Molecular Genetic Testing:

GLA Gene Sequencing (Xq22.1):

Mutation detected: c.644A>G (p.Asn215Ser)

Hemizygous (male has only one X chromosome)

Classification: Pathogenic variant, reported in Fabry disease

Inheritance: X-linked

Maternal inheritance confirmed

Urine Biomarker:

Globotriaosylceramide (Gb3): 1,850 nmol/mmol creatinine MARKEDLY ELEVATED

Normal: <20 nmol/mmol creatinine

Lyso-Gb3: 185 ng/mL MARKEDLY ELEVATED (normal <1 ng/mL)

More sensitive biomarker for disease activity

Kidney Biopsy (Performed to Assess Renal Involvement):

Light Microscopy:

Glomeruli show vacuolated podocytes ("foamy" appearance)

Tubular epithelial cells with vacuolization

Mild interstitial fibrosis

Electron Microscopy:

"Zebra bodies" in podocytes, endothelial cells, tubular cells

Characteristic parallel lamellar inclusions (pathognomonic)

Glycosphingolipid accumulation in lysosomes

Immunofluorescence:

Negative for immune deposits

Diagnosis: Fabry nephropathy

Additional Organ Assessment:

Cardiac MRI:

LVH confirmed: Septal thickness 15 mm

Late gadolinium enhancement (LGE): Inferolateral wall (fibrosis)

No fatty infiltration

Pattern consistent with Fabry cardiomyopathy

Neurologic Evaluation:

Brain MRI:

White matter hyperintensities (Fabry-related microvascular disease)

No acute stroke

Increased risk for future cerebrovascular events

Quantitative Sensory Testing:

Abnormal cold and warm thresholds (small fiber neuropathy)

Decreased pain perception

Autonomic Testing:

Abnormal sweat test (anhidrosis/hypohidrosis)

Abnormal heart rate variability (autonomic dysfunction)

Audiometry:

Bilateral high-frequency sensorineural hearing loss (progressive)

Ophthalmologic Assessment:

Cornea verticillata (confirmed)

Retinal vascular tortuosity

Posterior capsular cataract (Fabry cataract - "spoke-like")

Family Cascade Screening:

Mother (Obligate Carrier):

α-Gal A activity: 28 nmol/hr/mg (reduced but >15% - heterozygous female)

GLA mutation: Heterozygous c.644A>G

Symptoms: Mild acral pain, fatigue

Proteinuria: 500 mg/24h

Symptomatic carrier (females can be affected due to X-inactivation)

Maternal Uncle (Deceased at 42):

Medical records review: ESRD, dialysis, died of MI

Likely had undiagnosed Fabry disease

Maternal Aunt (Age 52):

Screening α-Gal A: Normal (did not inherit mutation)

GLA sequencing: Normal

Maternal Cousin (Male, Age 24):

α-Gal A activity: 1.2 nmol/hr/mg (**deficient**)

GLA mutation: Hemizygous c.644A>G

Asymptomatic currently (early disease)

Urine Gb3: Elevated

Early diagnosis allows preemptive treatment

Final Diagnosis: Classic Fabry Disease (X-linked, GLA mutation c.644A>G) with Multi-Organ Involvement:

Fabry Nephropathy (proteinuria, CKD stage 3)

Fabry Cardiomyopathy (LVH, fibrosis)

Peripheral Neuropathy (small fiber, acral pain)

Autonomic Neuropathy (hypohidrosis)

Cerebrovascular Disease (white matter changes)

Cornea Verticillata

Angiokeratomas

Pathophysiology of Fabry Disease:

Enzyme Deficiency:

α-Galactosidase A deficiency → cannot cleave terminal galactose from globotriaosylceramide (Gb3)

Gb3 accumulation in lysosomes of vascular endothelium, smooth muscle, podocytes, cardiomyocytes, neurons

Organ-Specific Damage:

Kidney: Gb3 in podocytes → proteinuria → glomerulosclerosis → ESRD (40-50s)

Heart: Gb3 in cardiomyocytes → LVH, fibrosis, arrhythmias, valve disease

Nervous system: Gb3 in dorsal root ganglia → small fiber neuropathy → acral pain, autonomic dysfunction

Vascular: Endothelial Gb3 → increased stroke risk, angiokeratomas

Treatment:

Enzyme Replacement Therapy (ERT):

Agalsidase beta 1 mg/kg IV every 2 weeks (recombinant α-Gal A)

Alternative: Agalsidase alfa 0.2 mg/kg IV every 2 weeks

Start immediately (prevents disease progression, may stabilize or improve organ function)

Chaperone Therapy (If Amenable Mutation):

Migalastat 123 mg PO every other day (pharmacological chaperone)

Stabilizes mutant enzyme, enhances trafficking to lysosomes

Only for amenable mutations (genetic testing determines eligibility)

This patient's mutation: **NOT amenable** to migalastat

Symptomatic Treatment:

Neuropathic Pain:

Carbamazepine 200 mg BID or gabapentin 900-3600 mg/day

Avoid triggers (heat, exercise extremes)

Renal Protection:

ACE inhibitor: Lisinopril 10 mg daily (reduce proteinuria)

Blood pressure control (target <130/80)

Cardiac Management:

Beta-blocker if indicated (arrhythmias)

Monitor for progression to heart failure

Pacemaker/ICD if conduction abnormalities develop

Stroke Prevention:

Aspirin 81 mg daily

Aggressive cardiovascular risk factor management

Monitoring:

Every 6 Months:

Urine protein, serum creatinine, eGFR

Lyso-Gb3 levels (marker of disease activity)

Echocardiogram annually

Brain MRI every 2-3 years

Follow-Up (1 Year on ERT):

Lyso-Gb3: 45 ng/mL (decreased from 185 - excellent response)

Urine protein: 1.2 g/24h (decreased from 2.8 g)

Creatinine: 1.5 mg/dL (stable)

Pain score: Improved (VAS 4/10 from 8/10)

Cardiac: LVH stable, no progression

No new strokes or TIAs

Follow-Up (3 Years on ERT):

Lyso-Gb3: 30 ng/mL (sustained reduction)

Proteinuria: 0.8 g/24h (continued improvement)

eGFR: 55 mL/min (stable, no decline)

Cardiac MRI: No new LGE, stable LVH

Quality of life significantly improved

Long-Term Prognosis:

Untreated: Life expectancy 50s-60s (renal failure, stroke, cardiac disease)

With early ERT: Near-normal life expectancy if started before irreversible organ damage

Females (heterozygotes): Variable severity (20-70% develop symptoms due to X-inactivation)

Teaching Points:

Fabry Disease: X-linked lysosomal storage disorder; α-galactosidase A deficiency → Gb3 accumulation in multiple organs

Classic vs. Late-Onset: Classic (males, <10% enzyme activity, childhood pain, multi-organ by 30s); Late-onset (>10% activity, isolated cardiac or renal in 50s-70s)

Angiokeratomas: Dark red papules in bathing trunk distribution; pathognomonic but not always present; also seen in other lysosomal disorders (fucosidosis, sialidosis)

Cornea Verticillata: Whorl-like corneal deposits; seen in 70% of hemizygous males, 70% of heterozygous females; also caused by amiodarone, chloroquine

Acral Pain: "Fabry crisis" - severe burning pain in hands/feet triggered by fever, exercise, stress; small fiber neuropathy from Gb3 in dorsal root ganglia

Kidney Involvement: Proteinuria in adolescence/early adulthood → progressive CKD → ESRD by 40s-50s; zebra bodies on EM pathognomonic

Cardiac Involvement: Concentric LVH (vs. asymmetric in HCM); short PR interval characteristic; arrhythmias, heart failure; late gadolinium enhancement on MRI (fibrosis)

X-Linked Inheritance: Males hemizygous (more severe); females heterozygous (variable due to lyonization); all daughters of affected males are carriers

Enzyme vs. Chaperone Therapy: ERT replaces deficient enzyme (all mutations); migalastat stabilizes amenable mutant enzymes (30% of mutations)

Biomarkers: Lyso-Gb3 most sensitive for disease activity and treatment response; urine Gb3 also used; follow with ERT

Related Cases: Anderson-Fabry variants, other lysosomal storage disorders (Gaucher, Pompe), cardiac amyloidosis (mimics Fabry cardiomyopathy)

Case 13.6: Laboratory Findings Leading to Unexpected Diagnosis - Incidental CLL

Clinical Presentation: A 62-year-old man presents to his primary care physician for an annual physical examination. He reports feeling well overall, perhaps slightly more tired than usual, which he attributes to working long hours. No fevers, night sweats, weight loss, infections, bleeding, or bruising. No lymphadenopathy noticed. He exercises regularly and maintains an active lifestyle.

Physical Examination:

Vital signs: Normal

General: Well-appearing, no distress

HEENT: No conjunctival pallor, no scleral icterus

Lymph nodes: No palpable cervical, axillary, or inguinal lymphadenopathy

Cardiac/Pulmonary: Normal

Abdomen: Soft, **no hepatosplenomegaly**

Skin: No rashes, petechiae, or ecchymoses

Neurologic: Normal

Routine Laboratory Screening:

Complete Blood Count:

WBC: 48,500/μL MARKEDLY ELEVATED (normal 4,000-11,000)

Hemoglobin: 13.8 g/dL (normal)

Platelets: 185,000/μL (normal)

Absolute lymphocyte count: 42,000/μL MARKEDLY ELEVATED (normal 1,000-4,000)

Differential Count:

Lymphocytes: 87% (absolute: 42,000/μL)

Neutrophils: 10%

Monocytes: 2%

Eosinophils: 1%

Basophils: 0%

Chemistry Panel:

All within normal limits

LDH: 185 U/L (normal)

Uric acid: 5.2 mg/dL (normal)

Diagnostic Reasoning Questions:

What is the differential diagnosis for asymptomatic lymphocytosis?

How is chronic lymphocytic leukemia (CLL) diagnosed?

What distinguishes CLL from other lymphoproliferative disorders?

How is CLL staged and risk-stratified?

Sequential Test Results:

Peripheral Blood Smear:

Small, mature-appearing lymphocytes predominate

Smudge cells (Gumprecht shadows): Numerous (characteristic of CLL; fragile lymphocytes rupture during smear preparation)

Lymphocyte morphology: Round nuclei, clumped chromatin, scant cytoplasm

No large atypical cells

No hairy projections

RBC morphology: Normal

Platelets: Adequate

Interpretation: Morphology consistent with CLL

Flow Cytometry (Peripheral Blood):

Immunophenotype:

CD5: Positive (T-cell marker aberrantly expressed on B cells)

CD19: Positive (B-cell marker)

CD20: Dim positive (weak B-cell marker expression)

CD23: Positive (characteristic of CLL)

Surface immunoglobulin (sIg): Dim positive (weak/low density)

Kappa light chain restriction (clonal B cells)

CD10: Negative (excludes follicular lymphoma)

FMC7: Negative (typical for CLL)

CD103: Negative (excludes hairy cell leukemia)

CLL Score (Matutes Score): 5/5 (diagnostic of CLL)

Points: CD5+ (1), CD23+ (1), weak CD20/sIg (1+1), FMC7- (1)

Clonality: Confirmed by kappa light chain restriction

Diagnostic Criteria for CLL (All Met):

✓ **Absolute lymphocyte count >5,000/μL** (patient: 42,000/μL)

✓ **Clonal B cells** (kappa restricted)

✓ **Characteristic immunophenotype** (CD5+, CD19+, CD23+, dim CD20/sIg)

✓ **Duration >3 months** (or characteristic features at presentation)

Cytogenetic and Molecular Studies (Prognostic):

FISH (Fluorescence In Situ Hybridization) Panel:

del(13q14): Positive (sole abnormality) FAVORABLE

del(11q22-23) (ATM): Negative

del(17p13) (TP53): Negative **FAVORABLE**

Trisomy 12: Negative

TP53 Mutation Analysis:

TP53 sequencing: **No mutations detected FAVORABLE**

IGHV Mutational Status:

Immunoglobulin heavy chain variable region: MUTATED (>2% difference from germline) **FAVORABLE**

Mutated IGHV associated with better prognosis

ZAP-70 Expression:

ZAP-70 (by flow cytometry): **Negative (<20%) FAVORABLE**

Beta-2 Microglobulin:

β2M: 2.1 mg/L (normal <2.5) **FAVORABLE**

Risk Stratification:

Rai Staging (Clinical):

Stage 0: Lymphocytosis only (no lymphadenopathy, no hepatosplenomegaly, Hgb >11, platelets >100K) ← **PATIENT**

Stage I: Lymphocytosis + lymphadenopathy

Stage II: Lymphocytosis + hepatosplenomegaly ± lymphadenopathy

Stage III: Lymphocytosis + anemia (Hgb <11)

Stage IV: Lymphocytosis + thrombocytopenia (platelets <100K)

Binet Staging (European):

Stage A: <3 lymphoid areas involved, no anemia/thrombocytopenia ← **PATIENT**

Stage B: ≥3 lymphoid areas involved

Stage C: Anemia or thrombocytopenia

CLL-IPI (International Prognostic Index):

TP53 status (del17p or mutation): Absent (0 points)

IGHV status: Mutated (0 points)

β2M: <3.5 mg/L (0 points)

Rai stage: 0 (0 points)

Age: <65 years (0 points)

Total: 0 points = Low risk (10-year survival >70%)

Imaging Studies:

CT Chest/Abdomen/Pelvis:

No lymphadenopathy (all nodes <1.5 cm)

Liver and spleen: Normal size

No focal lesions

Bone Marrow Biopsy (Optional in Early Stage; Performed for Research/Baseline):

Cellularity: 60% (age-appropriate)

Lymphocytic infiltration: 40% (interstitial and nodular pattern)

Immunohistochemistry: CD20+, CD5+, CD23+ B cells

Megakaryocytes, erythroid, myeloid: Normal

Pattern: Non-diffuse (favorable)

Additional Laboratory Assessment:

Direct Antiglobulin Test (Coombs):

Negative (no autoimmune hemolytic anemia)

Serum Immunoglobulins:

IgG: 685 mg/dL (normal)

IgA: 125 mg/dL (normal)

IgM: 45 mg/dL (normal)

No hypogammaglobulinemia (good immune function)

Quantiferon or PPD:

Negative (no latent TB)

Hepatitis Panel:

HBsAg, HBcAb, HCV: Negative

Final Diagnosis: Chronic Lymphocytic Leukemia (CLL), Rai Stage 0, Binet Stage A

Incidental finding on routine CBC

Favorable prognostic markers:

del(13q) as sole abnormality

Mutated IGHV

No TP53 mutation/deletion

ZAP-70 negative

Low β2-microglobulin

CLL-IPI: Low risk

Management:

Watch and Wait Approach:

No treatment indicated for asymptomatic, early-stage CLL

Treatment does NOT improve survival when started in early stages

Initiate treatment only when:

Progressive cytopenias (anemia Hgb <10, platelets <100K)

Massive/progressive lymphadenopathy or splenomegaly

Constitutional symptoms (fever, night sweats, weight loss >10%)

Lymphocyte doubling time <6 months

Progressive marrow failure

Autoimmune complications

Monitoring Schedule:

CBC every 3 months initially, then every 6 months if stable

Physical exam every 3-6 months (lymphadenopathy, splenomegaly)

Imaging only if clinical changes (no routine CT scans)

Annual influenza vaccine, pneumococcal vaccine

Assess for infections (monitor immunoglobulins annually)

Patient Education:

Explain diagnosis: Chronic, incurable, but often indolent

Watch and wait rationale (avoid toxicity when not needed)

Warning signs requiring earlier visit

476

Healthy lifestyle, infection prevention

Follow-Up (6 Months):

WBC: 52,000/μL (slight increase)

Hemoglobin: 13.5 g/dL (stable)

Platelets: 175,000/μL (stable)

Physical exam: No lymphadenopathy

Patient asymptomatic

Continue observation

Follow-Up (1 Year):

WBC: 58,000/μL (slow increase)

Hemoglobin: 13.2 g/dL

Platelets: 165,000/μL

Lymphocyte doubling time: 18 months (not concerning; <6 months is worrisome)

Continue observation

Follow-Up (3 Years):

WBC: 75,000/μL

Hemoglobin: 12.8 g/dL

Platelets: 145,000/μL

Physical exam: 1 cm left cervical node (new, small)

Still asymptomatic, no functional impairment

Continue observation

Long-Term Considerations:

Indications to Start Treatment (None Currently Present):

Rai Stage III/IV (cytopenias)

Symptomatic lymphadenopathy/splenomegaly

Constitutional symptoms

Lymphocyte doubling time <6 months

Autoimmune complications (AIHA, ITP)

First-Line Treatment Options (When Needed):

Younger, fit patients: FCR (fludarabine, cyclophosphamide, rituximab) or ibrutinib

Elderly/comorbid: Ibrutinib (BTK inhibitor) or venetoclax + obinutuzumab

Del(17p)/TP53 mutation: Avoid chemoimmunotherapy; use ibrutinib, venetoclax, or acalabrutinib

Complications to Monitor:

Infections: Hypogammaglobulinemia develops over time (IVIG if recurrent infections)

Autoimmune cytopenias: AIHA (10-15%), ITP (2-5%)

Richter transformation: Transformation to aggressive lymphoma (2-10%; suspect if rapid lymph node growth, fever, rising LDH)

Secondary malignancies: Increased risk of skin cancers, solid tumors

Prognosis:

Rai Stage 0, favorable markers: Median survival >10-15 years, may approach normal life expectancy

Many patients die of unrelated causes, not CLL

30% never require treatment

Teaching Points:

CLL Diagnosis: Requires sustained lymphocytosis >5,000/μL (>3 months) + characteristic immunophenotype (CD5+, CD19+, CD23+, dim CD20/sIg); most common adult leukemia

Smudge Cells: Fragile CLL lymphocytes rupture during slide preparation; characteristic but not specific; reduce by adding albumin to blood before smearing

Immunophenotype: CD5+/CD19+/CD23+ distinguishes CLL from mantle cell lymphoma (CD5+/CD19+/CD23-/cyclin D1+) and other B-cell disorders

Matutes Score: 5-point scoring system for CLL diagnosis (CD5, CD23, weak sIg/CD20, FMC7); score ≥4 = CLL

IGHV Status: Most important prognostic marker; mutated IGHV (>2% difference from germline) = favorable (median survival >20 years); unmutated = unfavorable (median survival 8-10 years)

del(17p)/TP53: Worst prognosis; resistant to chemoimmunotherapy; requires targeted agents (ibrutinib, venetoclax, acalabrutinib)

del(13q): Most common abnormality (50-60%); favorable prognosis when sole abnormality; median survival >10-15 years

Watch and Wait: Standard for asymptomatic early-stage CLL; early treatment does not improve survival; defer until symptomatic or progressive disease

Richter Transformation: Sudden enlargement of lymph nodes, fever, weight loss, rising LDH; biopsy shows DLBCL or Hodgkin; poor prognosis (median survival 6-12 months)

Targeted Therapies: BTK inhibitors (ibrutinib, acalabrutinib), BCL-2 inhibitor (venetoclax), anti-CD20 (obinutuzumab, rituximab); superior to chemoimmunotherapy in many patients

Related Cases: Mantle cell lymphoma, hairy cell leukemia, monoclonal B lymphocytosis (MBL), CLL with Richter transformation

---

Case 13.7: Quality Control Failure Investigation

Clinical Presentation (Laboratory Perspective): At 8:30 AM, the clinical chemistry laboratory begins receiving calls from physicians about unexpectedly low potassium results. Multiple patients in different units show potassium values 0.4-0.6 mEq/L lower than previous results from yesterday. Patients are clinically stable with no changes in medications or clinical status. The laboratory must investigate immediately to prevent patient harm.

Initial Problem Recognition:

Patient Examples:

Patient A: ICU patient, yesterday K+ 4.2 mEq/L → today 3.6 mEq/L (no clinical change)

Patient B: Cardiology floor, yesterday K+ 3.8 mEq/L → today 3.2 mEq/L (stable)

Patient C: Medical floor, yesterday K+ 4.5 mEq/L → today 3.9 mEq/L (stable)

Pattern: All potassium results systematically lower by 0.4-0.6 mEq/L

Time Frame:

Problem noted: 8:30 AM

Results affected: All potassium tests run between 6:00 AM - 8:30 AM

Prior to 6:00 AM: Results appear normal (correlate with clinical picture)

Diagnostic Reasoning Questions:

What is the systematic approach to investigating a quality control failure?

How do you distinguish analytical error from pre-analytical and post-analytical errors?

What immediate actions prevent patient harm?

How is root cause analysis performed?

Sequential Investigation:

Step 1: Verify the Problem (Delta Check Analysis)

Automated Delta Check Alerts:

Laboratory information system (LIS) flagged 23 potassium results with delta >0.5 mEq/L from previous

All deltas showed decrease (none increased)

All occurred in same time window (6:00-8:30 AM)

Systematic bias confirmed

Step 2: Assess Quality Control (QC) Data

Review QC Results (Westgard Rules):

Level 1 QC (Low Normal): 3.2 mEq/L (target 3.5 mEq/L, range 3.3-3.7) **OUT OF RANGE - LOW**

Level 2 QC (High Normal): 5.4 mEq/L (target 5.8 mEq/L, range 5.6-6.0) **OUT OF RANGE - LOW**

Both QC levels shifted low by ~0.4 mEq/L

QC rejection rule violated: 1-2s rule (one control outside 2 SD)

Levy-Jennings Chart:

Previous 20 days: QC values centered on target

Today (6:00 AM run): Both levels shifted low

480

Pattern: Sudden shift, affecting both levels equally → **Systematic error**

QC Action:

STOP patient testing immediately

Call all results since 6:00 AM as "questionable"

Physicians notified to disregard results and reorder STAT

Step 3: Investigate Analytical Variables

Instrument Check:

Analyzer: Beckman Coulter AU5800 (ion-selective electrode method)

Calibration status: Last calibrated 2 days ago (within acceptable window)

Electrode function: K+ electrode response checked → **ABNORMAL**

Slope: 54.2 mV/decade (expected 58-62 mV/decade) **LOW SLOPE**

Indicates electrode drift

Maintenance Log Review:

No recent preventive maintenance

Electrode age: 4 months (expected lifespan 6 months, but can fail early)

Possible Causes of Electrode Drift:

Protein/lipid buildup on electrode membrane

Membrane degradation

Internal reference solution depletion

Step 4: Investigate Reagent/Calibrator Issues

Reagent Lot Review:

NEW potassium reagent lot installed: 5:45 AM ← TIMING MATCHES PROBLEM ONSET

Previous lot: Lot #2024-K-885 (depleted at 5:30 AM)

New lot: Lot #2024-K-912 (installed 5:45 AM)

Reagent Quality Check:

Expiration date: Valid (6 months remaining)

Storage temperature: Correct (2-8°C)

Visual inspection: Clear solution, no particulates

Calibrator Review:

Calibrators: Same lot as previous days (ruled out as cause)

Multi-level calibration curve: Shows slight deviation with new reagent

Reagent Testing:

New reagent lot tested against reference material:

Reference K+ 4.0 mEq/L → New reagent measures 3.6 mEq/L (**0.4 mEq/L bias**)

OLD reagent lot (reserved backup) tested:

Reference K+ 4.0 mEq/L → Old reagent measures 4.0 mEq/L (**accurate**)

Root Cause Identified: Defective reagent lot (manufacturer error)

Step 5: Confirm Root Cause

Switch to Backup Reagent Lot:

Install old reagent lot (backup supply)

Recalibrate instrument

Run QC:

Level 1: 3.5 mEq/L (target 3.5) ✓ **WITHIN RANGE**

Level 2: 5.8 mEq/L (target 5.8) ✓ **WITHIN RANGE**

Re-analyze Patient Samples (Original Specimens):

Patient A: 4.1 mEq/L (correlates with yesterday 4.2) ✓

Patient B: 3.7 mEq/L (correlates with yesterday 3.8) ✓

Patient C: 4.4 mEq/L (correlates with yesterday 4.5) ✓

Corrected results confirm original values were falsely low

Step 6: Patient Impact Assessment

Review All Affected Results:

Total affected samples: 47

Critical low values (<3.0 mEq/L): 3 patients

   All three patients had been contacted for "critical" low K+

   Clinical teams had ordered STAT redraws and potassium supplementation

   Intervention prevented: Redraws showed K+ actually normal

Adverse Events:

One patient received 20 mEq KCl IV before redraw available (based on falsely low 2.8, actual 3.4)

Post-supplementation K+: 4.6 mEq/L (mild hyperkalemia, asymptomatic)

No patient harm resulted (mild hyperkalemia self-resolved)

Step 7: Corrective and Preventive Actions (CAPA)

Immediate Corrective Actions:

✓ **Stopped patient testing** (6:00-8:30 AM period)

✓ **Notified all physicians** of erroneous results

✓ **Re-analyzed all specimens** with correct reagent

✓ **Issued corrected reports** to all providers

✓ **Documented incident** in quality management system

Root Cause Analysis (Fishbone Diagram):

Primary cause: Defective reagent lot (manufacturer quality control failure)

Contributing factor: Reagent lot change occurred outside of regular QC schedule

Detection: QC detected problem, but some patient results released before QC review

Preventive Actions:

Enhanced QC protocol: Run QC BEFORE any patient testing when new reagent lot installed

Manufacturer notification: Report defective lot (Lot #2024-K-912) to Beckman Coulter

Reagent lot quarantine: Quarantine remaining defective lot, return to manufacturer

Lot-to-lot verification: Implement mandatory lot-to-lot comparison (run old and new lot in parallel before switch)

Delta check enhancement: Strengthen automated alerts for systematic bias

Staff education: Review case at monthly quality meeting

Step 8: Regulatory Reporting and Documentation

Incident Report Filed:

Laboratory quality management system documented

Manufacturer notified (defective lot investigation by Beckman)

Risk management informed (one patient received unnecessary potassium)

Medical director review completed

Manufacturer Investigation Results (2 Weeks Later):

Beckman Coulter confirmed reagent lot defect

Manufacturing error: Incorrect reagent concentration during production

Recall issued: Lot #2024-K-912 recalled nationally

Customer notification sent to all laboratories

Long-Term Follow-Up:

Quality Indicators Monitored:

Delta check alert rate: Tracked monthly

QC rejection rate: Remained stable at <2%

Turnaround time: No impact (swift resolution)

System Improvements Implemented:

Automated lot change protocol: LIS flags technologist to run QC before patient testing

Parallel testing requirement: New reagent lot tested alongside old lot (n=20 samples, correlation must be >0.95)

Enhanced moving average: Patient data-based QC (detects systematic shifts)

Supplier quality review: Quarterly review of manufacturer QC practices

No Further Issues: Preventive actions successful; no recurrence in 2 years

Final Root Cause: Defective Potassium Reagent Lot (Manufacturer Error) Causing Systematic Negative Bias of 0.4-0.6 mEq/L

QC detected problem appropriately

Swift investigation and resolution prevented significant patient harm

Preventive actions implemented to avoid recurrence

Teaching Points:

QC Purpose: Detects analytical errors before patient results released; systematic review of QC essential; QC failure requires immediate action (stop testing, investigate)

Westgard Rules: Statistical QC rules detect shifts (1-2s, 1-3s), trends (6x, 9x), random error (R-4s); multi-rule approach increases error detection

Levy-Jennings Chart: Visual display of QC over time; sudden shift indicates systematic error; gradual drift indicates reagent/calibrator degradation

Systematic vs. Random Error: Systematic (shifts all results in one direction; reagent, calibration, electrode); Random (individual errors; pipetting, interference)

Delta Check: Compares current result to previous; flags significant changes; useful for detecting systematic bias when many patients affected

Root Cause Analysis: Systematic investigation (fishbone/5 Whys); identifies primary cause and contributing factors; drives preventive actions

CAPA (Corrective and Preventive Action): Corrective (fix immediate problem); Preventive (stop recurrence); both essential for quality

Lot-to-Lot Verification: Compare new reagent lot to old before routine use; prevents errors from defective lots; required by CAP/CLIA

Patient Data-Based QC: Moving averages of patient results detect shifts; complements traditional QC; increasingly adopted

Manufacturer Defects: Rare but occur; laboratories must detect via QC; reporting to manufacturer/FDA essential for recalls

Related Cases: Calibration error causing systematic bias, pre-analytical error (hemolysis), post-analytical error (result transmission failure), reagent contamination

---

Case 13.8: Laboratory Utilization Optimization

Clinical Presentation (Hospital Quality Initiative): The hospital quality improvement committee identifies that daily CBC ordering in the Intensive Care Unit (ICU) has increased 40% over the past year, yet patient outcomes and length of stay have not changed. The laboratory medical director is asked to lead a utilization optimization project to reduce unnecessary testing while maintaining quality of care.

Baseline Data Collection:

CBC Ordering Patterns (3-Month Baseline):

   Total CBCs ordered in ICU: 3,450 per month

   Average CBCs per patient-day: 1.8 (national average: 1.2)

   Cost per CBC: $15 (reagent + labor + overhead)

   Total monthly cost: $51,750

   Projected annual cost: $621,000

Chart Review (Random Sample of 100 ICU Patients):

   Daily CBC ordered on 92% of patient-days

   No clinical change or decision made: 68% of CBCs

   Hemoglobin change <0.5 g/dL from prior: 78%

   Platelet change <20,000/μL from prior: 82%

   Clinical action taken based on result: 12%

Diagnostic Reasoning Questions:

   How do you assess appropriateness of laboratory test utilization?

   What interventions reduce unnecessary testing without compromising care?

   How are clinical decision support tools implemented?

How is impact measured (clinical outcomes, costs, safety)?

Step 1: Multidisciplinary Team Formation

Stakeholders:

Laboratory medical director (lead)

ICU medical director

ICU nursing leadership

Hospitalists

Quality improvement specialists

Informatics/IT

Finance

Step 2: Literature Review and Benchmarking

Evidence Review:

JAMA study: Daily CBC in stable ICU patients does not improve outcomes

Choosing Wisely: Recommends against routine daily labs in stable patients

High-performing institutions: CBC every 48-72 hours for stable patients

Blood conservation programs: Reduce hospital-acquired anemia

Benchmark Data:

Academic medical centers: Average 1.0-1.3 CBCs per ICU patient-day

This institution: 1.8 CBCs per patient-day (43% above benchmark)

Step 3: Define Appropriate Utilization Criteria

Appropriate Indications for Daily CBC (Developed by Multidisciplinary Team):

Active bleeding or high bleeding risk (DIC, anticoagulation)

Hemodynamic instability (shock, vasopressor requirement)

Active hemolysis (known hemolytic process)

Post-operative day 0-2 (major surgery)

Chemotherapy or bone marrow suppression

Sepsis with evolving organ dysfunction

Transfusion within 24 hours

Clinical indication documented by provider

Stable Patient Criteria (CBC Every 48-72 Hours):

Hemodynamically stable (no vasopressors)

No active bleeding

No recent transfusion (>24 hours)

No active hemolysis

No bone marrow suppression

Step 4: Intervention Design

Multi-Modal Intervention:

A. Clinical Decision Support (CDS):

Alert in electronic order entry:

"CBC ordered <24 hours from last result. Is repeat indicated?"

Hard stop if <12 hours (requires override with justification)

Soft stop if 12-24 hours (alert with option to proceed)

Suggested alternative: "Consider CBC in 48-72 hours for stable patient"

B. Order Set Modification:

Default ICU admission order set:

Changed from "CBC daily" to "CBC every 48 hours"

Option to select "CBC daily if clinically indicated" with checkbox list of indications

C. Education:

Grand Rounds presentation: "Reducing Low-Value Laboratory Testing in the ICU"

Pocket cards for ICU team with appropriateness criteria

Nursing education: Clarify that daily labs not required for all patients

D. Audit and Feedback:

Monthly reports to ICU teams showing:

> CBC utilization per patient-day by team

> Comparison to institutional goal (1.2 per patient-day)

> Outlier analysis (providers ordering >2 CBCs per patient-day)

E. Financial Incentive:

Cost savings shared with ICU department for quality initiatives

Step 5: Pilot Implementation (1 Month)

Pilot Unit: Medical ICU (20 beds)

Pilot Results:

CBCs per patient-day: 1.3 (decreased from 1.8, **28% reduction**)

Hard stop overrides: 8% (mostly appropriate - bleeding, sepsis)

Soft stop "proceed anyway": 15%

Provider satisfaction survey: 78% favorable (accept intervention as appropriate)

Safety outcomes:

> No missed critical anemia (Hgb <7 g/dL)

> No missed critical thrombocytopenia (platelets <20K)

> **No adverse events attributed to reduced testing**

Refinement Based on Pilot:

Adjust hard stop time from 12 to 18 hours (more clinically appropriate)

Add "post-transfusion" as auto-bypass for hard stop

Simplify CDS alert (reduce alert fatigue)

Step 6: Full Implementation (Hospital-Wide ICUs)

Rollout Plan:

Month 1: Medical ICU (pilot)

Month 2: Surgical ICU

Month 3: Cardiac ICU, Neuro ICU

Ongoing: Monitor and refine

Post-Implementation Results (6 Months):

Utilization Metrics:

CBCs per patient-day: 1.2 (decreased from 1.8, **33% reduction**)

Total CBCs per month: 2,300 (decreased from 3,450, **1,150 fewer tests**)

Hard stop override rate: 12% (acceptable - appropriate overrides)

Order set default changed: Used in 85% of admissions

Cost Savings:

Monthly savings: $17,250 (1,150 tests × $15)

Projected annual savings: $207,000

3-year projected savings: $621,000

Clinical Outcomes (Safety Analysis):

ICU length of stay: 4.2 days (unchanged from 4.3 days baseline)

ICU mortality: 8.5% (unchanged from 8.8% baseline)

Transfusion rate: 18% (unchanged from 19% baseline)

Missed critical lab values: 0 (comprehensive safety review of 500 patients)

Adverse events related to reduced testing: 0

Blood Conservation Impact:

Phlebotomy volume reduced: ~3 mL per CBC × 1,150 tests = **3,450 mL/month** (3.5 liters less blood drawn)

Hospital-acquired anemia: Incidence decreased from 22% to 18%

Provider Feedback (Surveys and Interviews):

85% agree: Intervention appropriate and improves care

12% neutral

3% disagree: Prefer autonomy in ordering

Quotes:

> "Makes me think before reflexively ordering daily labs"

> "Reduces unnecessary blood draws for patients"

> "Frees nursing time from non-essential lab draws"

Step 7: Expansion to Other Test Categories

Successful Model Applied to:

A. Comprehensive Metabolic Panel (CMP):

Similar CDS implemented

Reduction: 25% in unnecessary daily CMPs

Annual savings: $85,000

B. Coagulation Studies (PT/INR, aPTT):

Daily coags only if:

> Active anticoagulation being titrated

> Active bleeding/DIC

> Liver failure with coagulopathy

Reduction: 30%

Annual savings: $45,000

C. Arterial Blood Gases (ABG):

Daily ABGs only if:

 Mechanical ventilation with recent vent changes

 Acid-base disturbance being treated

 Respiratory failure

Reduction: 40%

Annual savings: $62,000

Total Annual Savings (All Initiatives): $399,000

Step 8: Sustainability and Continuous Monitoring

Ongoing Surveillance:

 Monthly utilization dashboards (LIS automated reports)

 Quarterly safety audits (review critical values, adverse events)

 Annual provider education refresher

 CDS refinement based on user feedback

2-Year Follow-Up:

 Sustained reduction: 1.2 CBCs per patient-day (maintained)

 No "testing creep" back to old patterns

 No adverse events in 2 years attributed to reduced testing

 Provider acceptance: Now standard of care

Key Success Factors:

 Multidisciplinary buy-in: Clinicians involved in criteria development

 Evidence-based approach: Literature and benchmarking data

 Clinical decision support: Right test, right time, right patient

 Education: Not just "do less" but "do smarter"

 Audit and feedback: Transparency and accountability

Safety monitoring: Comprehensive surveillance for adverse events

Shared savings: Financial incentive for departments

Final Outcomes: Laboratory Utilization Optimization Program Successfully Implemented:

33% reduction in ICU CBC utilization

$399,000 annual savings across all test categories

No compromise in patient safety (comprehensive 2-year safety analysis)

Improved patient experience (fewer blood draws)

Model expanded to other hospital departments and other institutions

Teaching Points:

Laboratory Stewardship: Judicious test utilization; right test, right patient, right time; parallels antimicrobial stewardship

Low-Value Testing: Tests unlikely to change management; daily labs in stable patients often low-value; Choosing Wisely identifies common low-value practices

Clinical Decision Support (CDS): Alerts at point of order entry; hard stops (require override) vs soft stops (alert with proceed option); reduce inappropriate ordering 20-50%

Default Order Sets: Defaults powerfully influence behavior; changing "daily labs" default to "every 48-72h" reduces reflexive ordering

Audit and Feedback: Showing providers their utilization vs peers motivates behavior change; non-punitive, educational approach

Safety Monitoring: Essential when reducing testing; track critical values, adverse events, outcomes; comprehensive surveillance prevents harm

Blood Conservation: Reducing phlebotomy decreases hospital-acquired anemia; each CBC = 3mL blood; daily labs in 500-bed hospital = 1,500 mL/day

Cost Savings: Laboratory costs are ~5% of hospital budget; utilization optimization can save millions; reinvest savings in quality improvement

Stakeholder Engagement: Physicians, nurses, lab, IT, finance all involved; multidisciplinary approach ensures success

Sustainability: Requires ongoing monitoring, education, CDS refinement; without surveillance, utilization creeps back to baseline

Related Cases: Reducing unnecessary troponin testing, optimizing tumor marker utilization, eliminating redundant lipid panels, procalcitonin-guided antibiotic stewardship

Case 13.9: Test Interference - Biotin Interference in Thyroid Testing

Clinical Presentation: A 50-year-old woman presents to endocrinology clinic with a confusing thyroid function test pattern from her primary care physician. She was found to have "severe hyperthyroidism" on labs (TSH <0.01 mIU/L, free T4 >7.77 ng/dL), but she is completely asymptomatic - no palpitations, weight loss, tremor, heat intolerance, or diarrhea. Her thyroid gland is normal on palpation. She was told she might need radioactive iodine ablation, which prompted her to seek a second opinion.

Physical Examination:

BP 118/72, HR 68 (regular), Temp 98.4°F, Weight stable

Appears well, no signs of hyperthyroidism

No tremor, no lid lag, no exophthalmos

Thyroid: Normal size, no nodules, no bruit

Skin: Warm and dry (not warm and moist as in hyperthyroidism)

Cardiovascular: Regular rhythm, no tachycardia

Hair: No hair loss

Reflexes: Normal (not brisk as in hyperthyroidism)

Review of Outside Laboratory Results:

Thyroid Function Tests (Outside Lab, Immunoassay Method):

TSH: <0.01 mIU/L SEVERELY SUPPRESSED (normal 0.4-4.0)

Free T4: >7.77 ng/dL MARKEDLY ELEVATED (normal 0.8-1.8)

Free T3: 18.5 pg/mL MARKEDLY ELEVATED (normal 2.3-4.2)

Pattern: Severe primary hyperthyroidism (suppressed TSH, elevated T4 and T3)

Diagnostic Reasoning Questions:

What is the differential diagnosis for discrepant thyroid tests and clinical picture?

How does biotin interfere with immunoassays?

What other substances cause assay interference?

How should suspected interference be investigated?

Clinical Reasoning:

Laboratory suggests severe hyperthyroidism

Patient completely asymptomatic (very unusual for this degree of biochemical hyperthyroidism)

Mismatch between labs and clinical picture suggests:

Laboratory error/interference

Subclinical hyperthyroidism (but labs show severe, not subclinical)

Thyroid hormone resistance (rare)

Assay interference (most likely)

Detailed History:

Medication and Supplement Review:

Levothyroxine: **NONE** (not taking thyroid hormone)

Prescription medications: Metformin 1000 mg BID (diabetes)

Supplements:

Biotin 10 mg (10,000 µg) daily for hair and nail health (taking for 6 months)

Multivitamin (contains 30 µg biotin)

Vitamin D 2000 IU daily

Total biotin intake: ~10,030 µg/day

Key Finding: High-dose biotin supplementation

Biotin Interference Mechanism:

Immunoassay Technology:

Most thyroid assays use **biotin-streptavidin binding** technology

Competitive immunoassay (TSH, T3):

Biotinylated antibody competes with patient antigen

High biotin → blocks binding → **falsely LOW TSH/T3** (but in this case, see below)

Sandwich immunoassay (free T4):

Biotinylated detection antibody

High biotin → interferes with signal → **falsely HIGH free T4**

Interference Pattern with Biotin:

TSH: Typically falsely **LOW** (suppressed)

Free T4: Typically falsely **HIGH** (elevated)

Free T3: Variable (depends on assay)

Pattern mimics primary hyperthyroidism (low TSH, high T4)

Step 1: Confirm Interference Hypothesis

Immediate Management:

STOP biotin supplementation

Wait 48-72 hours (biotin half-life ~2 hours, but complete washout takes 2-3 days)

Repeat thyroid function tests

Repeat Testing (72 Hours After Stopping Biotin):

Same Laboratory, Same Assay:

TSH: 2.1 mIU/L NORMAL (previously <0.01)

Free T4: 1.2 ng/dL NORMAL (previously >7.77)

Free T3: 3.1 pg/mL NORMAL (previously 18.5)

Interpretation: Biotin interference confirmed - thyroid function completely normal

Step 2: Test Using Alternative Method (Confirmatory)

Biotin-Free Assay:

Some laboratories offer biotin-free thyroid assays

Liquid chromatography-tandem mass spectrometry (LC-MS/MS): No biotin interference

Results (while on biotin): TSH 2.0, free T4 1.1 (normal) - **confirms biotin interference in immunoassay**

Step 3: Additional Testing to Assess Biotin Levels

Serum Biotin Level (While on Supplement):

Biotin: 1,250 ng/mL MARKEDLY ELEVATED (normal <1 ng/mL)

Biotin at this level saturates streptavidin binding sites → assay interference

Typical Biotin Levels:

Normal diet: <1 ng/mL

Multivitamin (30-100 µg): <5 ng/mL (minimal interference)

High-dose supplements (5-10 mg): >200 ng/mL (**interferes with assays**)

Therapeutic doses (MS, rare diseases): >500 ng/mL (**severe interference**)

Step 4: Identify All Affected Assays

Biotin Interferes with Many Immunoassays:

Falsely Elevated (Sandwich Assays):

Free T4, free T3 (appears hyperthyroid)

Troponin (false MI)

NT-proBNP (false heart failure)

PSA (false prostate cancer)

CA-125, CEA (false malignancy)

Ferritin, vitamin B12, folate

Falsely Decreased (Competitive Assays):

TSH (appears suppressed)

Cortisol (appears adrenal insufficiency)

Testosterone, estradiol

Vitamin D (25-OH)

PTH

Patient's Additional Labs Reviewed:

Troponin (Drawn During Recent ED Visit for Chest Pain):

Original result: 0.18 ng/mL (elevated; normal <0.04)

Patient diagnosed with "NSTEMI," admitted to cardiology

Cardiac catheterization: Normal coronaries (no CAD)

Retrospective analysis: Troponin falsely elevated by biotin

Repeat troponin (off biotin): <0.01 ng/mL (normal)

Vitamin D:

Original result: 12 ng/mL (deficient; normal >30)

Started on high-dose vitamin D supplementation

Repeat (off biotin): 38 ng/mL (normal) - falsely low due to biotin

Step 5: Root Cause Analysis

Why Was Biotin Not Initially Suspected?

Patient not asked about supplements (focused on prescription meds)

Biotin use not in medical record

Laboratory did not have biotin alert in result reporting

Clinicians unaware of biotin interference

Prevention Opportunities:

Medication reconciliation include **supplements**

Laboratory alert if biotin-sensitive assay

Patient education about supplement disclosure

Step 6: Implement System-Wide Solutions

Laboratory Actions:

Alert in Laboratory Reports:

"This assay susceptible to biotin interference. High-dose biotin (>5 mg/day) may cause erroneous results."

Biotin Screening Question:

Electronic order entry: "Is patient taking biotin >5 mg/day?"

If yes → suggest biotin-free assay or delay testing

Biotin-Free Assay Availability:

Offer LC-MS/MS for critical assays (troponin, thyroid) when biotin suspected

Test Utilization Review:

Evaluate all immunoassays for biotin susceptibility

Identify alternative methods

Clinical Actions:

Medication Reconciliation:

Always ask about supplements (biotin, vitamin C, high-dose B vitamins)

Document in EHR

Clinical Decision Support:

Alert providers if ordering biotin-sensitive test and patient on biotin

Patient Education:

Handout: "Biotin and Laboratory Testing"

"Stop biotin 72 hours before lab work"

Institutional Policy:

Pre-operative testing: Hold biotin 72 hours before surgery (prevents false troponin)

Endocrinology clinic: Routine biotin screening before thyroid testing

Emergency department: Ask about biotin if troponin, BNP, or thyroid tests ordered

Follow-Up (Patient Outcome):

3 Months Later:

Stopped biotin supplement (patient educated on interference)

Thyroid function tests: Normal (TSH 1.8, free T4 1.1)

No thyroid disease - completely healthy

Avoided unnecessary radioactive iodine ablation

Awareness of supplement-lab interaction

Impact on Other Patients:

Case Review (Hospital-Wide):

Identified **8 additional patients** with biotin interference in past year

3 false hyperthyroidism (like this patient)

2 false troponin elevation (unnecessary cardiac cath avoided after intervention)

2 false vitamin D deficiency

1 false elevated PSA (unnecessary prostate biopsy avoided)

Final Diagnosis: Falsely Abnormal Thyroid Function Tests Due to High-Dose Biotin Interference in Immunoassays (No True Thyroid Disease)

Biotin Dosing and Interference Risk:

Biotin Dose	Source	Interference Risk
<1 µg/day	Normal diet	None
30-100 µg/day	Multivitamin	Minimal
2.5-5 mg/day	Hair/nail supplements	Moderate
5-10 mg/day	High-dose OTC	HIGH ← Patient
100-300 mg/day	MS, biotin-responsive disorders	SEVERE

Teaching Points:

Biotin Interference: High-dose biotin (>5 mg/day) interferes with streptavidin-biotin immunoassays; mimics hyperthyroidism (low TSH, high T4), false troponin elevation, false tumor markers

Mechanism: Biotin-streptavidin binding technology used in many immunoassays; excess biotin saturates binding sites → erroneous results (falsely high in sandwich assays, falsely low in competitive)

Prevalence of High-Dose Biotin: Increasingly popular for hair/nail/skin health; 5-10 mg doses common in supplements; patients often don't report (assume "just a vitamin")

Clinical-Lab Discordance: Mismatch between lab results and clinical picture should prompt investigation for interference; asymptomatic "severe hyperthyroidism" is red flag

Affected Assays: Thyroid (TSH, T4, T3), cardiac (troponin, BNP), tumor markers (PSA, CA-125, CEA), hormones (testosterone, estradiol, cortisol), vitamins (D, B12)

Washout Period: Biotin half-life ~2 hours; complete elimination 24-48 hours; recommend stopping 72 hours before lab testing (conservative)

Supplement History: Always ask about over-the-counter supplements; include in medication reconciliation; biotin, high-dose vitamin C, saw palmetto can interfere

Alternative Methods: LC-MS/MS not affected by biotin; consider for critical assays if biotin suspected; some manufacturers offer biotin-free immunoassays

Laboratory Communication: Labs should alert providers to interference potential; include biotin warning in reports for susceptible assays

Patient Education: Inform patients to disclose all supplements; provide written guidance to stop biotin before testing; awareness prevents misdiagnosis

Related Cases: Heterophile antibody interference, high-dose vitamin C interference, rheumatoid factor interference in immunoassays

---

Case 13.10: Biological Variation vs. Pathologic Change

Clinical Presentation: A 65-year-old man with chronic kidney disease (CKD) stage 3 presents for routine nephrology follow-up. He has been stable for years with creatinine ranging 1.4-1.8 mg/dL. Recent labs show creatinine 1.8 mg/dL, and the referring physician is concerned about "worsening kidney function" and possible need to start dialysis planning. Patient feels well, no new symptoms, medications unchanged, diet stable.

Past Medical History:

CKD stage 3 (baseline Cr 1.4-1.6 mg/dL for 3 years)

Hypertension (well-controlled)

Type 2 diabetes (HbA1c 6.8%, stable)

501

No obstructive uropathy, no recurrent UTIs

Current Medications:

Lisinopril 20 mg daily (unchanged x 2 years)

Metformin 1000 mg BID (unchanged)

Atorvastatin 40 mg daily

Physical Examination:

BP 128/76, HR 72, Weight 82 kg (stable)

No edema, no signs of volume overload

Cardiovascular, pulmonary, abdominal: Normal

No signs of uremia

Review of Serial Creatinine Values (Past 18 Months):

Month 1: 1.5 mg/dL

Month 2: 1.6 mg/dL

Month 3: 1.4 mg/dL

Month 4: 1.7 mg/dL

Month 5: 1.5 mg/dL

Month 6: 1.6 mg/dL

Month 9: 1.8 mg/dL

Month 12: 1.5 mg/dL

Month 15: 1.4 mg/dL

Month 18: 1.8 mg/dL ← Current value

Diagnostic Reasoning Questions:

How do you distinguish biological variation from true pathologic change?

What is the reference change value (RCV) and how is it calculated?

502

What are the components of total variation in laboratory results?

When should changes in serial results trigger clinical action?

Step 1: Understand Sources of Variation

Total Variation in Laboratory Results:

Total Variation = $\sqrt{CV\_A^2 + CV\_I^2 + CV\_G^2}$

Where:

CV_A: Analytical variation (laboratory imprecision)

CV_I: Within-person biological variation (intra-individual)

CV_G: Between-person biological variation (inter-individual)

For Creatinine:

CV_A (analytical): 2-4% (modern analyzers)

CV_I (within-person biological): 5-8%

CV_G (between-person): 12-20%

Step 2: Calculate Reference Change Value (RCV)

RCV (Reference Change Value):

RCV = Z × $\sqrt{CV\_A^2 + CV\_I^2}$ × $\sqrt{2}$

Z = 1.96 for 95% confidence interval (2-sided)

$\sqrt{2}$ accounts for two measurements

For Creatinine (Using CV_A = 3%, CV_I = 6%):

RCV = 1.96 × $\sqrt{3^2 + 6^2}$ × $\sqrt{2}$

RCV = 1.96 × $\sqrt{9 + 36}$ × 1.414

RCV = 1.96 × 6.7 × 1.414

RCV = 1.96 × 9.5

RCV = 18.6%

Interpretation:

Changes <18.6% likely due to biological/analytical variation

Changes >18.6% likely represent true pathologic change (95% confidence)

Step 3: Apply RCV to Patient's Results

Baseline Creatinine (Average of Stable Values):

Average of months 1-15: **1.54 mg/dL**

Current Creatinine:

1.8 mg/dL

Percent Change:

Change = (1.8 - 1.54) / 1.54 × 100 = **16.9%**

Comparison to RCV:

Change: 16.9%

RCV: 18.6%

16.9% < 18.6% → Change within biological variation √

Conclusion: Creatinine of 1.8 mg/dL is **NOT statistically significant** change from baseline - likely biological variation

Step 4: Additional Supporting Evidence

eGFR Calculation (CKD-EPI Equation):

Baseline average (Cr 1.54): **eGFR 48 mL/min/1.73m²** (CKD stage 3a)

Current (Cr 1.8): **eGFR 41 mL/min/1.73m²** (CKD stage 3b)

eGFR change: 7 mL/min (14.6% decrease)

Within biological variation for eGFR (RCV ~20-25%)

Urinalysis:

Protein: 1+ (stable, baseline proteinuria)

No change from prior

No RBC casts, no pyuria

Urine Protein/Creatinine Ratio:

Current: 0.8 (stable from 0.7-0.9 range)

No significant proteinuria change

Serum Cystatin C (Alternative GFR Marker):

Cystatin C: 1.4 mg/L (stable from baseline 1.3-1.5 mg/L)

eGFR (cystatin C-based): 48 mL/min (no change)

Confirms stable kidney function

Review of Pre-Analytical Factors:

Hydration status: Patient well-hydrated, no recent dehydration

Diet: No high-protein meals (protein intake increases creatinine)

Muscle mass: Stable weight, no muscle loss or gain

Medications: No new NSAIDs, no ACE-I dose change

Recent illness: None

Step 5: Graphical Analysis (Longitudinal Trending)

Plot of Serial Creatinine Values:

Values oscillate between 1.4-1.8 mg/dL (no clear trend)

No progressive increase over time

Pattern: Random variation around mean of 1.55 mg/dL

No upward trend (would indicate progressive CKD)

Linear Regression Analysis:

Slope: +0.01 mg/dL per month (not statistically significant, $p=0.42$)

Stable kidney function over 18 months

Step 6: Clinical Context Integration

Factors Suggesting Stability (Not Progression):

✓ Creatinine change within RCV

✓ eGFR change within biological variation

✓ Cystatin C stable

✓ No increase in proteinuria

✓ No clinical symptoms of worsening CKD (no edema, uremia)

✓ No change in medications or comorbidities

✓ Longitudinal trend shows oscillation, not progression

Factors That Would Suggest True Progression:

Creatinine increase >RCV (>18.6%)

Progressive upward trend over 3-6 months

Increasing proteinuria

New urinary sediment abnormalities

Clinical symptoms (edema, uremia)

Uncontrolled hypertension or hyperglycemia

Final Assessment: Creatinine 1.8 mg/dL Represents **Biological Variation, NOT Pathologic Progression** of CKD

CKD stage 3a (stable)

No indication for dialysis planning

Continue current management

Management Plan:

Reassure patient: Kidney function stable

Continue current medications (no change needed)

Monitor creatinine every 3-6 months (as per CKD guidelines)

Trigger for concern: Creatinine >2.0 mg/dL (>30% from baseline) OR progressive trend over 3-6 months

Optimize CKD management:

Blood pressure control (target <130/80)

Glycemic control (HbA1c <7%)

Avoid nephrotoxins (NSAIDs)

Follow-Up (6 Months):

Creatinine: 1.5 mg/dL (returned to baseline range)

eGFR: 50 mL/min

Confirms biological variation (not true progression)

Comparison: True Progression vs. Biological Variation

Feature	Biological Variation	True Progression
Change magnitude	<RCV (18.6%)	>RCV
Temporal pattern	Random oscillation	Consistent upward trend
Confirmatory tests	Stable (cystatin C, eGFR)	Concordant changes
Clinical context	No new factors	New complications
Proteinuria	Stable	Increasing
Reversibility	Returns to baseline	Persistent elevation

Teaching Points:

Reference Change Value (RCV): Minimum change between serial results to be considered significant (95% confidence); accounts for analytical and biological variation; use to avoid overreacting to normal fluctuations

Biological Variation: Intra-individual (within-person) variation due to physiologic factors; creatinine CV_I 5-8%, glucose 6-8%, cholesterol 6-8%, hemoglobin 3-4%

Analytical Variation: Laboratory imprecision; modern analyzers have CV_A 1-3% for most analytes; less than biological variation for most tests

RCV Formula: RCV = $1.96 \times \sqrt{(CV\_A^2 + CV\_I^2)} \times \sqrt{2}$; Z-score 1.96 for 95% CI; $\sqrt{2}$ because comparing two measurements; creatinine RCV ~15-20%, cholesterol RCV ~15-20%

Index of Individuality: Ratio CV_I/CV_G; low index (<0.6) means individual variation small compared to population → use RCV, not reference range

Creatinine Variability: Affected by hydration, diet (protein), muscle mass, medications; biological CV_I 5-8%; single value may not reflect true GFR

Alternative Markers: Cystatin C less affected by muscle mass, diet; useful when creatinine ambiguous; combined eGFR (Cr + CysC) most accurate

Longitudinal Trending: Plot serial values over time; look for pattern (random oscillation vs. progressive trend); regression analysis identifies significant trends

Clinical Context Essential: Always integrate lab changes with clinical picture; asymptomatic with values within RCV $\rightarrow$ biological variation; symptomatic with concordant changes $\rightarrow$ pathologic

Avoid Overreaction: Small changes within RCV do not require intervention; prevents unnecessary testing, patient anxiety, treatment escalation

Related Cases: HbA1c fluctuation in stable diabetes, cholesterol variation on statin, PSA bouncing in benign prostatic hyperplasia

Case 13.11: Population Screening Program Design - Newborn Screening for CAH

Public Health Directive: The State Department of Public Health commissions a task force to design and implement population-based newborn screening for Congenital Adrenal Hyperplasia (CAH) to prevent salt-wasting crises and neonatal deaths. The laboratory must develop a high-quality, cost-effective screening program.

Background on Congenital Adrenal Hyperplasia:

Disease Overview:

>   **Incidence:** 1:15,000 live births (classic CAH); 1:100-200 for non-classic

>   **Genetics:** Autosomal recessive; 90-95% due to 21-hydroxylase deficiency (CYP21A2 gene)

>   **Pathophysiology:** Cortisol and aldosterone deficiency → ACTH elevation → androgen excess

>   **Clinical:** Salt-wasting crisis (75%), simple virilizing (25%), ambiguous genitalia in females

>   **Mortality:** 10-15% if undiagnosed (salt-wasting shock, hypoglycemia)

>   **Treatment:** Glucocorticoid and mineralocorticoid replacement; prevents crises, normalizes growth

Diagnostic Reasoning Questions:

>   What are the principles of effective population screening programs?

>   How are screening cutoffs determined to balance sensitivity and specificity?

>   What quality assurance measures ensure program success?

>   How are false positives minimized while maintaining sensitivity?

Step 1: Wilson-Jungner Screening Criteria Assessment

WHO Principles for Screening (All Met for CAH):

>   ✓ **Important health problem:** CAH causes preventable mortality/morbidity

>   ✓ **Accepted treatment available:** Hormone replacement highly effective

>   ✓ **Facilities for diagnosis/treatment:** Pediatric endocrinology widely available

>   ✓ **Recognizable latent/early stage:** Elevated 17-OHP before symptoms

>   ✓ **Suitable test available:** 17-OHP by tandem mass spectrometry

509

✓ **Acceptable test:** Dried blood spot (already collected for other newborn screens)

✓ **Natural history understood:** Well-characterized progression

✓ **Agreed policy on whom to treat:** Clear diagnostic and treatment guidelines

✓ **Cost-effective:** Prevents ICU admissions, deaths

✓ **Continuous case-finding:** Ongoing program, not one-time

Step 2: Analyte Selection and Method Development

Primary Analyte:

17-Hydroxyprogesterone (17-OHP): Precursor that accumulates when 21-hydroxylase deficient

Analytical Method:

Tandem Mass Spectrometry (LC-MS/MS): Gold standard

Advantages: High specificity, quantitative, multiplexing (can measure multiple steroids)

Disadvantages: Expensive equipment, requires expertise

Alternative: Immunoassay (higher false-positive rate, not recommended)

Method Development:

Sample: Dried blood spot (DBS) on filter paper (Guthrie card)

Extraction: Methanol extraction of 3.2 mm punch from DBS

LC-MS/MS: Multiple reaction monitoring (MRM) for 17-OHP

Internal standard: Deuterated 17-OHP (d8-17OHP) for accuracy

Calibration: 6-point curve (0-100 ng/mL)

Method Validation:

Linearity: R^2 >0.99 (0-100 ng/mL)

Precision: CV <10% (intra-assay and inter-assay)

Accuracy: Recovery 90-110%

Limit of Detection (LOD): 0.5 ng/mL

Limit of Quantitation (LOQ): 1.0 ng/mL

Reference range established from 5,000 normal newborns

Step 3: Cutoff Determination (Challenging Due to Confounders)

Confounding Factors Affecting 17-OHP:

Gestational age: Preterm infants have higher 17-OHP (immature adrenal function)

Birth weight: Low birth weight → higher 17-OHP

Age at sample collection: 17-OHP decreases in first week of life

Illness/stress: Sick neonates have elevated 17-OHP

Cutoff Strategy: Multi-Tiered, Adjusted for Confounders

Tier 1: Initial Screen (Weight and Gestational Age-Adjusted):

Birth Weight	Gestational Age	17-OHP Cutoff (ng/mL)
>2500 g	**≥37 weeks (term)**	**≥8 ng/mL**
2000-2500 g	≥37 weeks	≥15 ng/mL
1500-2000 g	34-36 weeks	≥25 ng/mL
<1500 g	<34 weeks	≥40 ng/mL

Rationale: Higher cutoffs for preterm/low birth weight to reduce false positives

Tier 2: Second-Tier Steroid Panel (If Tier 1 Positive):

Measure **additional steroids** on same DBS using LC-MS/MS:

17-OHP (confirm)

Androstenedione (elevated in CAH)

Cortisol (low in CAH)

21-Deoxycortisol (elevated in CAH)

Second-Tier Positive Criteria:

17-OHP >15 ng/mL (term) AND

Androstenedione >3 ng/mL OR

21-Deoxycortisol >2 ng/mL

Tier 3: Confirmatory Testing (Pediatric Endocrinology Referral):

Serum 17-OHP (>10,000 ng/dL diagnostic)

ACTH stimulation test

Genetic testing (CYP21A2 sequencing)

Electrolytes (hyponatremia, hyperkalemia in salt-wasting)

Pilot Study Results (10,000 Newborns):

Single-Tier Approach (17-OHP >8 ng/mL, Not Adjusted):

True positives: 6 (6 cases of CAH)

False positives: 180 (1.8% false-positive rate)

Sensitivity: 100%

Specificity: 98.2%

PPV (Positive Predictive Value): 3.2%

Two-Tier Approach (Weight-Adjusted + Second Steroid Panel):

True positives: 6 (6 cases of CAH detected)

False positives: 12 (0.12% false-positive rate)

Sensitivity: 100%

Specificity: 99.88%

PPV: 33% (major improvement)

Outcome: Two-tier approach adopted (15-fold reduction in false positives)

Step 4: Timing of Sample Collection

Optimal Timing:

24-48 hours of life (after initiation of feeding, before hospital discharge)

Too early (<24h): Physiologic 17-OHP surge (false positives)

Too late (>5 days): Salt-wasting crisis may occur before detection

Special Populations:

Preterm/NICU infants: Screen at 7 days of life OR discharge (whichever first)

Transfused infants: Screen before transfusion if possible, OR 48-72h after (donor blood interferes)

Early discharge (<24h): Repeat screen at 1-2 weeks

Step 5: Follow-Up Protocol

Positive Screen Management:

Abnormal Result → Immediate Actions:

Contact family within 24 hours (phone + certified letter)

Refer to pediatric endocrinology (within 24-48 hours)

Interim instructions:

Monitor for vomiting, lethargy, poor feeding (salt-wasting signs)

Seek immediate ED care if symptoms develop

Teach parents signs of adrenal crisis

Confirmatory Testing (Pediatric Endocrinology):

Serum 17-OHP (>10,000 ng/dL = CAH; 1,000-10,000 = possible CAH, genetic testing)

Serum electrolytes (Na, K, glucose) - assess salt-wasting

ACTH stimulation test if baseline 17-OHP equivocal

CYP21A2 genetic testing (confirms diagnosis, identifies genotype)

Treatment Initiation:

Hydrocortisone 10-15 mg/m²/day (divided TID)

Fludrocortisone 0.1-0.2 mg/day (if salt-wasting)

Sodium chloride supplementation (infants)

Stress-dose steroids during illness (prevent crisis)

False Positive Management:

Confirmatory serum 17-OHP normal → Reassure family, no CAH

Counsel: False positives common in preterm, ill infants

No further follow-up needed

Step 6: Quality Assurance

Internal QC:

Daily QC: Run low, medium, high controls with each batch

Westgard rules: 1-2s, 1-3s, 2-2s, R-4s, 4-1s, 10x

Proficiency testing: CAP/CDC quarterly challenges

External Validation:

CDC Newborn Screening Quality Assurance Program (NSQAP)

Blind split samples to reference labs

Inter-laboratory comparison: Participate in national CAH QC program

Performance Monitoring:

Sensitivity: Track missed cases (false negatives)

Specificity: Track false-positive rate (target <0.5%)

PPV: Target >20% (two-tier approach achieves 33%)

Turnaround time: Screen-to-result <5 days (target <3 days)

Outcome Surveillance:

Long-term follow-up: Track all screen-positive and diagnosed cases

Sensitivity assessment: Identify false negatives (cases missed by screening)

Incidence calculation: Validate expected 1:15,000 incidence

Step 7: Cost-Effectiveness Analysis

Program Costs (Annual, State with 100,000 Births/Year):

LC-MS/MS equipment: $500,000 (one-time capital)

Reagents/consumables: $3 per test × 100,000 = $300,000

Personnel: 2 FTE technologists = $150,000

Follow-up coordinator: 1 FTE = $75,000

Confirmatory testing: $200 per positive × 120 positives = $24,000

Total annual cost: $549,000

Cost per Case Detected:

Expected cases per year: 100,000 births ÷ 15,000 = **7 cases**

Cost per case: $549,000 ÷ 7 = **$78,000**

Cost Savings (Prevented):

Neonatal ICU admission for salt-wasting crisis: $150,000 per case × 5 cases (75% of classic CAH) = **$750,000**

Mortality prevention: 1 death prevented (15% mortality) = Priceless

Long-term growth/development: Normal outcomes vs. delays from uncontrolled CAH

Net savings: $750,000 - $549,000 = **$201,000 per year**

Cost-effectiveness: Program is cost-saving (prevents more costs than it incurs)

Step 8: Implementation and Rollout

Phase 1: Pilot (6 Months, 2 Hospitals):

Test workflow, refine protocols

Train hospital staff on sample collection

Establish endocrinology referral pathways

Phase 2: Regional Expansion (6 Months, 10 Hospitals):

Scale up operations

Monitor quality metrics

Address logistical challenges

515

Phase 3: Statewide Implementation (Year 2):

All birthing hospitals participate

Centralized laboratory processing

24/7 result reporting

Continuous quality improvement

Education and Training:

Hospital staff: Sample collection, timing, documentation

Primary care providers: Interpretation of results, referral protocols

Endocrinologists: Confirmatory testing, treatment initiation

Families: Condition education, emergency management

Step 9: Program Outcomes (5-Year Data)

Screening Volume:

Screened: 500,000 newborns over 5 years

Cases detected: 35 (1:14,285 incidence - close to expected 1:15,000)

Performance Metrics:

Sensitivity: 100% (no missed cases identified through follow-up)

False-positive rate: 0.15% (two-tier approach)

PPV: 32%

Turnaround time: 2.8 days (mean screen-to-result)

Clinical Outcomes:

Salt-wasting crises prevented: 26 (75% of 35 cases would have presented with crisis)

Deaths prevented: 5 (estimated 15% mortality without screening)

All diagnosed infants: Started treatment within 7 days of birth

Growth and development: Normal in treated patients

Challenges Encountered:

Preterm false positives: Addressed with higher cutoffs

Late discharge follow-up: Implemented repeat screen protocol

Rural access to endocrinology: Telemedicine consultations added

Family anxiety: Enhanced counseling for false positives

Final Program Design: Statewide Newborn Screening for Congenital Adrenal Hyperplasia Successfully Implemented:

Two-tier LC-MS/MS approach (weight-adjusted 17-OHP + steroid panel)

Sensitivity 100%, PPV 32% (15-fold improvement over single-tier)

Cost-effective: Net savings $200K/year

35 cases detected, 26 salt-wasting crises prevented, 5 deaths prevented

National model for CAH screening programs

Teaching Points:

Newborn Screening Principles: Identify serious, treatable conditions before symptoms; CAH meets all Wilson-Jungner criteria; prevents mortality and morbidity

Two-Tier Screening: Initial screen (sensitive) → second-tier test (specific) reduces false positives; CAH second tier includes androstenedione, 21-deoxycortisol

Confounder Adjustment: Preterm/low birth weight infants have higher 17-OHP; weight/gestational age-adjusted cutoffs essential to reduce false positives

Tandem Mass Spectrometry: Gold standard for steroid measurement; allows multiplexing (multiple steroids from one sample); superior to immunoassay for newborn screening

Timing Critical: Screen 24-48 hours (after feeding, before discharge); too early = false positives; too late = miss salt-wasting crisis

Positive Predictive Value (PPV): Proportion of positive screens with true disease; single-tier CAH screening PPV 3-5%; two-tier improves to 25-35%

Follow-Up Essential: Rapid communication (<24h), endocrinology referral (<48h), interim monitoring instructions; prevents adverse outcomes

Quality Assurance: Daily QC, proficiency testing, outcome surveillance; sensitivity monitoring (track missed cases) essential for program credibility

Cost-Effectiveness: CAH screening cost-saving (prevents ICU admissions >$100K each); $78,000 cost per case detected vs. $150,000 per crisis

False Negatives: Rare but devastating; non-classic CAH, late-onset may be missed; genetic testing for symptomatic patients with negative screen

Related Cases: Newborn screening for PKU, SCID screening (TREC assay), critical congenital heart disease (pulse oximetry screening)

Case 13.12: Cost-Effective Test Algorithm Development - Iron Deficiency Anemia Diagnosis

Hospital Quality Initiative: The hospital utilization committee notes that the current approach to diagnosing iron deficiency anemia (IDA) involves ordering a comprehensive iron panel (serum iron, TIBC, ferritin, soluble transferrin receptor) for every patient with anemia. This results in high costs and often provides redundant information. The laboratory is tasked with developing a cost-effective diagnostic algorithm that maintains accuracy while reducing unnecessary testing.

Current State Analysis:

Existing Approach:

All anemic patients (Hgb <12 women, <13 men) → comprehensive iron panel

Tests ordered reflexively: Iron, TIBC, % saturation, ferritin, sTfR (soluble transferrin receptor)

Cost per complete panel: $150

   Ferritin: $25

   Iron: $20

   TIBC: $25

   % Saturation: Calculated (no added cost)

   sTfR: $80

Annual volume: 12,000 panels per year

Total annual cost: $1,800,000

Diagnostic Yield:

Chart review of 500 cases:

   Ferritin <15 ng/mL: 280 cases (56%) → Diagnosed as IDA based on ferritin alone

518

Ferritin 15-100 ng/mL: 150 cases (30%) → Required additional testing

Ferritin >100 ng/mL: 70 cases (14%) → IDA unlikely, other causes investigated

Observation: 56% of patients could be diagnosed with ferritin alone (rest of panel unnecessary)

Diagnostic Reasoning Questions:

What is the sensitivity and specificity of ferritin for iron deficiency?

How can a stepwise algorithm reduce costs without missing diagnoses?

What are the causes of falsely elevated ferritin?

How should algorithm performance be validated?

Step 1: Evidence Review

Ferritin Diagnostic Performance:

Ferritin <15 ng/mL: Sensitivity 59%, **Specificity 99%** for IDA (highly specific)

Ferritin <30 ng/mL: Sensitivity 92%, Specificity 98%

Ferritin >100 ng/mL: IDA very unlikely (NPV 98%)

Limitations of Ferritin:

Acute phase reactant: Falsely elevated in inflammation, infection, malignancy, liver disease

Anemia of chronic disease (ACD): Ferritin normal/elevated despite functional iron deficiency

Other Iron Tests:

Transferrin saturation (<20%): Sensitive for IDA but less specific (affected by inflammation)

Soluble transferrin receptor (sTfR): Distinguishes IDA from ACD; expensive

sTfR/log ferritin ratio: Most accurate for ACD vs IDA; high cost

Step 2: Algorithm Development (Stepwise Approach)

Proposed Algorithm:

Step 1: Ferritin ONLY (Initial Test)

Order: Ferritin as first test for all anemic patients

Cost: $25

Interpretation:

Ferritin <15 ng/mL → Diagnose IDA, START TREATMENT

No further testing needed

High specificity (99%), sufficient for diagnosis

Ferritin 15-100 ng/mL → REFLEX to Iron/TIBC

Equivocal range (could be IDA with inflammation, or ACD)

Measure iron and TIBC on same sample (reflex testing)

Calculate % saturation

Added cost: $45 (iron $20 + TIBC $25)

Ferritin >100 ng/mL → IDA UNLIKELY

Consider anemia of chronic disease, other causes

If clinical suspicion high for functional iron deficiency:

Reflex to sTfR and calculate sTfR/log ferritin ratio

Added cost: $80

Step 2A: Iron/TIBC Interpretation (If Ferritin 15-100)

% Saturation <20% AND TIBC >400 μg/dL → Diagnose IDA

Treat with iron supplementation

Stop testing

% Saturation ≥20% OR TIBC <300 μg/dL → Consider ACD

If differentiation critical: Reflex to sTfR

Added cost: $80

Step 2B: sTfR Interpretation (If Needed)

sTfR >28 nmol/L → IDA likely (increased erythropoietic demand)

sTfR/log ferritin ratio >2 → IDA

sTfR/log ferritin ratio <1 → ACD

Final Algorithm Summary:

All patients: Ferritin ($25)

If ferritin 15-100: Reflex iron/TIBC ($45 added)

If still unclear: Reflex sTfR ($80 added)

Step 3: Cost Analysis (Projected)

Expected Test Utilization (Based on Pilot Data):

Ferritin alone sufficient: 56% of cases

Cost per case: $25

Ferritin + Iron/TIBC: 30% of cases

Cost per case: $70 ($25 + $45)

Ferritin + Iron/TIBC + sTfR: 14% of cases

Cost per case: $150 ($25 + $45 + $80)

Weighted Average Cost per Case:

$(0.56 \times \$25) + (0.30 \times \$70) + (0.14 \times \$150)$

$= \$14 + \$21 + \$21$

$= \textbf{\$56 per case}$ (vs. $150 current approach)

Annual Cost Savings (12,000 Cases/Year):

Current cost: $12,000 \times \$150 = \$1,800,000$

Proposed cost: $12,000 \times \$56 = \textbf{\$672,000}$

Savings: $\$1,800,000 - \$672,000 = \textbf{\$1,128,000 per year (63\% reduction)}$

Step 4: Pilot Implementation (3 Months, 1,000 Patients)

Pilot Results:

Test Utilization:

  Ferritin only: 58% (580 patients) - diagnosed IDA or excluded IDA

  Ferritin + Iron/TIBC: 28% (280 patients) - needed additional testing

  Ferritin + Iron/TIBC + sTfR: 14% (140 patients) - complex cases

Diagnostic Accuracy:

  Sensitivity for IDA: 96% (no missed cases vs. comprehensive panel)

  Specificity: 98% (minimal false positives)

  Agreement with comprehensive panel: 98% (kappa 0.96)

Cost Performance:

  Average cost per patient: $58 (close to projected $56)

  Pilot period savings: 1,000 × ($150 - $58) = **$92,000 in 3 months**

Clinical Outcomes:

  Time to diagnosis: Unchanged (same day for 58% with low ferritin)

  Treatment initiation: No delays

  Provider satisfaction: 88% favorable (appropriate algorithm)

Step 5: Refinement Based on Pilot

Algorithm Adjustments:

  Ferritin cutoff optimized:

    Changed <15 to **<30 ng/mL** for IDA diagnosis (increased sensitivity to 92%, minimal cost impact)

  Inflammation marker integration:

    If CRP >10 mg/dL or ESR >30 mm/hr → Flag ferritin result

    Alert: "Ferritin may be falsely elevated (acute phase reactant); interpret with caution"

  Clinical decision support:

    EMR alert if comprehensive panel ordered: "Consider stepwise algorithm to reduce costs"

Link to algorithm pathway

Step 6: Full Implementation (Hospital-Wide)

Rollout:

Month 1: Internal medicine wards

Month 2: Hematology/oncology (excluded from algorithm - need comprehensive panels)

Month 3: Emergency department

Month 4: Outpatient clinics

Education:

Grand rounds presentation

Pocket cards with algorithm

EMR integration with reflex testing automation

Post-Implementation Results (1 Year):

Utilization:

Annual cases: 12,000

Ferritin only: 6,960 (58%)

Ferritin + Iron/TIBC: 3,360 (28%)

Ferritin + Iron/TIBC + sTfR: 1,680 (14%)

Cost Outcomes:

Total annual cost: $696,000 (58% × $25 + 28% × $70 + 14% × $150)

Savings vs. old approach: $1,104,000 per year

5-year projected savings: $5.5 million

Quality Metrics:

Diagnostic accuracy: 97% sensitivity, 98% specificity (maintained)

False negatives: 3 cases in 12,000 (0.025%) - all had inflammatory conditions masking ferritin

Adverse events: None (all false negatives identified on follow-up, treated)

Provider Feedback:

92% satisfaction with algorithm

Perceived benefits: Cost savings, reduced unnecessary testing, streamlined workflow

Concerns: 8% prefer "comprehensive panel" (mostly hematologists treating complex patients)

Step 7: Expansion to Other Algorithms

Successful Model Applied to Other Conditions:

Vitamin B12 Deficiency:

Step 1: Serum B12 ($30)

<200 pg/mL → Diagnose B12 deficiency

400 pg/mL → Deficiency unlikely

200-400 pg/mL → Reflex to MMA and homocysteine ($90)

Savings: 55% annual reduction

Thyroid Disorders:

Step 1: TSH ($25)

Normal → Stop

Abnormal → Reflex free T4 ($35)

If T4 abnormal → Reflex free T3, thyroid antibodies ($80)

Savings: 48% annual reduction

Celiac Disease Screening:

Step 1: tTG-IgA + total IgA ($50)

If IgA deficient → Reflex tTG-IgG, DGP-IgG ($60)

If tTG negative → Stop

Savings: 40% annual reduction

Total Hospital-Wide Savings (All Algorithms): $2.8 million annually

Step 8: Continuous Quality Improvement

Ongoing Monitoring:

Monthly utilization reports (track adherence to algorithm)

Quarterly diagnostic accuracy audits (review false negatives/positives)

Annual cost analysis (validate savings)

Provider feedback surveys (assess satisfaction, identify barriers)

Algorithm Updates:

Literature review annually (new biomarkers, diagnostic thresholds)

Refinement based on performance data

Expansion to additional clinical scenarios

Final Algorithm: Cost-Effective Stepwise Algorithm for Iron Deficiency Anemia Diagnosis Successfully Implemented:

Step 1: Ferritin alone (58% of cases, $25)

Step 2: Iron/TIBC if ferritin equivocal (28% of cases, $70 total)

Step 3: sTfR if still unclear (14% of cases, $150 total)

Average cost: $58 (vs. $150 prior, **63% reduction**)

Annual savings: $1.1 million

Diagnostic accuracy maintained (97% sensitivity, 98% specificity)

No adverse patient outcomes

Model expanded to B12, thyroid, celiac (total savings $2.8M/year)

Teaching Points:

Stepwise Algorithms: Start with high-yield, low-cost test; reflex to additional tests only if needed; reduces unnecessary testing while maintaining accuracy

Ferritin for IDA: Ferritin <30 ng/mL highly specific (99%) for IDA; sufficient for diagnosis in most cases; ferritin >100 makes IDA unlikely

Acute Phase Reactant: Ferritin elevated in inflammation, infection, malignancy; can mask iron deficiency; consider CRP/ESR to identify inflammatory states

Reflex Testing: Automated add-on testing based on initial result; improves efficiency, reduces repeat venipuncture; requires laboratory information system integration

Cost-Effectiveness: Comprehensive panels often contain redundant tests; stepwise approach reduces costs 40-70% without sacrificing accuracy

sTfR (Soluble Transferrin Receptor): Distinguishes IDA (elevated sTfR) from ACD (normal sTfR); expensive ($80), reserve for equivocal cases; sTfR/log ferritin ratio >2 = IDA

Clinical Decision Support: EMR alerts guide appropriate test ordering; reduce reflexive comprehensive panel orders; "alert fatigue" risk requires thoughtful implementation

Pilot Testing: Validate algorithm in small cohort before full rollout; assess diagnostic accuracy, cost savings, provider acceptance; refine based on data

Stakeholder Engagement: Involve clinicians in algorithm design; education essential for adoption; shared savings incentivize participation

Continuous Monitoring: Track utilization, accuracy, costs; quarterly audits identify false negatives (patient safety); annual updates ensure evidence-based practice

Related Cases: Stepwise lipid screening algorithm, PSA reflex to free PSA, troponin serial testing protocols

---

Case 13.13: Laboratory-Driven Diagnosis in Asymptomatic Patient - Paget's Disease

Clinical Presentation: A 62-year-old man presents to his primary care physician for an annual physical examination. He feels well and has no specific complaints. He is physically active, walks daily, and has no pain or functional limitations. Routine laboratory screening is performed as part of preventive care.

Physical Examination:

Vital signs: Normal

General: Well-appearing, no distress

Musculoskeletal: Full range of motion all joints, no tenderness, no deformity

Neurologic: Normal gait, normal strength, normal sensation

Cardiovascular, pulmonary, abdominal: Normal

Skin: No abnormalities

Past Medical History:

Hypertension (well-controlled on lisinopril)

Hyperlipidemia (well-controlled on atorvastatin)

No history of fractures, bone pain, or skeletal abnormalities

Routine Laboratory Screening:

Comprehensive Metabolic Panel:

Alkaline phosphatase: 385 U/L MARKEDLY ELEVATED (normal 40-120 U/L)

All other chemistries normal:

Calcium: 9.6 mg/dL (normal)

Phosphorus: 3.8 mg/dL (normal)

Albumin: 4.2 g/dL (normal)

Liver enzymes (AST, ALT, bilirubin): Normal

Creatinine, electrolytes: Normal

Initial Finding: Isolated alkaline phosphatase elevation in asymptomatic patient

Diagnostic Reasoning Questions:

What is the differential diagnosis for isolated alkaline phosphatase elevation?

How is alkaline phosphatase isoenzyme fractionation used?

What imaging studies identify Paget's disease?

When should asymptomatic Paget's disease be treated?

Step 1: Differential Diagnosis for Elevated Alkaline Phosphatase

Sources of Alkaline Phosphatase:

Liver: Cholestasis, hepatobiliary disease

Bone: Increased osteoblastic activity (Paget's, hyperparathyroidism, bone metastases, fracture healing)

Intestine: Minimal contribution

527

Placenta: Pregnancy (not applicable)

Initial Differentiation:

Liver Disease Excluded:

AST, ALT, bilirubin, GGT: All normal

No hepatomegaly, no jaundice

Liver origin unlikely

Step 2: Alkaline Phosphatase Isoenzyme Fractionation

Isoenzyme Analysis (Electrophoresis):

Bone-specific alkaline phosphatase (BSAP): 345 U/L MARKEDLY ELEVATED (normal <20 U/L)

Liver alkaline phosphatase: 40 U/L (normal)

Interpretation: Bone origin confirmed

Step 3: Evaluate Causes of Elevated Bone Alkaline Phosphatase

Additional Laboratory Testing:

Parathyroid Hormone (PTH):

PTH: 42 pg/mL (normal 10-65 pg/mL)

Excludes hyperparathyroidism (would be elevated)

Calcium and Vitamin D:

Calcium: 9.6 mg/dL (normal)

25-OH Vitamin D: 32 ng/mL (normal)

Excludes vitamin D deficiency, hypercalcemia

Prostate-Specific Antigen (PSA):

PSA: 1.2 ng/mL (normal for age)

Prostate cancer unlikely (bone metastases would elevate PSA)

Serum Protein Electrophoresis (SPEP):

No monoclonal protein

Excludes multiple myeloma

Bone Turnover Markers:

C-terminal telopeptide (CTX): 0.8 ng/mL ELEVATED (normal <0.6)

N-terminal propeptide of type I procollagen (P1NP): 125 ng/mL ELEVATED (normal <80)

Interpretation: High bone turnover (increased formation and resorption)

Pattern: Isolated bone alkaline phosphatase elevation + high bone turnover markers → **Consider Paget's Disease**

Step 4: Imaging Studies

Plain Radiographs (Skeletal Survey):

Skull X-ray:

"Cotton wool" appearance: Areas of sclerosis and lucency (mixed lytic-sclerotic pattern)

Thickened calvarium: Increased density

Findings consistent with Paget's disease

Pelvis X-ray:

Right ilium: Cortical thickening, sclerotic changes

Left femur: Normal

Tibia X-ray:

Anterior bowing of right tibia

Cortical thickening

"Blade of grass" lucency (V-shaped advancing lytic front)

Spine X-ray:

L3 vertebra: "Picture frame" appearance (thickened cortical margins, central lucency)

Bone Scan (Technetium-99m MDP):

Increased uptake: Skull, right ilium, right tibia, L3 vertebra

Polyostotic Paget's disease (multiple bones involved)

Confirms extent of disease

Step 5: Confirm Diagnosis

Diagnosis: Paget's Disease of Bone (Osteitis Deformans)

Diagnostic Criteria (All Met):

✓ **Elevated bone-specific alkaline phosphatase** (345 U/L)

✓ **Characteristic radiographic findings** (cotton wool skull, blade of grass tibia, picture frame vertebra)

✓ **Increased bone turnover markers** (CTX, P1NP elevated)

✓ **Bone scan shows polyostotic involvement**

Paget's Disease Overview:

Pathophysiology: Abnormal bone remodeling; excessive osteoclast activity → osteoblast overcompensation → disorganized bone (woven bone)

Epidemiology: Prevalence 1-2% over age 55; more common in males, Northern Europeans

Etiology: Unknown; genetic (SQSTM1 mutations in familial cases); possible viral trigger (paramyxovirus)

Step 6: Assess Disease Activity and Complications

Clinical Assessment:

Pain: None (asymptomatic)

Deformity: Mild tibial bowing (not causing disability)

Fractures: None

Neurologic: No hearing loss, no nerve compression

Cardiac: No high-output heart failure (rare complication)

Audiometry:

Bilateral high-frequency sensorineural hearing loss (mild)

May be early Paget's involvement of temporal bone

530

Neurologic Examination:

No spinal stenosis symptoms

No radiculopathy

No complications at this time

Complications of Paget's Disease (None Present):

Bone pain: Most common symptom

Fractures: Pathologic fractures through pagetic bone (femur, tibia)

Osteoarthritis: Secondary to bone deformity (hips, knees)

Neurologic:

Hearing loss (skull base involvement, CN VIII compression)

Spinal stenosis (vertebral involvement)

Nerve root compression

High-output heart failure: Rare, from increased vascularity of pagetic bone

Osteosarcoma: <1% (malignant transformation, very poor prognosis)

Hypercalcemia: If immobilized

Step 7: Treatment Decision

Indications for Treatment:

Symptomatic disease: Bone pain attributed to Paget's

Complications:

Pathologic fracture or impending fracture

Neurologic complications (hearing loss, spinal stenosis)

High-output heart failure

Hypercalcemia

High-risk sites:

Skull involvement (risk of hearing loss, neurologic complications)

Weight-bearing bones (risk of fracture, deformity)

Vertebrae adjacent to spinal cord (risk of stenosis)

Active disease:

Alkaline phosphatase >2x upper limit normal

Rapidly progressive disease on imaging

This Patient:

Asymptomatic (no pain, no functional limitation)

Mild complications: Early hearing loss (may be age-related vs. Paget's)

High-risk sites involved: Skull, tibia, pelvis

Alkaline phosphatase 385 U/L (>3x upper limit of normal)

Decision: TREAT (high-risk site involvement + markedly elevated alkaline phosphatase)

Step 8: Treatment Initiation

Bisphosphonate Therapy:

Zoledronic acid 5 mg IV single infusion (first-line)

Alternative: Risedronate 30 mg PO daily x 2 months

Mechanism: Inhibits osteoclast-mediated bone resorption → reduces bone turnover → normalizes bone remodeling

Pre-Treatment:

Vitamin D and calcium: Ensure adequate (prevent hypocalcemia post-bisphosphonate)

Dental evaluation: Rule out active infection (risk of osteonecrosis of jaw)

Renal function: Adequate (CrCl >35 for zoledronic acid)

Zoledronic Acid Infusion Given:

Pre-treatment: Calcium 1,200 mg + vitamin D 2,000 IU daily x 1 week

Infusion: 5 mg IV over 15 minutes

Post-infusion: Continue calcium/vitamin D

Step 9: Monitoring and Follow-Up

Biochemical Monitoring:

3 Months Post-Infusion:

Alkaline phosphatase: 145 U/L (decreased from 385 - **62% reduction**)

Bone-specific alkaline phosphatase: 42 U/L (decreased from 345)

CTX: 0.3 ng/mL (normalized)

6 Months Post-Infusion:

Alkaline phosphatase: 98 U/L (near-normal, **75% reduction from baseline**)

Patient remains asymptomatic

Excellent biochemical response

Radiographic Follow-Up (12 Months):

X-rays: Stable (no progression of lytic areas, no new deformity)

Bone scan: Decreased uptake in affected bones (reduced disease activity)

Clinical Follow-Up:

Pain: Still asymptomatic (no bone pain)

Hearing: Stable (no further decline)

Fractures: None

Quality of life: Unchanged (remains active)

Long-Term Management:

Monitoring Schedule:

Alkaline phosphatase: Every 6-12 months

Radiographs: Only if symptomatic or alkaline phosphatase rising

Bone scan: Not routinely repeated

Retreatment Criteria:

Alkaline phosphatase rises >25% from nadir OR

Develops symptoms (pain, complications) OR

New lytic lesions on imaging

Prognosis:

Zoledronic acid: Single dose provides 2-5 years of disease control in 60-90%

This patient: Likely 3-5 years before retreatment needed

Complications prevented: Treatment reduces fracture risk, pain, hearing loss

Final Diagnosis: Asymptomatic Polyostotic Paget's Disease of Bone (Skull, Pelvis, Tibia, Spine) Discovered Incidentally by Elevated Alkaline Phosphatase

Successfully treated with zoledronic acid

Alkaline phosphatase normalized

No disease-related complications

Remains asymptomatic 2 years post-treatment

Teaching Points:

Isolated Alkaline Phosphatase Elevation: Always fractionate (bone vs. liver); liver tests normal + elevated bone-specific alk phos → bone disease (Paget's, hyperparathyroidism, bone metastases, osteomalacia)

Paget's Disease Diagnosis: Elevated bone alkaline phosphatase + characteristic X-ray findings (cotton wool skull, blade of grass, picture frame vertebra); bone scan determines extent

Radiographic Findings: Mixed lytic-sclerotic pattern; cotton wool (skull), blade of grass (long bones), picture frame (vertebrae); cortical thickening, bone expansion

Asymptomatic Paget's: 70-90% asymptomatic; discovered incidentally (elevated alk phos, X-ray for other reason); treatment recommended if high-risk sites or very active disease

Bone Turnover Markers: Alkaline phosphatase (formation), CTX/NTX (resorption); elevated in Paget's; track response to treatment (goal >50% reduction)

Treatment Indications: Symptomatic disease, complications (fracture, neuro), high-risk sites (skull, spine, weight-bearing), alk phos >2x ULN, rapidly progressive

Bisphosphonates: First-line; zoledronic acid single 5 mg IV infusion most effective (2-5 year remission); alternative: risedronate, alendronate (daily/weekly for months)

Complications: Fracture (most common), hearing loss (skull base), spinal stenosis, osteoarthritis, high-output heart failure (rare), osteosarcoma (<1%, poor prognosis)

Monitoring: Alkaline phosphatase every 6-12 months; retreatment if rises >25% from nadir or symptoms develop; X-rays only if clinically indicated

Prevention: Early treatment may prevent complications (fracture, deformity, hearing loss); asymptomatic patients with high-risk involvement benefit from treatment

Related Cases: Hyperparathyroidism with elevated alk phos, bone metastases, osteomalacia, fibrous dysplasia

References

Andes, D. R., Safdar, N., Baddley, J. W., Playford, G., Reboli, A. C., Rex, J. H., ... & Kullberg, B. J. (2012). Impact of treatment strategy on outcomes in patients with candidemia and other forms of invasive candidiasis: A patient-level quantitative review of randomized trials. Clinical Infectious Diseases, 54(8), 1110-1122. https://doi.org/10.1093/cid/cis021

Asgari, M. M., & Begos, D. G. (1997). Spontaneous splenic rupture in infectious mononucleosis: A review. Yale Journal of Biology and Medicine, 70(2), 175-182. https://www.ncbi.nlm.nih.gov/pmc/articles/PMC2589234/

Baddour, L. M., Wilson, W. R., Bayer, A. S., Fowler, V. G., Tleyjeh, I. M., Rybak, M. J., ... & Taubert, K. A. (2015). Infective endocarditis in adults: Diagnosis, antimicrobial therapy, and management of complications. Circulation, 132(15), 1435-1486. https://doi.org/10.1161/CIR.0000000000000296

Baron, E. J., Miller, J. M., Weinstein, M. P., Richter, S. S., Gilligan, P. H., Thomson, R. B., ... & Pritt, B. S. (2013). A guide to utilization of the microbiology laboratory for diagnosis of infectious diseases: 2013 recommendations by the Infectious Diseases Society of America (IDSA) and the American Society for Microbiology (ASM). Clinical Infectious Diseases, 57(4), e22-e121. https://doi.org/10.1093/cid/cit278

Benoit, S. R., Zhang, Y., Geiss, L. S., Gregg, E. W., & Albright, A. (2018). Trends in diabetic ketoacidosis hospitalizations and in-hospital mortality—United States, 2000–2014. MMWR Morbidity and Mortality Weekly Report, 67(12), 362-365. https://doi.org/10.15585/mmwr.mm6712a3

Bhutani, V. K., Johnson, L., & Sivieri, E. M. (1999). Predictive ability of a predischarge hour-specific serum bilirubin for subsequent significant hyperbilirubinemia in healthy term and near-term newborns. Pediatrics, 103(1), 6-14. https://doi.org/10.1542/peds.103.1.6

Bilezikian, J. P., Brandi, M. L., Eastell, R., Silverberg, S. J., Udelsman, R., Marcocci, C., & Potts, J. T. (2014). Guidelines for the management of asymptomatic primary hyperparathyroidism. Journal of Clinical Endocrinology & Metabolism, 99(10), 3561-3569. https://doi.org/10.1210/jc.2014-1413 [Year corrected from 2018]

Bizzaro, N. (1995). EDTA-dependent pseudothrombocytopenia: A clinical and epidemiological study of 112 cases, with 10-year follow-up. American Journal of Hematology, 50(2), 103-109. https://doi.org/10.1002/ajh.2830500206

Bolton-Maggs, P. H., Langer, J. C., Iolascon, A., Tittensor, P., & King, M. J. (2012). Guidelines for the diagnosis and management of hereditary spherocytosis—2011 update. British Journal of Haematology, 156(1), 37-49. https://doi.org/10.1111/j.1365-2141.2011.08921.x

Bonkovsky, H. L., Maddukuri, V. C., Yazici, C., Anderson, K. E., Bissell, D. M., Bloomer, J. R., ... & Desnick, R. J. (2014). Acute porphyrias in the USA: Features of 108 subjects from porphyrias consortium. American Journal of Medicine, 127(12), 1233-1241. https://doi.org/10.1016/j.amjmed.2014.06.036

Bornemann, M., Hill, L., & Patel, R. (2018). Acid-base disorders. Disease-a-Month, 64(8), 437-471. https://doi.org/10.1016/j.disamonth.2018.04.003

Bosch, X., Poch, E., & Grau, J. M. (2009). Rhabdomyolysis and acute kidney injury. New England Journal of Medicine, 361(1), 62-72. https://doi.org/10.1056/NEJMra0801327

Boyce, J. M., & Pittet, D. (2002). Guideline for hand hygiene in health-care settings: Recommendations of the Healthcare Infection Control Practices Advisory Committee and the HICPAC/SHEA/APIC/IDSA Hand Hygiene Task Force. Morbidity and Mortality Weekly Report, 51(RR-16), 1-45.

Brandow, A. M., & Panepinto, J. A. (2010). Monitoring pain in sickle cell disease. Current Opinion in Hematology, 17(3), 199-205. https://doi.org/10.1097/MOH.0b013e328337b99f

Callum, J. L., Waters, J. H., Shaz, B. H., Sloan, S. R., & Murphy, M. F. (2014). The PROPPR trial: A story of blood and blood components. Transfusion, 54(7), 1716-1718. https://doi.org/10.1111/trf.12730

Camaschella, C. (2019). Iron deficiency. Blood, 133(1), 30-39. https://doi.org/10.1182/blood-2018-05-815944

Carlotti, A. P., Bohn, D., Mallie, J. P., Ejike, J. C., & Halperin, M. L. (2013). Tonicity balance, and not electrolyte-free water calculations, more accurately guides therapy for acute changes in natremia. Intensive Care Medicine, 39(7), 1109-1117. https://doi.org/10.1007/s00134-013-2954-4

Castaman, G., & Linari, S. (2017). Diagnosis and treatment of von Willebrand disease and rare bleeding disorders. Journal of Clinical Medicine, 6(4), 45. https://doi.org/10.3390/jcm6040045

Cepeda, N. J., Pashler, H., Vul, E., Wixted, J. T., & Rohrer, D. (2006). Distributed practice in verbal recall tasks: A review and quantitative synthesis. Psychological Bulletin, 132(3), 354-380. https://doi.org/10.1037/0033-2909.132.3.354

Cohen, S. H., Gerding, D. N., Johnson, S., Kelly, C. P., Loo, V. G., McDonald, L. C., ... & Wilcox, M. H. (2010). Clinical practice guidelines for Clostridium difficile infection in adults: 2010 update by the Society for Healthcare Epidemiology of America (SHEA) and the Infectious Diseases Society of America (IDSA). Infection Control & Hospital Epidemiology, 31(5), 431-455. https://doi.org/10.1086/651706

Conter, V., Bartram, C. R., Valsecchi, M. G., Schrauder, A., Panzer-Grümayer, R., Möricke, A., ... & Schrappe, M. (2010). Molecular response to treatment redefines all prognostic factors in children and adolescents with B-cell precursor acute lymphoblastic leukemia. Blood, 115(16), 3206-3214. https://doi.org/10.1182/blood-2009-10-248146

DeFronzo, R., Fleming, G. A., Chen, K., & Bicsak, T. A. (2016). Metformin-associated lactic acidosis: Current perspectives on causes and risk. Metabolism, 65(2), 20-29. https://doi.org/10.1016/j.metabol.2015.10.014

Delaney, M., Wendel, S., Bercovitz, R. S., Cid, J., Cohn, C., Johnson, S. T., ... & Ziman, A. (2016). Transfusion reactions: Prevention, diagnosis, and treatment. The Lancet, 388(10061), 2825-2836. https://doi.org/10.1016/S0140-6736(15)01313-6

Dellinger, R. P., Levy, M. M., Rhodes, A., Annane, D., Gerlach, H., Opal, S. M., ... & Moreno, R. (2013). Surviving sepsis campaign: International guidelines for management of severe sepsis and septic shock: 2012. Critical Care Medicine, 41(2), 580-637. https://doi.org/10.1097/CCM.0b013e31827e83af

Doshi, S. M., Shah, P., Lei, X., Lahoti, A., & Salahudeen, A. K. (2008). Hyponatremia in hospitalized cancer patients and its impact on clinical outcomes. American Journal of Kidney Diseases, 52(3), 487-494. https://doi.org/10.1053/j.ajkd.2008.04.029

Duntas, L. H. (2002). Thyroid disease and lipids. Thyroid, 12(4), 287-293. https://doi.org/10.1089/10507250252949405

Ebell, M. H. (2004). Epstein-Barr virus infectious mononucleosis. American Family Physician, 70(7), 1279-1287. https://www.aafp.org/pubs/afp/issues/2004/1001/p1279.html

Freeman, S., Eddy, S. L., McDonough, M., Smith, M. K., Okoroafor, N., Jordt, H., & Wenderoth, M. P. (2014). Active learning increases student performance in science, engineering, and mathematics. Proceedings of the National Academy of Sciences, 111(23), 8410-8415. https://doi.org/10.1073/pnas.1319030111

Gaddey, H. L., & Riegel, A. M. (2016). Unexplained lymphadenopathy: Evaluation and differential diagnosis. American Family Physician, 94(11), 896-903. https://www.aafp.org/pubs/afp/issues/2016/1201/p896.html

Garber, J. R., Cobin, R. H., Gharib, H., Hennessey, J. V., Klein, I., Mechanick, J. I., ... & Woeber, K. A. (2012). Clinical practice guidelines for hypothyroidism in adults. Endocrine Practice, 18(6), 988-1028. https://doi.org/10.4158/EP12280.GL

Gladwin, M. T., & Vichinsky, E. (2008). Pulmonary complications of sickle cell disease. New England Journal of Medicine, 359(21), 2254-2265. https://doi.org/10.1056/NEJMra0804411

Gosmanov, A. R., Gosmanova, E. O., & Kitabchi, A. E. (2014). Hyperglycemic crises: Diabetic ketoacidosis and hyperglycemic hyperosmolar state. Endotext. MDText.com. https://www.ncbi.nlm.nih.gov/books/NBK279052/

Gupta, K., Hooton, T. M., Naber, K. G., Wullt, B., Colgan, R., Miller, L. G., ... & Soper, D. E. (2011). International clinical practice guidelines for the treatment of acute uncomplicated cystitis and pyelonephritis in women. Clinical Infectious Diseases, 52(5), e103-e120. https://doi.org/10.1093/cid/ciq257

Hamdi, T., Latta, S., Jallad, B., & Kheetan, M. (2019). Rhabdomyolysis: A review of clinical presentation, etiology, diagnosis, and management. Cureus, 11(8), e5567. https://doi.org/10.7759/cureus.5567

Harteveld, C. L., & Higgs, D. R. (2010). Alpha-thalassaemia. Orphanet Journal of Rare Diseases, 5, 13. https://doi.org/10.1186/1750-1172-5-13

Hendrickson, J. E., & Tormey, C. A. (2016). Understanding red blood cell alloimmunization triggers. Hematology, 2016(1), 446-451. https://doi.org/10.1182/asheducation-2016.1.446

Hew-Butler, T., Rosner, M. H., Fowkes-Godek, S., Dugas, J. P., Hoffman, M. D., Lewis, D. P., ... & Verbalis, J. G. (2015). Statement of the third international exercise-associated hyponatremia consensus development conference. Clinical Journal of Sport Medicine, 25(4), 303-320. https://doi.org/10.1097/JSM.0000000000000221

Holcomb, J. B., Tilley, B. C., Baraniuk, S., Fox, E. E., Wade, C. E., Podbielski, J. M., ... & Cotton, B. A. (2015). Transfusion of plasma, platelets, and red blood cells in a 1:1:1 vs a 1:1:2 ratio and mortality in patients with severe trauma: The PROPPR randomized clinical trial. JAMA, 313(5), 471-482. https://doi.org/10.1001/jama.2015.12

Huang, C. L., & Kuo, E. (2007). Mechanism of hypokalemia in magnesium deficiency. Journal of the American Society of Nephrology, 18(10), 2649-2652. https://doi.org/10.1681/ASN.2007070792

Hunt, J. R. (2003). Bioavailability of iron, zinc, and other trace minerals from vegetarian diets. American Journal of Clinical Nutrition, 78(3), 633S-639S. https://doi.org/10.1093/ajcn/78.3.633S

Jameson, J. L., & De Groot, L. J. (2015). Endocrinology: Adult and Pediatric (7th ed.). Elsevier Saunders. https://www.elsevier.com/books/endocrinology-adult-and-pediatric-7e/jameson/978-0-323-18907-1

Joly, B. S., Coppo, P., & Veyradier, A. (2017). Thrombotic thrombocytopenic purpura. Blood, 129(21), 2836-2846. https://doi.org/10.1182/blood-2016-10-709857

Kalil, A. C., Metersky, M. L., Klompas, M., Muscedere, J., Sweeney, D. A., Palmer, L. B., ... & Brozek, J. L. (2016). Management of adults with hospital-acquired and ventilator-associated pneumonia: 2016 clinical practice guidelines by the Infectious Diseases Society of America and the American Thoracic Society. Clinical Infectious Diseases, 63(5), e61-e111. https://doi.org/10.1093/cid/ciw353

Kaplan, M., Bromiker, R., & Hammerman, C. (2014). Hyperbilirubinemia, hemolysis, and increased bilirubin neurotoxicity. Seminars in Perinatology, 38(7), 429-437. https://doi.org/10.1053/j.semperi.2014.08.006

Kitabchi, A. E., Umpierrez, G. E., Miles, J. M., & Fisher, J. N. (2009). Hyperglycemic crises in adult patients with diabetes. Diabetes Care, 32(7), 1335-1343. https://doi.org/10.2337/dc09-9032

Kleinman, S., Caulfield, T., Chan, P., Davenport, R., McFarland, J., McPhedran, S., ... & Slinger, P. (2004). Toward an understanding of transfusion-related acute lung injury: Statement of a consensus panel. Transfusion, 44(12), 1774-1789. https://doi.org/10.1111/j.0041-1132.2004.04347.x

Kujovich, J. L. (2011). Factor V Leiden thrombophilia. Genetics in Medicine, 13(1), 1-16. https://doi.org/10.1097/GIM.0b013e3181faa0f2

Landolfi, R., Marchioli, R., Kutti, J., Gisslinger, H., Tognoni, G., Patrono, C., & Barbui, T. (2004). Efficacy and safety of low-dose aspirin in polycythemia vera. New England Journal of Medicine, 350(2), 114-124. https://doi.org/10.1056/NEJMoa035572

Leebeek, F. W., & Eikenboom, J. C. (2016). Von Willebrand's disease. New England Journal of Medicine, 375(21), 2067-2080. https://doi.org/10.1056/NEJMra1601561

Levi, M., & Ten Cate, H. (1999). Disseminated intravascular coagulation. New England Journal of Medicine, 341(8), 586-592. https://doi.org/10.1056/NEJM199908193410807

Liamis, G., Milionis, H., & Elisaf, M. (2008). A review of drug-induced hyponatremia. American Journal of Kidney Diseases, 52(1), 144-153. https://doi.org/10.1053/j.ajkd.2008.03.004

Liu, C., Bayer, A., Cosgrove, S. E., Daum, R. S., Fridkin, S. K., Gorwitz, R. J., ... & Chambers, H. F. (2011). Clinical practice guidelines by the Infectious Diseases Society of America for the treatment of methicillin-resistant Staphylococcus aureus infections in adults and children. Clinical Infectious Diseases, 52(3), e18-e55. https://doi.org/10.1093/cid/ciq146

Lopez, A., Cacoub, P., Macdougall, I. C., & Peyrin-Biroulet, L. (2016). Iron deficiency anaemia. The Lancet, 387(10021), 907-916. https://doi.org/10.1016/S0140-6736(15)60865-0

Malcovati, L., Karimi, M., Papaemmanuil, E., Ambaglio, I., Jädersten, M., Jansson, M., ... & Cazzola, M. (2020). SF3B1 mutation identifies a distinct subset of myelodysplastic syndrome with ring sideroblasts. Blood, 126(2), 233-241. https://doi.org/10.1182/blood-2015-03-633537

Marchioli, R., Finazzi, G., Specchia, G., Cacciola, R., Cavazzina, R., Cilloni, D., ... & Barbui, T. (2013). Cardiovascular events and intensity of treatment in polycythemia vera. New England Journal of Medicine, 368(1), 22-33. https://doi.org/10.1056/NEJMoa1208500

Marino, P. L. (2014). Marino's The ICU Book (4th ed.). Wolters Kluwer Health/Lippincott Williams & Wilkins. https://www.lww.com/Product/9781451121186

McDonald, L. C., Gerding, D. N., Johnson, S., Bakken, J. S., Carroll, K. C., Coffin, S. E., ... & Wilcox, M. H. (2018). Clinical practice guidelines for Clostridium difficile infection in adults and children: 2017 update by the Infectious Diseases Society of America (IDSA) and Society for Healthcare Epidemiology of America (SHEA). Clinical Infectious Diseases, 66(7), e1-e48. https://doi.org/10.1093/cid/cix1085

Miller, J. M., Binnicker, M. J., Campbell, S., Carroll, K. C., Chapin, K. C., Gilligan, P. H., ... & Yao, J. D. (2018). A guide to utilization of the microbiology laboratory for diagnosis of infectious diseases: 2018 update by the Infectious Diseases Society of America and the American Society for Microbiology. Clinical Infectious Diseases, 67(6), e1-e94. https://doi.org/10.1093/cid/ciy381

Moe, S. M. (2008). Disorders involving calcium, phosphorus, and magnesium. Primary Care: Clinics in Office Practice, 35(2), 215-237. https://doi.org/10.1016/j.pop.2008.01.007

Moise, K. J. (2008). Management of rhesus alloimmunization in pregnancy. Obstetrics & Gynecology, 112(1), 164-176. https://doi.org/10.1097/AOG.0b013e31817d453c

Mount, D. B. (2014). Disorders of potassium balance. In K. Skorecki, G. M. Chertow, P. A. Marsden, M. W. Taal, & A. S. L. Yu (Eds.), Brenner and Rector's The Kidney (10th ed., pp. 640-688). Elsevier. https://www.elsevier.com/books/brenner-and-rectors-the-kidney-2-volume-set/skorecki/978-0-323-53186-3

Muñoz, M., Breymann, C., García-Erce, J. A., Gómez-Ramírez, S., Comin, J., & Bisbe, E. (2017). Efficacy and safety of intravenous iron therapy as an alternative/adjunct to allogeneic blood transfusion. Vox Sanguinis, 94(3), 172-183. https://doi.org/10.1111/j.1423-0410.2007.01014.x

Neunert, C., Lim, W., Crowther, M., Cohen, A., Solberg, L., & Crowther, M. A. (2011). The American Society of Hematology 2011 evidence-based practice guideline for immune thrombocytopenia. Blood, 117(16), 4190-4207. https://doi.org/10.1182/blood-2010-08-302984

Ng, A. K., Mauch, P. M., & LaCasce, A. S. (2017). Treatment of classical Hodgkin lymphoma. UpToDate. https://www.uptodate.com/contents/treatment-of-classical-hodgkin-lymphoma

Palmer, B. F., & Clegg, D. J. (2016). Electrolyte disturbances in patients with chronic alcohol-use disorder. New England Journal of Medicine, 377(14), 1368-1377. https://doi.org/10.1056/NEJMra1604202

Panel on Antiretroviral Guidelines for Adults and Adolescents. (2023). Guidelines for the use of antiretroviral agents in adults and adolescents with HIV. Department of Health and Human Services. Available at https://clinicalinfo.hiv.gov/en/guidelines

Patterson, T. F., Thompson III, G. R., Denning, D. W., Fishman, J. A., Hadley, S., Herbrecht, R., ... & Bennett, J. E. (2016). Practice guidelines for the diagnosis and management of aspergillosis: 2016 update by the Infectious Diseases Society of America. Clinical Infectious Diseases, 63(4), e1-e60. https://doi.org/10.1093/cid/ciw326

Peeling, P., Blee, T., Goodman, C., Dawson, B., Claydon, G., Beilby, J., & Prins, A. (2008). Effect of iron injections on aerobic-exercise performance of iron-depleted female athletes. International Journal of Sport Nutrition and Exercise Metabolism, 17(3), 221-231. https://doi.org/10.1123/ijsnem.17.3.221

Pham, H. P., & Shaz, B. H. (2013). Update on massive transfusion. British Journal of Anaesthesia, 111(suppl_1), i71-i82. https://doi.org/10.1093/bja/aet376

Pickering, J. W., Than, M. P., Cullen, L., Aldous, S., Ter Avest, E., Body, R., ... & Greenslade, J. H. (2018). Rapid rule-out of acute myocardial infarction with a single high-sensitivity cardiac troponin T measurement below the limit of detection. Annals of Internal Medicine, 166(10), 715-724. https://doi.org/10.7326/M16-2562

Pui, C. H., & Evans, W. E. (2006). Treatment of acute lymphoblastic leukemia. New England Journal of Medicine, 354(2), 166-178. https://doi.org/10.1056/NEJMra052603

Rasouli, M. (2016). Basic concepts and practical equations on osmolality: Biochemical approach. Clinical Biochemistry, 49(12), 936-941. https://doi.org/10.1016/j.clinbiochem.2016.06.001

Rodeghiero, F., Stasi, R., Gernsheimer, T., Michel, M., Provan, D., Arnold, D. M., ... & George, J. N. (2009). Standardization of terminology, definitions and outcome criteria in immune thrombocytopenic purpura of adults and children. Blood, 113(11), 2386-2393. https://doi.org/10.1182/blood-2008-07-162503

Rose, B. D., & Post, T. W. (2001). Clinical Physiology of Acid-Base and Electrolyte Disorders (5th ed.). McGraw-Hill Medical. https://accessmedicine.mhmedical.com/book.aspx?bookid=1316

Sabatine, M. S. (2017). Pocket Medicine: The Massachusetts General Hospital Handbook of Internal Medicine (6th ed.). Wolters Kluwer. https://www.lww.com/Product/9781496349613

Scully, M., Cataland, S. R., Peyvandi, F., Coppo, P., Knöbl, P., Kremer Hovinga, J. A., ... & Liebman, H. (2019). Caplacizumab treatment for acquired thrombotic thrombocytopenic purpura. New England Journal of Medicine, 380(4), 335-346. https://doi.org/10.1056/NEJMoa1806311

Seifter, J. L. (2005). Acid-base disorders. In A. S. Fauci, E. Braunwald, D. L. Kasper, S. L. Hauser, D. L. Longo, J. L. Jameson, & J. Loscalzo (Eds.), Harrison's Principles of Internal Medicine (19th ed.). McGraw-Hill. https://accessmedicine.mhmedical.com/book.aspx?bookid=2129

Shanbhag, S., & Ambinder, R. F. (2018). Hodgkin lymphoma: A review and update on recent progress. CA: A Cancer Journal for Clinicians, 68(2), 116-132. https://doi.org/10.3322/caac.21438

Srinivasan, M., Wilkes, M., Stevenson, F., Nguyen, T., & Slavin, S. (2007). Comparing problem-based learning with case-based learning: Effects of a major curricular shift at two institutions. Academic Medicine, 82(1), 74-82. https://doi.org/10.1097/01.ACM.0000249963.93776.aa

Steinberg, M. H., Barton, F., Castro, O., Pegelow, C. H., Ballas, S. K., Kutlar, A., ... & Terrin, M. (2003). Effect of hydroxyurea on mortality and morbidity in adult sickle cell anemia. JAMA, 289(13), 1645-1651. https://doi.org/10.1001/jama.289.13.1645

Sterns, R. H. (2015). Disorders of plasma sodium—Causes, consequences, and correction. New England Journal of Medicine, 372(1), 55-65. https://doi.org/10.1056/NEJMra1404489

Tefferi, A., & Barbui, T. (2020). Polycythemia vera: 2020 update on diagnosis, risk-stratification, and management. American Journal of Hematology, 95(12), 1599-1613. https://doi.org/10.1002/ajh.26008

Thistlethwaite, J. E., Davies, D., Ekeocha, S., Kidd, J. M., MacDougall, C., Matthews, P., ... & Clay, D. (2012). The effectiveness of case-based learning in health professional education: A BEME systematic review. Medical Teacher, 34(6), e421-e444. https://doi.org/10.3109/0142159X.2012.680939

Thongprayoon, C., Cheungpasitporn, W., & Erickson, S. B. (2016). Admission calcium levels and risk of acute kidney injury in hospitalised patients. International Journal of Clinical Practice, 70(2), 181-188. https://doi.org/10.1111/ijcp.12779

Tormey, C. A., & Stack, G. (2019). The characterization and classification of concurrent blood group antibodies. Transfusion, 59(7), 2472-2479. https://doi.org/10.1111/trf.15304

Tunkel, A. R., Hartman, B. J., Kaplan, S. L., Kaufman, B. A., Roos, K. L., Scheld, W. M., & Whitley, R. J. (2004). Practice guidelines for the management of bacterial meningitis. Clinical Infectious Diseases, 39(9), 1267-1284. https://doi.org/10.1086/425368

Unwin, R. J., Luft, F. C., & Shirley, D. G. (2011). Pathophysiology and management of hypokalemia: A clinical perspective. Nature Reviews Nephrology, 7(2), 75-84. https://doi.org/10.1038/nrneph.2010.175

Urrechaga, E., Borque, L., & Escanero, J. F. (2015). Biomarkers of hypochromia: The contemporary assessment of iron status and erythropoiesis. BioMed Research International, 2015, 603786. https://doi.org/10.1155/2015/603786

Verbalis, J. G., Goldsmith, S. R., Greenberg, A., Korzelius, C., Schrier, R. W., Sterns, R. H., & Thompson, C. J. (2013). Diagnosis, evaluation, and treatment of hyponatremia. Journal of the American Society of Nephrology, 24(10), 1889-1905. https://doi.org/10.1681/ASN.2013010038

Vlaar, A. P., & Juffermans, N. P. (2013). Transfusion-related acute lung injury: A clinical review. The Lancet, 382(9896), 984-994. https://doi.org/10.1016/S0140-6736(12)62197-7

Weatherall, D. J. (2010). The inherited diseases of hemoglobin are an emerging global health burden. Blood, 115(22), 4331-4336. https://doi.org/10.1182/blood-2010-01-251348

Weiner, I. D., & Wingo, C. S. (2014). Hypokalemia—Consequences, causes, and correction. Journal of the American Society of Nephrology, 8(7), 1179-1188. https://doi.org/10.1681/ASN.V871179

Weisberg, L. S. (2008). Management of severe hypernatremia. Critical Care Medicine, 36(12), 3246-3251. https://doi.org/10.1097/CCM.0b013e31818f222a

Workowski, K. A., Bachmann, L. H., Chan, P. A., Johnston, C. M., Muzny, C. A., Park, I., ... & Bolan, G. A. (2021). Sexually transmitted infections treatment guidelines, 2021. MMWR Recommendations and Reports, 70(4), 1-187. https://dx.doi.org/10.15585/mmwr.rr7004a1

Wu, A. H. B. (2006). Tietz Clinical Guide to Laboratory Tests (4th ed.). Elsevier Saunders. https://www.elsevier.com/books/tietz-clinical-guide-to-laboratory-tests/wu/978-0-7216-0561-6

Zaidi, M., & Yuen, T. (2016). Hypercalcemia of malignancy. In K. R. Feingold, B. Anawalt, A. Boyce, G. Chrousos, W. W. de Herder, K. Dhatariya, et al. (Eds.), Endotext. MDText.com. https://www.ncbi.nlm.nih.gov/books/NBK279049/

Zerra, P. E., & Josephson, C. D. (2019). Transfusion in neonatal patients: Review of evidence-based guidelines. Clinics in Laboratory Medicine, 39(4), 573-594. https://doi.org/10.1016/j.cll.2019.07.007

Zilberberg, M. D., Exuzides, A., Spalding, J., Foreman, A., Jones, A. G., Colby, C., & Shorr, A. F. (2008). Epidemiology, clinical and economic outcomes of admission hyponatremia among hospitalized patients. Current Medical Research and Opinion, 24(6), 1601-1608. https://doi.org/10.1185/03007990802081675

Zufferey, A., Kapur, R., Semple, J. W., Provan, D., Arnold, D. M., & Berchtold, P. (2017). Pathogenesis and therapeutic mechanisms in immune thrombocytopenia. Journal of Thrombosis and Haemostasis, 15(7), 1246-1258. https://doi.org/10.1111/jth.13705